TEACHING
HEALTH SCIENCE

in middle and secondary schools

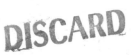

About the Authors

Ms. Linda Brower Meeks is an Assistant Professor of Health Education at The Ohio State University. She is the co-author of several health textbooks including *Education for Sexuality, Toward A Healthy Lifestyle Through Elementary Health Education,* and *Group Strategies in Understanding Human Sexuality: Getting in Touch.* Professor Meeks is the co-author with Phil Heit of *Health: Focus on You,* a textbook series for middle and secondary school students, and *Human Sexuality.* Professor Meeks consults with school districts throughout the country in the area of curriculum and program planning. She is committed to a healthy lifestyle through running, playing competitive tennis, and low calorie cooking. She is divorced and the mother of Kristen.

Dr. Phil Heit is an Associate Professor of Health Education at The Ohio State University. He is Project Director of the Ohio State University Teacher Training Institute for the School Health Curriculum Project and the Primary Grades Curriculum Project. His fitness interests are compatible with his lifestyle. He has run the Boston and New York marathons. Phil is married to Sheryl Heit and is the father of Yve and Gay.

Ms. Sharon Mitchell Pottebaum is the Director of Education at Family Hospital in Milwaukee, Wisconsin. She is the co-author of *Toward A Healthy Lifestyle Through Elementary Health Education.* Sharon has been very active in curriculum development in health education as well as the development of media. Her overlays, games, and teaching strategies are used in numerous school systems. Sharon is married to Joseph Pottebaum.

TEACHING
HEALTH SCIENCE
in middle and secondary schools

Linda Brower Meeks
Ohio State University

Philip Heit
Ohio State University

Sharon Mitchell Pottebaum
Family Hospital, Milwaukee, Wisconsin

ωcb

Wm. C. Brown Company Publishers
Dubuque, Iowa

Cover credits: Allen Ruid and David S. Strickler

Consulting Editor

Health

Robert Kaplan
The Ohio State University

We dedicate this book to our immediate families who lovingly examine with us alternatives to healthy, happy living.

Kristen Ann Meeks

Sheryl Wynn Heit
Yve Bari Heit
Gay Leah Heit

Joseph Raymond Pottebaum

Contents

Preface

Teaching Health Science in Middle and Secondary Schools is a methods textbook designed for teachers of health by teachers of health. Section 1. Preparing to Teach Health Science contains a comprehensive discussion of the teaching of middle and secondary schools students as well as the teaching of the health education curriculum. The instructor is provided a philosophy of health education from which (s)he can develop his or her own. Techniques for assuring a positive classroom environment are co-ordinated with strategies for disciplining and counseling middle and secondary school students.

The teacher is familiarized with his or her role in the total school health program and exposed to a variety of health education curricula. Special emphasis is placed on implementing curricula with the selection of creative methods, materials, and media. Evaluation is covered comprehensively, and the teacher is furnished a list of resources for obtaining free or inexpensive health education aids.

Section 2. Creative Lessons for Teaching Health in Middle and Secondary Schools describes the characteristics of the students; this section contains selected topics and activities for teaching health, which have been field tested with middle and secondary school students and teachers. The major areas of the curriculum were identified by examining the health requirements in each state. The areas were: mental health and self concept; the human body; cardiovascular fitness and health; nutrition and weight control; the use and abuse of drugs; tobacco and health, diseases and disorders; communicable diseases; first aid and safety; human sexuality and family life; consumer health and medical care; environment; aging, dying, and death.

After specifying the major curriculum areas, we developed a needs assessment survey and administered it to students, parents, teachers, school administrators, counselors, and health education experts, in order to select lesson topics for each area. An outline of the topics for lesson plans is included within each of the curriculum areas covered in Section 2. In addition to selected learning activities for each subject area, the authors have included three sample lesson plans. Each sample lesson plan contains the unit title, topics, objectives, sources, content and procedures, materials, and evaluation. Although there are many other important topics that could be covered, if the teacher implemented all three lessons for each of the thirteen areas the students would receive a well-balanced and remunerative health education.

In addition to the simple writing style, *Teaching Health Science in Middle and Secondary Schools* is organized in outline form with marginal headings and subheadings that help the teacher to locate rapidly whatever is needed. Thus the instructor has confidence that the health program will be stimulating and motivating. The topical outline of lessons for each area is thorough, and the three lessons provided are varied in approach to provide a creative, exciting classroom. However, the style or format of each lesson remains the same, allowing the teacher to have (1) a clear perception of the objectives, (2) an outline of the content needed to reach the stated goals, (3) a technique for teaching involving both methods and materials, and (4) an effective means of evaluation. Many of the lessons contain student handouts or overlays which can easily be reproduced by the teacher. Thus, the instructor has everything that is needed for the health education program.

Finally, the materials in this book have been field tested by teachers in middle and secondary schools. We are confident that you will be able to utilize these materials in a classroom dedicated to the enrichment of your students' lifestyles through the examination and selection of positive health behaviors.

Linda Brower Meeks

Phil Heit

Sharon Mitchell Pottebaum

Acknowledgments

There are many individuals without whose help this text would not have been completed. Dr. Robert Kaplan deserves special thanks. His role served a dual purpose. First, as Health Education Editor at Wm. C. Brown, Dr. Kaplan added many constructive comments which added to the quality of this text. Second, as our Chairman in the Health Education Division at The Ohio State University, he encouraged and supported this project.

We are also indebted to Rick Bond, Curriculum Coordinator for Health Education in the Grandview Heights, Ohio School System, who permitted us to field test the many activities used in this text.

Our reviewers also provided us with many useful insights. Grateful acknowledgment is due D. A. Hicks-University of Florida, Glen Gilbert-Portland State University, Nicholas Iammarino-Rice University, and Charles W. Worland-California State University-Hayward. In particular, we would like to thank Dr. William L. Yarber of Purdue University for his extra efforts in assuring that the content of this text is meaningful and current.

Special thanks to Ted Cyphert, former Dean of The Ohio State University College of Education and currently Professor on the Foundations and Research Faculty at the same institution, and Don Anderson, Associate Dean of the College of Education at The Ohio State University for their efforts in establishing a productive environment.

Two other individuals helped in many ways; Kathy Jarvis and Claudia Spencer, our secretaries at The Ohio State University assisted us by taking care of often asked favors.

Finally, much appreciation to Judith A. Clayton, our editor at Brown Publishing Company for arriving half way through the writing of this book and taking us to completion.

And to the users of this text, we hope the outcome is a healthier you.

Section 1

Preparing to Teach Health Science

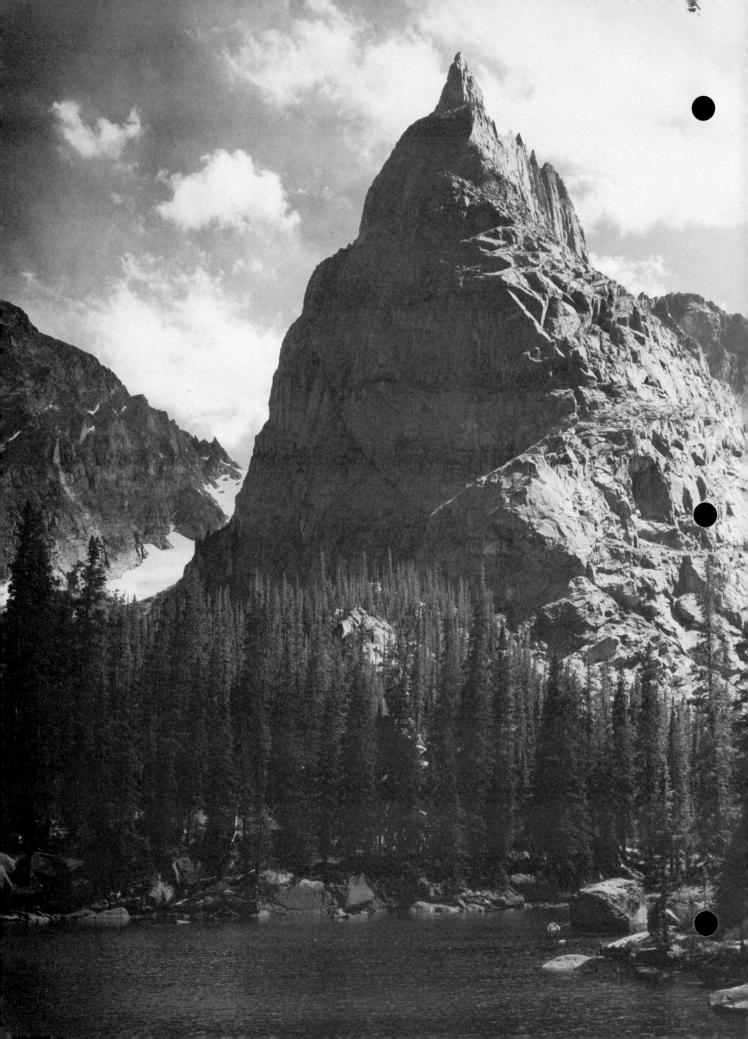

Quality Living
A Philosophy of Health Education for the Middle and Secondary Schools

1970s: Decade of Accomplishment

The United States experienced a decade of accomplishment in the 1970s in the area of health. Consider the decade's progress:

Life expectancy for the average American jumped 2.5 years, nearly as much as it increased over the preceding two decades.

Deaths from stroke decreased 31% between 1972 and 1978.

Heart-disease mortality fell 18% between 1970 and 1977, more than during the previous 20 years.

The infant-mortality rate was reduced from 20.0 deaths per 1,000 live births in 1970 to 13.1 in 1979.

Leukemia, Hodgkin's disease and other lymphomas, and osteogenic sarcoma ceased being early death sentences for youngsters.

Chemotherapy and radiotherapy gave breast-cancer patients more years of life. Testicular cancer yielded to cis-platinum, duodenal ulcers to cimetidine.

Rabies vaccination improved dramatically.

Amniocentesis and ultrasound made possible the accurate prenatal diagnosis of such genetic disorders as Down's syndrome.

The invention and widespread adoption of CT scanning and radioimmunoassay revolutionized much of diagnostic medicine.

Microsurgery led to routine replantation of severed limbs that regained a remarkable degree of function.

Treatment for diabetes, epilepsy, and end-stage kidney disease improved impressively, and treatment for the last was made available to everyone.

Nine out of 10 children between five and 14 were immunized against the major childhood infectious diseases; dreaded rubella epidemics all but disappeared.

Exposure to environmental carcinogens declined sharply.

The health status of minorities improved and their use of health services increased; the long decline in the number of primary care doctors was reversed; progress was made in distributing physician manpower better.[1]

A Look At Youth The 70s

Certainly these vast accomplishments in medicine are impressive. And their result, an increased 2.5 years of life expectancy, would lead us to believe that the health of our nation is greatly improving.

Unfortunately, statistics which describe the health status of youth in the United States during the late 1970s present a different picture.

United States Department of the Interior National Park Service Photo—George A. Grant

Death Rate

For example, the death rate of 15–24 year olds, our "young adults" was twenty times greater in 1977 than twenty years previously. In 1960, 15–24 year olds had a death rate of 106 per 100,000. By 1970, the rate was up to 128. By 1976, it had dropped to 113, but the next year climbed to 117, representing nearly 48,000 deaths in 1977.[2]

Causes of Death

The three major causes of deaths in this age group were accidents, homicides, and suicides.

> Accidents, homicides, and suicides account for about three fourths of all deaths in this age group. Responsibility has been attributed to behavior patterns characterized by judgmental errors, aggressiveness, and, in some cases, ambivalence about wanting to live or die. Certainly greater risk taking occurs in this period of life.[3]

Accidents

Accidents were the major cause of death during this period. Of these, motor accidents were the greatest single cause of death, accounting for 37% of all 15–24 year old deaths in 1977. Motorcycle accidents killed 1200 youth under the age of 20 in 1977.[4]

These data indicate the need for education about traffic safety in this age group. This data would also emphasize the need for education in earlier age groups such as the middle school, where important preventive steps can be taken.

Homicides

The second leading cause of death in the 15–24 year old age group in 1977 was homicide. Among blacks homicide is the leading cause of death, ranking slightly ahead of accidents. Young blacks are five times as likely to be murdered as whites. An overall American rate of 10.2 homicides per 100,000 per year in the 15–24 age group can be compared to other industrialized nations such as France, with 0.9, Britain, with 1.0, and Japan with 1.3.[5]

What factors in the American lifestyle might be altered to prevent such aggressive behavior, conduct that indicates a lack of value of the human life? Are there preventive measures and educational efforts that might be made in our middle and secondary schools which would lead to better adjusted young adults?

Suicide

Suicide ranked behind accidents and homicides in the 15–24 year old age group in 1977. Suicide accounted for 5600 deaths.[6]

Again we might ask what preventive measures and educational efforts might have been made in our middle and secondary schools to assist these youth in finding life worthwhile.

Health Problems

In addition to the statistics compiled for the 15–24 year old age group for which education in the middle and secondary schools might afford preventive measures, we might examine the health of adolescents.

Adolescence is the period of life ranging from ages 12 to 18. Examining the health behavior of adolescents in the late 70s we might focus on the following areas of concern:

teen-age pregnancy
alcohol consumption
tobacco smoking
marihuana usage
overweight and underweight

Teen Pregnancies

Teen-age pregnancy is certainly an area of concern and worth examining closely in the 80s. In 1977, one fourth of all teen-age girls had had at least one pregnancy by the age of 19.[7]

Teen pregnancies have an effect on the lifestyle of the mother as well as that of the unborn child. The children of teen mothers face increased risks in delivery and in birth defects. The teen mother often has her schooling interrupted, and if she marries she is six times as likely to become divorced. An examination of teen pregnancy in the middle and secondary school might alleviate this problem.

Alcohol, Tobacco, Marijuana

Other areas of concern focus are the use of alcohol, tobacco, and marijuana.

According to Grace Kovar, Statistician of the National Center for Health Statistics "Among all adolescents aged 12–17, it is estimated that 53% have tried alcohol, 47% have tried tobacco, and 28% have tried marijuana."[8]

Additional points made about the usage of alcohol, tobacco, and marijuana:

More than 90% of the class of 1977 in high school have tried alcohol at least one time.

Those who had tried cigarettes at least once constituted 76% of the senior class, and 56% had tried marijuana.

Sixteen percent had used marijuana within 30 days.[9]

A 1977 report from the Department of Health, Education and Welfare indicated that the number of young people aged 12–17 who were current users of marijuana jumped by almost one third from 1976 to 1977. In 1977, 16.1% of adolescents reported current use. Nine per cent of high school seniors used marijuana daily.[10]

"Although there were few new developments in research on human effects of marijuana during 1977, HEW stated that the increased use among adolescents was of concern since it is believed that this group may be more at risk than others because of their stage of psychological and physical development."[11]

Weight

In addition to the health problems that might result from the usage of drugs, we might note the problems that manifest themselves because of the increased consumption of foods. Weight is another factor that is affecting the health status of our adolescent population.

A Gallup poll in October of 1979 indicated that only one fourth of teens are happy with their present weight. One half of the teens polled wanted to lose weight, and one fourth would like to gain weight. An amazing 65% of teen girls want to lose weight, while 35% of teen boys want to do the same. Fourteen percent of girls want to gain and 35% of boys.[12]

It would appear that education in the middle and secondary schools might assist the adolescent in planning for weight control. When left to their own devices, "Boys who want to lose, exercise, girls often pick diet, but 18% of overweight boys and 13% of overweight girls do nothing."[13]

Lifestyle

In the same Gallup poll of 13–18 year olds in October of 1979, teens had some interesting comments about selecting a quality lifestyle.

When asked if they wanted a lifestyle similar to their parents:

54% wanted something different
42% wanted a lifestyle similar to what they have grown up with
 4% aren't sure what they want[14]

An examination of lifestyle and of alternate behaviors and styles that can contribute to quality living can and should be a part of the elementary, middle, and secondary curriculum.

The Role of Counselors, Teachers, Principals

The vast number of choices that a youngster can make need careful examination. A fortunate finding of another Gallup poll in 1979 indicated that teens have confidence in adults when examining problems.

During 1979, at least one American teenager in three sought help or advice for a disciplinary, academic, or personal problem, and 36% went to the school guidance counselor, 28% to a teacher, and 18% to someone else. The survey also found that 29% of teenagers indicated that they had had a private meeting with their school principal in the past year.[15]

The school can and should have a role in helping youth to examine the alternatives in lifestyle available. A careful examination of these alternatives may be helpful in solving some of the problems that adolescents encountered in the 70s and in promoting quality living in the 80s.

The Health Curriculum

We believe that an organized, sequential study of health should begin in the elementary school and continue in the middle and secondary schools.

In order for this type of education to have the greatest chance for success, each teacher will need an adequate preparation in health science.

The purpose of this text is to assist you, the middle and secondary teacher, in the careful preparation needed to teach health science. An additional purpose of this text is to provide you with some teaching materials that can be used successfully with middle and secondary school students.

As you begin to prepare yourself to teach health science, it is important to have a grasp on what is meant by the term "health" and what it means to have a "quality lifestyle."

What Is Health?

What is health? What is a healthy life style? How would you describe to someone else what a healthy life style means? How would you encourage someone to exhibit healthy behavior? How would you motivate or guide someone to change poor human habits?

These are some of the questions that the health educator faces in the 80's. Because of the difficulties experienced when attempting to provide answers, these questions have often been ignored. But if we are to influence the quality of life in the 80's we will have to pay close attention to these problems.

Defining health and health education, then establishing a philosophy of teaching are necessary and challenging tasks for the health educator. Thoughtful answers to these questions provide the groundwork for us to devise a framework for influencing, directing, and changing patterns of living.

Thus, we begin your book with an essential question: What Is Health?

Define *Health* in the space provided.

_____

_____

_____

Was this the first time that you examined and defined health? Have you always had the same feelings about what it means to be healthy?

A definition and philosophy are not static but dynamic. This means that your definitions of health and the philosophy you hold are most likely in a constant state of change. As you experience and learn more, you alter and add to your definition and philosophy.

One of the meaningful experiences in our professional life as health educators is the opportunity we have to share our definitions and our philosophies. These meaningful discussions and challenges of the mind through dialogue with other health educators help us to clarify what we are attempting to do and to become as professionals. We share our viewpoints with others, not to force these views upon them but to help them clarify their views.

Definitions of Health

Just how do people in our profession define health? Let us examine some explanations, beginning with the dictionary definitions. Immediately we will notice that there are many definitions for the word health. In the American Heritage Dictionary[16] we find the following:

> Health . . . the state of an organism with respect to functioning, disease, and abnormality at any given time.
> Health . . . the state of an organism functioning normally without disease or abnormality.
> Health . . . optimal functioning with freedom from disease and abnormality.
> Health . . . broadly, any state of optimal functioning, well being, or progress.

Next, we might turn to professional health organizations for descriptions of health. We will find a slightly different definition that deals with more than the absence of disease.

According to the World Health Organization, health is "a state of complete physical, mental, and social well-being and not merely the absence of disease or infirmity."

Examining the prominent authorities on the subject of health will enable us to further expand our definition of the meaning of health. René Dubos discusses man's ability to adapt to change as it relates to a concept of health. In his book *Man, Medicine, and Environment,* Dubos states his viewpoint on what it means to be healthy. Dubos considers health as a way of life which enables imperfect human beings "to achieve rewarding and not too painful existence while they cope with an imperfect world."[17]

Who Is Responsible for Health

It is important to us as professionals that each of us should examine the existing definitions of health, then formulate a definition that we can use with confidence. After defining health, the next logical question might be "Who is responsible for health?"

Who is responsible for *health*?

_____

_____

_____

_____

The Individual

Most of us would agree that the ultimate responsibility for health lies with the individual. However, the health of each individual is influenced by several environmental factors before the individual has any voice in the decision-making process. For example, the unborn child may experience alterations in environment such as the Rubella virus or the nicotine of the mother's cigarette. The unborn child has no choice as to the quality of his or her life. The small child may also experience environmental factors which influence that individual's health. The child's mother or father might brush his/her teeth until an age where the child can be responsible for his/her own dental health. In addition, rules might be set up for playing in the yard rather than near the street, in order to protect the child from traffic.

Returning to the question "Who is responsible for health?" we see that it cannot be simply answered with—"the individual." Although ultimately this person is in the driver's seat and has the right to make decisions about health, there are other factors to be considered.

In an article discussing the health educator's role, Phil Belcastro clarifies the responsibility for one's health. Belcastro[18] distinguishes between the obligation to protect health and the responsibility to promote health. For purposes of clarity, let us examine the following definitions:

> Protect: to cover or shield from danger or injury; to defend; to guard; to preserve in safety.[19]
> Protection: preservation from loss, injury or annoyance.[20]
> Promote: to forward; to advance; to contribute to the growth, engagement or excellence.[21]
> Promotion: the stirring up of interest in an enterprise.[22]

When we examine who is responsible for health, there is a clear distinction between being responsible for protecting health and being responsible for promoting health.

The Parent or Guardian

When we refer to the responsibility for protecting health, we think immediately of the mother of the unborn child and of the guardian of the small child. Because the unborn child and the small child are not yet mature enough to make decisions about the quality of their life, the person who is responsible for them also has the responsibility of protecting the child's health. As the child matures, this "protective role" shifts to the new identity of "promotion."

In other words, until the child can start making decisions for himself/ herself about health, the parent or guardian either makes the decisions or assists the child in making them. Eventually the parent shifts the responsibility to the child. At this point the older person is in the role of "promoting" health—contributing to the growth, arousing interest. The guardian (parent) realizes that the child is responsible for himself/herself and that the earlier the child assumes responsibility the better. We can see that it is necessary and desirable for the guardian (parents) of small children to protect and promote health.

The Community

Who else is responsible for the "protection" and "promotion" of health? Going back to our first answer, we said that ultimately the individual is responsible. At times, however, it becomes necessary to designate other safeguards. If each of us is responsible for protecting his or her health and making decisions that protect and promote health, we might select patterns of behaviors which infringe on the rights of others to protect their health. To safeguard the welfare of the community and the right of the individual to a healthy environment, we make laws that "protect" the health of the majority of people. For example, we make it mandatory that children be immunized prior to entering school. This "protects" school age children from a variety of diseases that would interfere with good health. We also enforce no smoking in public buildings to reduce the risk of a fire hazard. We designate crosswalks and enact traffic regulations.

We can see that it is necessary and desirable to have community "protection" for our health. But what about health "promotion?" Who assists the individual in advancing his/her health? Who assumes the role of "stirring up interest" and "contributing to the growth?"

What Is Health Education?

When the President's Committee on Health Education met in 1973, the Joint Committee on Health Education Terminology defined health education as a process with intellectual, psychological, and social dimensions relating to activities which increase the abilities of people to make informed decisions affecting their personal, family, and community well-being. This process, based on scientific principles, facilitates learning and behavioral change in both personnel and consumers, including children and youth.[3]

We can certainly say that the health educator has the role of "promoting" health. The definition of the Joint Committee is certainly compatible with the description of "promoting"— "stirring up interest" and "contributing to growth."

We might now ask "What does the health educator promote?" This is a very important, basic question. It is essential that each of us is able to answer this question so that we have some idea what our profession is all about.

What does the health educator promote?

_____

_____

_____

_____

Dr. John Burt, professor and chairman of Health Education at the University of Maryland, has advocated the idea that there are at least two very salient factors that contribute to the health of the individual. First, the individual needs to know "how to be healthy." In order to advance health, the person needs a knowledge base. This knowledge base provides useful information when the individual is engaged in making decisions which will effect life style.

Second, Burt discusses the notion of "something to be healthy for." He contends that individuals are much more likely to desire to protect and promote their health if they have "something to be healthy for." This latter aspect is certainly involved in achieving positive mental health.

Your Authors' Philosophy

We are in agreement with Dr. Burt. We feel that as health educators we need to look at the individual with at least two questions in mind:

1. What information does this individual require in order to know "how to be healthy?"

2. Does this individual have "something to be healthy for?"

We ask one question which helps further to clarify our purpose: What is a healthy life style?

A Healthy Life Style

We believe that "a healthy lifestyle" can be described in the words of Emmanuel Kant: *The three grand essentials to happiness in this life are something to do, someone to love, and something to hope for.*[24]

What differentiates those who select balanced, healthy life styles from those who develop poor human habits? What differentiates the periods in our lives when we make optimal healthy decisions from the times when our decisions are unhealthy or self-defeating?

We believe that most persons are engaged in balanced, healthy living when their life style includes:

1. Something to do: worthwhile projects that contribute to self esteem.

2. Someone to love: satisfying interpersonal relationships.

3. Something to hope for: a meaningful philosophy of life that makes the future worthwhile.

A Health Triangle

We have designed a health triangle depicting these three aspects of health with the center being the balance of these dimensions. The center symbolizes *the healthy life style.* A healthy life style is one in which there is an equilibrium of body, mind, and spirit, and where there is a balance of something to do, someone to love, and something to hope for.

We will discuss each dimension of the health triangle and relate it to how it serves to promote health. Let us begin by talking about two sides of the triangle: *Something to do* and *someone to love.*

It is interesting to note how many different researchers mention these two needs as being fundamental to the promotion of health.

For example, Zick Rubin, Harvard Researcher, in his book *Liking and Loving*[25] identifies the need for affection and the need for respect. We can relate the research of Rubin to *something to do* and *something to hope for.*

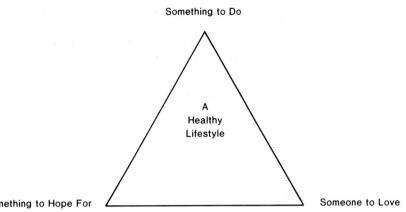

Something to Do

A Healthy Lifestyle

Something to Hope For

Someone to Love

1. Rubin said that each of us has a need for respect and therefore we need to do something to earn that respect. Our need for respect focuses on the evaluation of dimensions such as adjustment, maturity, good judgement, and intelligence.[26]

2. Rubin also points to the need we have for affection, for satisfying interpersonal relationships. The affectionate aspect of each person comprises different attachment components. This side of us seeks someone to care for, to confide in, to be close to.[27]

Do you have a need for respect and affection? How do you meet these needs? Complete the following sentences.

People respect me _____

_____

_____

_____

The people that care for me _____

_____

_____

_____

Rollo May in his book *Love and Will*[28] also discusses these two aspects of man. He describes life as a blending of wish and will.

May refers to *wish* as the imaginative, feeling part of man, and he uses *will* as the more logical plan for putting wish into action. May states indirectly that it is this plan (something to do) and the whimsical loving nature (someone to love) that blend together to form an integrated personality and optimal living.

Looking further, we can examine basic physiological processes and substantiate to our premise that healthy life style is dependent upon *something to do* and *someone to love*.

The brain is divided into two hemispheres, with dramatic distinctions in their functions.

The left hemisphere works like a computer. By stringing together linear messages into a logical chain of thought and filtering out sensory messages that do not apply to solving the problem at hand, the left section acts as an abstract deductor center.[29]

The right hemisphere operates intuitively. It allows a person to link external and internal qualities so that the self can be experienced as interrelated with nature, with others, with the chain of existence. It has the capacity to fantasize, which makes possible leaps of imagination and invention.[30]

There seems to be a point of equilibrium which functions to promote health. This is the balance of the need to be alone, productive, and logical with the need to be close, attached, and warm.

Let us further examine each side of the triangle to further clarify our concept of what acts to promote health.

Something to Do

If something to do is important in the promotion of health and in the development of a healthy life style, then we believe that there is a need to assist very young children find things to do to help them develop the respect which they need to function fully and enjoy optimal health.

The influence of projects and the attitude toward projects contribute significantly to self esteem. Studs Terkel in a book called *Working*[31] interviewed several people who had the same job and discovered how a person's perception of "something to do" greatly influenced happiness.

Isn't this perception related to our need for respect, especially self respect? It is disturbing to learn that a person does not like his job, his school major, his leisure projects—*the something to do.*

Some of the comments made during interviews which appear in Terkel's book:

> Bank Teller: You're never noticed or introduced. I don't even know who the president of the bank is. I don't even know what he looks like.[32]
>
> Farm Worker: If I had enough money I would take busloads of people out to the fields and into the labor camps. Then they'd know how that fine salad got on their table.[33]

We believe that *something to do* is essential to the promotion of health and that there are two underlying premises associated with this need.

First, we believe that each of us needs to have meaningful projects which give purpose to our lives. Second, we believe that sharing of these efforts promotes a healthy life style. The interest that we have and that others have in our projects, and the recognition which we convey in supporting the efforts of others, contribute to optimal health.

The farmer and the bank teller are examples of persons who are frustrated because their projects lack meaning for others. Thus, feedback is important in the promotion and development of healthy life style.

When was the last time that someone helped you to see something good about yourself? What was it? How did you feel?

_____

_____

_____

_____

When was the last time that you helped someone to see something good in himself or herself? Did you feel good when you shared this with that individual? How did the other person feel?

_____

_____

_____

_____

Someone to Love

Our projects are important to promoting and maintaining health. People are also very important in influencing our health. The impact of people might be described as follows:

> The people I love give meaning to my existence beyond simply feeding my gut, feeding my vanity, or giving me pleasure. I treasure them. They help me remain inspirited, "turned on" to my life. And when they need help, I abandon the projects on which I was then engaged and use my time and resources to help them live more fully, joyously, and meaningfully.[34]

We believe *someone to love* is important in the promotion and development of a healthy life style; to promote or advance health each of us needs to love and to be loved, to be loving and loveable.

Something to Hope For

A discussion of the third dimension of the health triangle, *something to hope for*, is frightening to many. Many persons believe that man's spiritual health is not a topic to be discussed in a public or professional setting.

We feel quite differently about the need for each health educator to examine *something to hope for*. By disclosing to others how we feel about *something to hope for* we draw closer to our fellow man rather than being alienated from that person, or indifferent to who he is, how he feels, and what he lives for.

According to Sidney Jourard, psychologist, "a person lives as long as he experiences his life as having meaning and value and as long as he has something to live for—meaningful projects that inspirit him and invite him to move into his future."[35]

His message is easily explained. A positive assessment of one's present existence and future horizons is an essential ingredient of health promotion and high level personal soundness.

There are two underlying premises which clarify *something to hope for*. First, we believe that each of us needs to take personal responsibility for our spiritual growth and needs. Second, we believe that each of us needs to respect the spiritual growth of our fellow man.

The neglect of this second premise may be what is responsible for the lack of discussion and communication about spiritual health.

It is our belief that *something to hope for* is not the same for everyone just as *something to do* (our projects) and *someone to love* (our relationships), which imply freedom of choice and individual responsibility.

What is common to health promotion and to the development of a healthy lifestyle is the need for *something to hope for*, and not the specific way of acting it out.

The health educator as health promoter assists the student in acting out in his own way *something to do, someone to love,* and *something to hope for.* The health educator promotes individual decisions and responsibility for those decisions. This is a specific type of teaching and sharing.

A Healthy Life Style: The Center

"Leading you to the threshold of your own mind" is another way of saying that when we promote health in the classroom we are concerned with assisting the student in making health decisions that promote a quality life style.

We have identified and discussed the three sides of equilateral triangle which we feel are important in promoting health. Those were: something to do, someone to love, and something to hope for. In the center of the triangle are the words "a healthy lifestyle."

About Your Textbook

Throughout this book we will be dealing with factors that we believe influence life style. Our approach to health education will be process oriented. We view the quality life style as specific to an individual's capabilities. The student is not indoctrinated with specific health behaviors but learns to take responsibility for making choices. This individual is taught a process that can be used throughout life to make decisions that will be conducive to a balanced lifestyle. The student assumes responsibility for health.

Health Education as a Process

It is our belief that the health education teacher promotes health in the student by assisting in the following process:

1. Identifying life-style dimensions that promote harmony and balance. The life-style dimensions which we have identified for study in middle and secondary schools are concerned with mental health and self concept, body systems, cardiovascular health and fitness, nutrition and weight control, drugs, tobacco, disease control and prevention, communicable and noncommunicable diseases, first aid and safety, human sexuality, consumer health and medical care, environmental health, and death, dying, and aging.

2. For each life-style dimension studied, alternative health behaviors are identified. For example, while studying nutrition and weight control several diets would be identified—low carbohydrate, grapefruit, vegetarian, etc.

3. After identifying the possible alternative health behaviors, each line of conduct is evaluated carefully. For example, how would we evaluate a low carbohydrate diet? How fast would one lose weight? Are there any health risks? What kinds of foods are available while on this type of diet?

4. The student then selects the health behavior pattern of his choice after he has evaluated each alternative carefully. Thus, the individual is accountable for the consequences and benefits of the behavior of his choice.

5. The student reassesses his behavior at intervals, evaluating the effects, and continuing behavior which positively influences lifestyle, while abandoning behavior that interferes with quality living.

The most important aspect of this approach is that by teaching the importance of quality living by means of a process for examining behavior, we give the student a process to use after leaving the classroom.

Chapter Summary

The health of the American public was advanced by the accomplishments of medicine in the 1970s. Although there were many encouraging advances, the health behavior patterns of adolescents in the 1970s were disappointing. For health to be improved in the adolescent, 12 to 18 year old population, in the 80s we will need to examine the components of a quality lifestyle.

Adolescents will need to consider health and to assume personal responsibility for health. The middle and secondary school teacher can:

1. Assist the student in finding worthwhile projects and developing self respect. (*Something to do*)

2. Help the student communicate openly in interpersonal relationships. (*Someone to love*)

3. Encourage the student to develop a philosophy of life. (*Something to hope for*)

4. Teach the student a process for selecting healthy behaviors and for evaluating and reevaluating these behaviors as they promote quality living. (*A healthy lifestyle*)

Notes

1. Dorsey W. Woodson, "The 1970s: decade of accomplishment," *Medical World News.* Vol. 21, No. 1, page 4, 1980.
2. "Death Rate Leaps for Youths 15–24," *Columbus Dispatch.* August 5, 1979, page 12. (excerpts from "Healthy People: The Surgeon Generals Report on Health Promotion and Disease Prevention," July, 1979.).
3. *IBID.*
4. *IBID.*
5. *IBID.*
6. *IBID.*
7. *IBID.*
8. "More Youths Try Alcohol Than Tobacco," *The Nation's Health.* June, 1979, page 16.
9. *IBID.*
10. "Use of Marijuana Rises Among Young," *The Nation's Health.* June, 1979, page 16.
11. *IBID.*
12. George Gallup, "Half of All Teens Want to Reduce," October, 1979.
13. *IBID.*
14. Gallup Youth Survey, "Different Lives Sought By Teens," *Columbus Dispatch.* Wednesday, March 5, 1980, A-11.
15. *IBID.*
16. *The American Heritage Dictionary.* New York: Houghton Mifflin, 1973.
17. Rene Dubos. *Man, Medicine, and Environment.* New York: Praeger, 1968, p. 67.
18. Phil Belcastro, "The Coalescence of Philosophy and Process in Health Education."
19. *Webster's New Twentieth Century Dictionary.* New York: World Publishing Company, 1975 (second edition).
20. *Webster's New Twentieth Century Dictionary.* New York: World Publishing Company, 1975 (second edition).
21. *Webster's New Twentieth Century Dictionary.* New York: World Publishing Company, 1975 (second edition).
22. *Webster's New Twentieth Century Dictionary.* New York: World Publishing Company, 1975 (second edition).
23. President's Committee on Health Education—The Joint Committee on Health Education Terminology. *The Report of the President's Committee on Health Education.* October, 1973, pg. 65–66.

24. Saying of Emmanuel Kant appears on plaques and cards.

25. Zick Rubin. *Liking and Loving: An Invitation to Social Psychology*. New York: Holt, Rinehart, and Winston, 1973.

26. Zick Rubin. *Liking and Loving: An Invitation to Social Psychology*. New York: Holt, Rinehart, and Winston, 1973.

27. Zick Rubin. *Liking and Loving: An Invitation to Social Psychology*. New York: Holt, Rinehart, and Winston, 1973.

28. Rollo May. *Love and Will*. New York: W. W. Norton Company, 1969.

29. Rollo May. *Love and Will*. New York: W. W. Norton Company, 1969.

30. Rollo May. *Love and Will*. New York: W. W. Norton Company, 1969.

31. Studs Terkel. *Working*. New York: Pantheon Books, 1972.

32. Studs Terkel. *Working*. New York: Pantheon Books, 1972,4.

33. Studs Terkel. *Working*. New York: Pantheon Books, 1972,4.

34. Sidney M. Jourard. *The Transparent Self*. New York: D. Van Nostrand Company, 1971.

35. *IBID*.

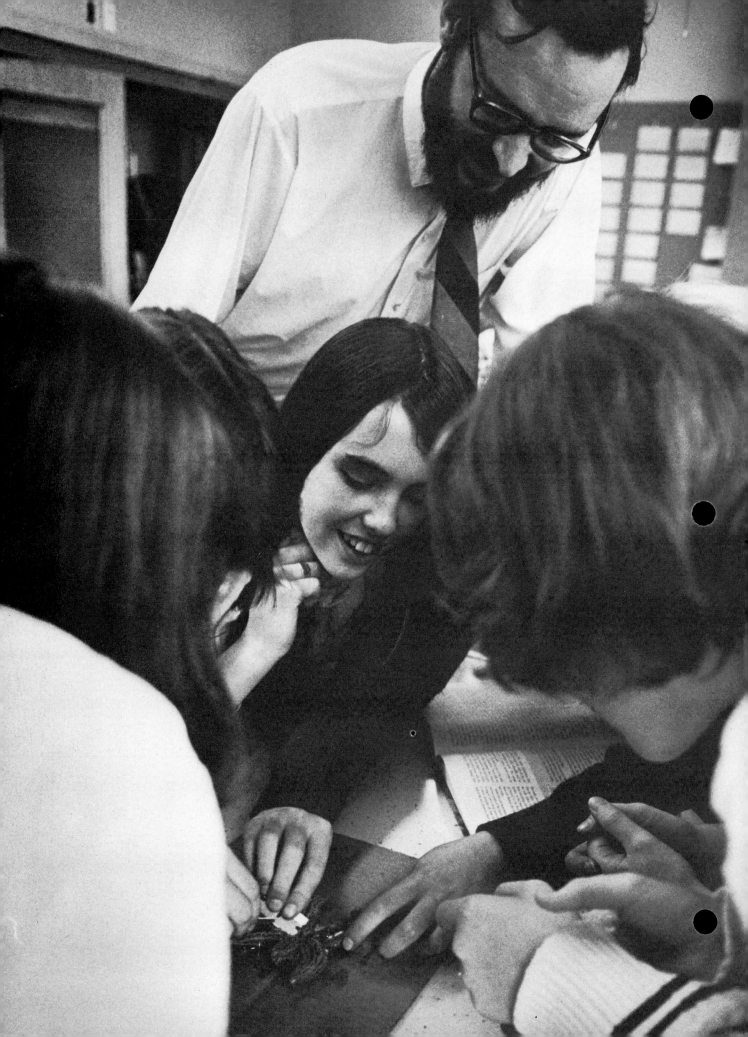

Classroom Atmosphere
Mental Health, Communication, and Discipline

The Learning Environment

Careful consideration of your philosophy of teaching is important in deciding the direction of learning that will take place in the classroom. The direction which you define will indicate to you what you want for your students.

As we mentioned in Chapter One, the direction or goal in which we wish to move is one that furnishes to the students a process for selecting their health behavior, of accountability for the consequences and benefits of the health behavior that they select.

We could state further that we want students to possess the skills of self-direction, self-responsibility, self-determination, self-control, and self-evaluation.

In this approach to education, the classroom becomes a laboratory where students learn to become an authority on their own life styles, as well as to learn and practice the skills mentioned above.

The learning environment is critical in this type of experience; it can promote or enhance this approach or flatly "kill it."

Consider the effect on learning that the following classroom environment poses:

About School[1]

He always wanted to say things. But no one understood.
He always wanted to explain things. But no one cared.
So he drew.

Sometimes he would just draw and it wasn't anything. He wanted to carve it in stone or write it in the sky.
He would lie out on the grass and look up in the sky, and it would be only he and the sky and the things inside that needed saying.

And it was after this that he drew the picture. It was a beautiful picture. He kept it under the pillow and would let no one see it.
And he would look at it every night and think about it. And when it was dark, and his eyes were closed, he could still see it.
And it was all of him. And he loved it.

When he started school he brought it with him. Not to show anyone, but just to have with him like a friend.

It was funny about school.

He sat in a square, brown desk like all the other square, brown desks and he thought it should be red.

And his room was a square, brown room. Like all the other rooms. And it was tight and close. And stiff.

He hated to hold the pencil and the chalk with his arm stiff and his feet flat on the floor, stiff, with the teacher watching and watching.

And then he had to write numbers. And they weren't anything. They were worse than the letters that could be something if you put them together.

And the numbers were tight and square and he hated the whole thing.

The teacher came and spoke to him. She told him to wear a tie like all the other boys. He said he didn't like them and she said it didn't matter.

After that they drew. And he drew all yellow and it was the way he felt about morning. And it was beautiful.

The teacher came and smiled at him. "What's this?" she said. "Why don't you draw something like Ken's drawing? Isn't that beautiful?"

It was all questions.

After that his mother bought him a tie and he always drew airplanes and rocket ships like everyone else. And he threw the old picture away.

And when he lay out alone looking at the sky, it was big and blue and all of everything, but *he* wasn't anymore.

He was square inside and brown, and his hands were stiff and he was like anyone else. And the thing inside him that needed saying didn't need saying anymore.

It had stopped pushing. It was crushed. Stiff.

Like everything else.

The classroom environment described in this poem is the antithesis of the environment that students need to practice and learn the skills of self-direction, self-responsibility, self-determination, self-control, and self-evaluation.

The classroom atmosphere and the relationship between the teacher and the student must focus on the development of these skills. The teacher-student relationship can promote self-direction, self-responsibility, and self-confidence when it has:[2]

The Teacher-Student Relationship

1. Openness or transparency, so each is able to risk directness and honesty with the other.

2. Caring, when each knows that he is valued by the other.

3. Interdependence (as opposed to dependency) of one on the other.

4. Separateness, to allow each to grow and to develop his uniqueness, creativity, and individuality.

5. Mutual Needs meeting so that neither's needs are met at the expense of the other's needs.

Schools that seem to have a positive classroom atmosphere, promote mental health, establish open communication, and foster creative discipline tend to have a significant number of teachers who "consciously strive to create school practices that teach students to think for themselves, to accept responsibility for themselves, and for life within the school, and to behave appropriately even when adults or rules are absent."[3]

Teaching Mental Health, Communication and Creative Discipline

Thus, mental health, communication, and creative discipline are learned in the classroom by means of a process.

How can we go about the difficult task of teaching this very important process? We might offer the following suggestions:

1. Establish an atmosphere of trust in the classroom so that the student can try out or risk ways of behaving to learn these skills.

2. Develop communication skills that foster openness, honesty, and responsibility for feelings and beliefs.

3. Plan classroom sessions which focus on the skills of problem solving at work.

4. Have a clear model to examine when conflict arises, a model with a multitude of alternatives from which to choose a creative approach to discipline.

An Atmosphere of Trust

In a classroom dealing with self-direction, self-responsibility, self-determination, self-control, and self-evaluation students need the opportunity to test out behaviors to experience and gain important self-knowledge.

This "testing out" process is a risky business for the novice. It means revealing things about oneself rather than hiding one's beliefs and feelings.

Establishing an atmosphere of trust in your classroom is the first step in facilitating the process of learning and furthering the opportunity to gain self-knowledge.

Definitions of Trust

What is trust? The following statements were made by our students when asked this question:[4]

1. "Trust is when I feel free to let myself go without worrying or being concerned with the consequences."

2. "Trust is when I accept myself and believe that others accept me."

3. "When I don't have any unresolved fears or blocks and I am able to communicate my true feelings to those individuals around me."

4. "Trust is a climate set up between individuals which provides for open and honest communication."

5. "Trust is when individuals can give me feedback about myself without me being overly defensive."

6. "When trust exists I am ready to risk a self-disclosure in a group situation."

How do you feel about trust? What is your definition? We liked the statements made by our students, especially the last one about the willingness to risk self-disclosure.

"Disclosure means to unveil, to make manifest, or to show. Self-disclosure is the act of making yourself manifest, showing yourself so others can perceive you."[5]

In the process which we outlined for making healthy decisions we talked about identifying alternatives to behavior, evaluating each alternative, selecting an alternative, being responsible for the consequences of the behavior, and at a later point, re-evaluating the behavior to see whether it fosters harmony and balance.

In order to have this process operating in the classroom, students need to share feelings, beliefs, and values in an atmosphere where they will not be judged, devalued, ridiculed, or feel ashamed.

Many students are afraid to disclose their thoughts in the classroom. John Powell, author of *Why Am I Afraid To Tell You Who I Am?* discusses this fear in his book. He says "I am afraid to tell you who I am, because if I tell you who I am, you may not like who I am, and it's all I have."[6]

Acceptance through Verbal and Nonverbal Behavior

For the student to have trust the teacher must be accepting of himself or herself and accepting of the student. The teacher can give the student indications of acceptance through verbal and nonverbal behavior.

Verbal Clues

The teacher can use verbal clues to show acceptance of the student. These clues and verbal patterns of response are discussed below in the section on communication skills.

The teacher can also discuss the concept of acceptance with students. We feel that a frank discussion of acceptance facilitates teacher-student understanding and sets the stage for open communication.

What is acceptance? Although there are several definitions of this term we especially liked the one which said "to take as it comes" and also "to acknowledge."

We liked these two definitions because we think it is important to acknowledge our students and to take them as they are. We do want to point out one thing that we share with them, however.

In a classroom where alternative behaviors are to be discussed, the teacher needs to clarify the difference between accepting the student as a person and accepting all behaviors. It is important for healthy living and for a classroom with an atmosphere of trust, that we as teachers accept, acknowledge, and allow our students to be themselves.

It is not always possible or desirable to acknowledge all student behavior acceptable. In other words, I can like and accept you, but your behavior may at times be displeasing to me.

It is important to discuss this notion with students so that when they receive feedback from you about displeasing behavior they do not feel that it is an attack on them personally.

Nonverbal Clues

Another means that teachers can use to convey acceptance of the student is in the realm of nonverbal. A smile, a sigh, or positive nod of the head can convey understanding, warmth, and encouragement.

In addition to these gestures, the teacher can employ touch to show the student that he is accepted.

In a recent survey conducted by one of your authors, students were asked to write down any question that they had regarding human sexuality. Questions were collected from several thousand students grades K–12, with the younger children being given assistance.

One of the most interesting findings in the survey was the most typical question asked by students in the third grade. It was "Can I kiss the teacher?"

It made us do some thinking about the needs that students have and how the teacher handles these needs. Why was this question asked repeatedly?

We felt that it was important and revealed a great deal about education and the need for acceptance at all grade levels, and not just the third grade students.

It had two implications for us. The first implication had to do with the students' attitude toward the teacher. It implied to us that the students had a warm, caring feeling. By stating "Can I kiss the teacher?" the student was sharing this warmth and desire to demonstrate his or her feelings.

We also felt that the students expressed a need for a gesture from the teacher. We were not concerned with whether or not kissing a third grade student was a desirable behavior for a third grade teacher, but we asked ourselves "In what ways can the teacher respond appropriately at each of the different grade levels with a physical gesture implying trust and acceptance?"

Sidney Jourard, psychologist, says, "But if I touch him or if he touches me, he takes on a dimension of reality more real than if I just see him or hear him."[7]

If the teacher is more "real" and the student is more "real" with touch, then the student-teacher relationship will be more real if touch is used in the classroom.

A pat on the back, a hand-shake, hug, or the latest "give me five" with an outspread hand may generate positive feelings in the classroom; this may facilitate the sharing and discussion of feelings that are necessary in a course on healthy living.

Acceptance, the act of acknowledging the student, can take many forms; acceptance facilitates communication.

Communication Skills

Communication is the process by which we send and receive messages. In the classroom setting, sometimes the teacher is sending messages and the student is in the role of receiver, while at other times the student is sending messages and the teacher assumes the receiving role.

When a message is sent there is usually a degree or level of comprehension on the part of the receiver. High level communication between teacher and student results from an open and honest transmission of ideas and a nonevaluative system of receiving messages.[8]

The sending and receiving skills necessary for high level communication need to be demonstrated in the classroom. These skills are necessary for communication. They are also necessary to reach one of our major goals—self-direction, self-responsibility, self-determination, self-control and self-evaluation.

Sending Messages

First we will consider sending messages. We are sitting in a classroom discussing the many alternatives to healthy behavior, asking our students to evaluate these alternatives and to account for their selection. We can anticipate two kinds of messages will be sent with a great frequency.

First, in order to evaluate behavior the student will need information about how certain behaviors influence his health. Student and teacher will be examining content or factual information. This type of sending focuses on messages that are conveyed objectively. They are sent without added feelings of the teacher or student, in their purely factual presentation. The data is transmitted for the purposes of gathering information to make wise decisions.

We then move to a second kind of message in the classroom. The student is going to evaluate at a personal level this information which he has gathered, reflecting his attitudes, beliefs, and values. After all, his next task is to select behavior and stand accountable for the consequences of the behavior that he selected.

I Messages

"One technique used to process and to effectively communicate at this level is through the use of *I* messages. Another word for an *I* message is 'responsibility message.' *I* messages are statements about the self, revelations of inner feelings and needs, information not processed by others. *I* messages entail three risks: self-disclosure, self-modification, responsibility."[9]

To have the greatest impact, an *I* message must have three components:[10]*

1. The first component involves the identification of a specific behavior.

2. The second component of a three part *I* message pins down the tangible or concrete effect of the specific behavior described in the message's first part.

3. The third part of the *I* message states the feelings generated by the effect.

Simply stated, *I* messages contain a behavior, an effect, and a feeling. We can examine examples of *I* messages to clarify these components.

I Messages to Describe Behavior

I messages can be used when discussing life-style dimensions. For example, if we were in a classroom discussing our nutritional style and the goal of the discussion was for the student to accept responsibility for his nutritional choices, we might hear the following *I* messages:

1. When I eat too many desserts, I gain weight and I don't feel very good about myself.

2. When I attempt to starve myself, I am very tired and irritable and I am not happy.

3. When someone tempts me to go off my diet, I usually begin to overeat and I get angry with myself for not having more self-control.

When students use *I* messages in the evaluation of life-style alternatives they learn to accept responsibility for their behavior, its effect, and the feelings generated.

I Messages Describe Student-Teacher Needs

I messages are also used in a classroom to communicate needs between teacher and student. Earlier we said that in a healthy classroom there was "mutual needs meeting" so that neither the teacher's or the students' needs are met at the expense of the other.

The following *I* messages convey messages sent for the purposes of mutual needs meeting:

1. (teacher) When the first aid box is left out, some of the contents are misplaced and I get angry trying to find them.

2. (student) When I am criticized in front of the class, some of the students laugh at me and I feel dumb and worthless.

3. (teacher) When we are studying a new lesson and no one asks a question I am unsure whether you understand me and I feel very uneasy.

---

*From *Teacher Effectiveness Training* by Thomas Gordon, © 1974, Published by Peter Wyden. Reprinted by permission of David McKay Company, Inc.

Receiving Messages

After messages are sent, it is important to make certain that they are received. We need only to sit in a circle and pass a secret around the classroom having the last person repeat it, to show how we misinterpret what we hear.

Active Listening or Feeding Back

Each of us needs some effective receiving tools to complete the communication process. In his book on *Teacher Effectiveness Training,* Dr. Thomas Gordon discusses the process of active listening or feeding back.

Gordon says:

> Most messages people send are uniquely coded. This means that the content of the message may be related to the feeling, but the feeling itself is not clearly expressed.
>
> Because most young people's messages are uniquely coded and therefore difficult to understand, it is foolish for teachers to respond only to the code. To do so results in misunderstanding the real meaning of the youngster's message.
>
> While the decoding process is critical in the communication process, you do not know whether you are right or wrong. Equally important, the student cannot know whether you have decoded his message correctly or incorrectly.
>
> The process of 'feeding back' is what we call 'active listening.' It is the last step that completes an effective communication process.[11]

Discipline: Problem Solving At Work

Thus far we have concerned ourselves with building a classroom with a trusting atmosphere, developing and practicing communication skills which enhance the teacher-student and student-student relationship.

We have focused on these skills sequentially because we believe that these are the tools for a creative approach to discipline, a major concern of the American public.

> According to seven of the last eight Annual Gallup Polls of the Public's Attitudes Toward the Public Schools, the American public considers "lack of discipline" the biggest problem for public schools.

The October, 1976, poll showed that:

> 22% of the respondents were concerned about discipline—7% more than the second place concern.
>
> Responding to related questions, 50% reported that enforcing stricter discipline would do the most to improve the quality of public education.
>
> 49% felt that test scores had declined because society is becoming too permissive.
>
> 47% said they would like to serve on a committee working on "discipline and related problems.[12]

Interestingly, Dr. William Wayson, well known designer of creative approaches to discipline at The Ohio State University, describes discipline as a process which closely parallels the process that we teach for selecting health behaviors. According to Wayson "Discipline is the ability to size up a situation and to see what needs to be done; to see several ways of behaving in a situation, to choose one of them, and to learn what happens. The measure of success is whether students conduct themselves in a productive way when there is no authority present to catch or correct them."[13]

Examining Dr. Wayson's statements we felt that he was saying that discipline is a process. Thus, we can also say that discipline is learned and that it can and should be taught. We also felt that Dr. Wayson's approach to discipline is philosophically compatible with the end results we desire—

that the student possesses the skills of self-direction, self-responsibility, self-determination, self-control, and self-evaluation.

Discipline and the skills needed for the process can be examined, tested, and practiced in the classroom by means of classroom sessions that focus on the skills of problem solving.

Role Simulation

Role simulation is a technique which makes it possible for students and teachers to experience what they are feeling while trying to cope with assigned problem situations similar to those they face in the regular classroom.

"Through role simulation, teachers and students can learn how to cope, how to make better choices, how to become aware and honest in the expression of feelings. The emphasis is on their doing rather than their thinking and on becoming aware that the key to their being is within themselves and not without."[14] Thus, role simulation can help develop the skills of self-direction, self-responsibility, self-determination, self-control, and self-evaluation.

Dr. George Borelli, author of *Role Simulation* and well known Gestalt psychologist, travels nationwide to utilize role simulation in the training of professionals in the mental health and education field. Dr. Borelli outlines four techniques for the design of role simulation in his book:[15]

1. The simplest way that role simulation can be set up is to give simple instructions to both participants at the same time.

2. A second technique is to give instructions to one participant in the room while the other participant is outside the room or not within hearing.

3. A third and slightly more difficult way is to set up a role where the conflict or problem is clearly known.

4. When individuals are more timid or less responsive, a fourth and still more difficult approach to role simulation is to ask an individual to talk to an empty chair so that only that person's side of the dialogue is characterized and identified.

The following education simulations can be found in Dr. Borelli's book. We suggest that you try these with your classmates. When you are teaching, utilize these simulations with your students as a problem solving technique.

Education Simulations

Aggressive Student
General: A person is to act the role of an aggressive student in a classroom by pushing, poking, shoving, and provoking the teacher.
To The Aggressive Student: You are to be aggressive toward the teacher. Poke him, push him, and pay little attention to his requests. Grab his wristwatch, pencil or paper, and refuse to give it back.
To The Teacher: Cope with this student.

Uncooperative Student
General: No matter what the teacher asks of the student, the student does not respond in a cooperative fashion.
To The Uncooperative Student: You are to play the role of an uncooperative student who does not respond positively but often negatively and contrary to whatever is asked or expected of him.
To The Teacher: You are to ask this particular student to participate in a series of activities or projects.

Smart Alecky Student

General: A student in the classroom is a smart aleck and is always saying things out loud in a crude, obnoxious, and abusive way.

To The Smart Aleck: You are to play the role of a smart aleck who always has something nasty, abusive, or obnoxious to say because of the response you get from the rest of the class. You really get a kick out of teasing your teacher.

To The Teacher: This particular student in your class has been having difficulties at home, and you've noticed a change in his behavior. Cope with him.

After the simulations, utilize the following discussion questions:[16]

How do you feel now?

Did you communicate what you wanted to?

Did you follow instructions or deviate? In what way? For what reason?

What did you leave unsaid? What nonverbal communication did you perceive?

What did the nonverbal communication say?

What prevented you from saying what you wanted to say?

What were your feelings during the role? After finishing the role?

Did you resolve the conflict to your satisfaction? Describe the conflict resolution.

Are you in a better or worse place? Describe how you feel.

Encourage classmates to share their feelings and reservations.

When acting out these simulations, allow the students to participate in the role of the teacher, as well as you, the teacher, participating in the student role. Thus, the roles can help to discover means of meeting mutual needs in the classroom.

Psychosocial Drama

Another method or technique used to focus on the skills of problem solving at work is the development of psycho-social drama.

Psycho-social drama is similar to role playing, but the roles are presented to the students rather than by them. One of the strengths of psycho-social drama is that it is a tool that students can relate to, but it is not threatening. Each situation presented is familiar, but moved from real life into a commentary.[17]

Developers of psycho-social drama, Dee Mason and Jim Million of The Institute for Human Awareness have identified nine steps to prepare psycho-social drama material. These steps are described in the following outline.

Nine Steps to Prepare Psycho-Social Drama Material[18]

Step One: Pick a target population for the psychosocial drama (for our purposes the target population will most likely be the school). However, there are other target populations associated with students of junior and senior high school age:

a. service clubs

b. churches

c. athletic teams

d. classroom

e. home

Step Two: Design the content of the drama to be presented. When designing content ask the following questions:
   a. What is it we want to say?
   b. What questions do we want them to ask themselves?
   c. What responses might we expect?

Step Three: Organize your psycho-social drama team. Your team might consist of other teachers in your school, volunteer parents, community resource personnel, or students from another class, etc. Get the psycho-social team together and create a setting (home, school, party, etc.) and characters (husband and wife with student, school-students in a classroom, friends, etc.).
   a. Setting
   b. Characters in Setting

Step Four: Role-play immediately a desired setting or situation. Example:
   a. Student hands in a term paper late to the teacher
   b. Student enters the classroom who has been using a drug (marijuana, or alcohol).
   c. Student is tardy frequently. Teacher is calling the parents.

Use a tape recorder for the first role-play session.

Step Five: With the desired target population and desired content of presentation in mind, extract and add to initial role play ideas that will add to the situation.
   a.
   b.
   c.
   d.
   e.
   f.

Step Six: With additions to material, run scene again using tape recorder.

Step Seven: When you have run the scene several times—examine the questions below on "How to Analyze A Character" to see it the characters you are playing are consistent.

How to Analyze a Character
Since no actor can express what he does not understand, ask yourself these questions as you attempt your characterization for any new role:
   1. Who am I?
   2. In what country do I live?
   3. What is the period or time of this play?
   4. How old am I?
   5. Am I single, married or divorced?
   6. Have I any unusual physical features?
   7. Do I dress neatly or carelessly?
   8. What is my habitual posture?
   9. Am I in good health?
   10. What is my disposition? Do I have any unusual traits or mannerisms?
   11. What is my position in society?
   12. What education do I have?
   13. Do I use good English? Do I have a dialect or accent?
   14. In what kind of house do I live?
   15. What have my environment and background been?
   16. What kind of life have I led?
   17. In what things am I most deeply interested?
   18. At the outset of the play how do I feel toward other characters?

19. Why do I feel that way?
20. How do other characters feel toward me?
21. During the play does my feeling toward others change? Why and how?
22. As the play progresses do the other characters treat me differently? How and why?
23. How is the audience supposed to feel about me . . . sympathy, distrust, admiration or disapproval?

Step Eight: Rehearse Again.

Step Nine: Once the scene is ready, put the scene together into the context of a program for the classroom (or Parent Teacher Meeting, etc.) and build processing material. How do you want the students to deal with the material presented?

Creative Discipline: A Model of Alternatives

Through classroom sessions, including role simulations and psycho-social drama, students experience problem-solving techniques which develop self-direction, self-responsibility, self-determination, self-control, and self-evaluation.

In addition to fostering the development of these skills in students, the teacher needs to have a clear model to examine when conflict arises, a model with a multitude of alternatives from which to choose a creative approach to discipline.

According to Dr. William Wayson "Ineffective disciplinary techniques are often used because as teachers explain 'I didn't know what else to do.' "[19]

Seven Approaches to Discipline

Dr. Wayson has identified seven different approaches[20] to dealing with discipline:

1. Punishment and Control: Techniques which utilize the authority of the school to control students (expulsion, corporal punishment, etc.).
2. Treatment of Individual Student Needs: Techniques which attempt to fulfill or counteract perceived deficiencies within individual students (dietary modifications, drugs, positive reinforcement, etc.).
3. Interactive Strategies: Techniques which bring the student's world and the school world together (behavior contracts, rap sessions, appeal boards, etc.).
4. Support Systems: Techniques which link human resources to help individuals (peer counseling, adult teams to help students).
5. Training Strategies: Techniques which seek to improve discipline problems through increasing the knowledge and skills of the people involved (case study).
6. Rule Systems: Techniques which attempt to solve discipline problems by improving the effectiveness of written rules and guidelines (discipline codes, bill of rights).
7. Alternative Educational Settings: Strategies which seek to improve discipline problems and help individuals by providing for student and parent choice (quiet places, work-study alternatives).

These seven approaches and the techniques to achieve each approach are described in detail at the end of this chapter. The advantages and disadvantages of each technique are discussed. In a classroom focusing on problem-solving skills, it is desirable to examine a model of alternatives to discipline and the probable effects of each choice.

The Teacher

Another way that students can experience and acquire the skills of self-direction, self-responsibility, self-determination, self-control, and self-evaluation is by observing the behavior of the teacher. The importance of teacher behavior in promoting these skills is expressed in the following poem:

I

I'd rather see a sermon
    Than hear one any day;
I'd rather one should walk with me
    Than merely show the way.
The eye's a better pupil,
    And more willing than the ear;
Fine counsel is confusing,
    But example's always clear.

II

I soon can learn to do it,
    If you'll let me see it done;
I can see your hands in action,
    But your tongue too fast may run.
And the lectures you deliver
    May be very fine and true,
But I'd rather get my lesson
    By observing what you do.
For I may misunderstand you
    And the high advice you give,
But there's no misunderstanding
    How you act and how you live!

Anonymous

The teacher needs to demonstrate certain behaviors in the classroom to let the students know that his or her behavior matches desired student behavior.

Chapter Summary

In summary, our discussion of classroom atmosphere, mental health, communication, and discipline in middle and secondary schools focuses on the teacher

1. encouraging the student to demonstrate self direction, self responsibility, self determination, self control, and self evaluation;

2. providing an atmosphere where the student can be self accepting, self disclosing, and trusting;

3. demonstrating acceptance of others through verbal and nonverbal communication as well as by the use of touch;

4. utilizing and encouraging student use of *I* messages when sending messages and active listening when receiving messages;

5. assisting the students in the development of problem solving skills by using techniques such as role simulation and psychosocial drama;

6. examining a model of alternatives for creative discipline with the students whenever conflict arises that is not alleviated by using problem solving skills.

Appendix
Approaches for Improving School Discipline

I. Punishment and Control: Techniques which utilize the authority of the school to control students.

Approach	Definition	Advantages	Disadvantages
Corporal punishment	The student is physically punished in some way (paddling, pinching, shaking, slapping, "swatting," smacking hands, etc.).	Immediate and concrete punishment is applied. Corporal punishment may be the only method some students respect. (Doubtful) Can clear the air and terminate the event.	Often used as outlet for adult frustration. May not be effective in changing behavior in desired direction. Students often do not understand the reason for punishment. Teachers that "might makes right" rather than the solving of problems. Violence is antiethical to the educational process and human dignity. Legal implications may make it impractical. Often unfairly administered to innocent parties. Often disproportionately administered to minority and poor students. Doesn't address school causes for problems.
Expulsion	Student must leave school for more than 10 days. May not be applied without • written notice to parent, • written reasons, • notification of opportunity for hearing, • notification of time and place for hearing.	Gets the disruptive student out of the school. Can improve group behavior by removing the "troublemaker." (Doubtful in most cases.) Removes disruptive elements before they spread. (Doubtful in most cases.)	Forces out students rather than dealing with the problem. Effects are the same as suspension except more severe. Doesn't address school causes for problems.
Suspension or variations such as sending home or extended "cooling off"	Student must leave school for a designated period of time. (Ohio law stipulates up to 10 school days.) May not be applied without • written notice prior to suspension, • written statement of reasons, • opportunity for informal hearing.	Gets the disruptive student out of the classroom and school. The disruptive student cannot disturb others. May get parents to come to school for a conference. (Generally poor method for doing so.)	Can teach that power is absolute and arbitrary. Without due process, teaches students a sense of helplessness. Has little positive educational value. Gives students official approval to be out of school. Encourages school officials to deny responsibility. Often disproportionately applied to minority groups. Students are denied education; time is not used productively. May put student irreparably behind in school work.

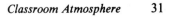

Approach	Definition	Advantages	Disadvantages
			Does not rehabilitate the student; does not get to the source of the problem; denies treatment. Often used for trivial or nondisruptive purposes. Gives students a "record"; often leads to repeated suspensions. In many cases, no parent conference is held. Often alienates students and parents. Doesn't address school causes for problems.
Security forces and precautions	Security officers are on duty in the school. Security aides such as locks and bars on windows are utilized. A promising variation is to have a person or a family live on school premises to discourage burglary or after-hours vandalism.	Security personnel can prevent vandalism. Security personnel sometimes deter potential discipline problems. Makes teachers feel more secure. Security personnel sometimes take personal interest in students. Security can save equipment, etc., from theft.	Often exacerbates problems, requires increasing effort. Can reinforce idea that students "don't belong." Security forces and equipment are expensive. Sets up a prison-like atmosphere in which students have little chance of developing self-discipline. Indicates fear and distrust on the part of school officials. May "turn off" staff, students, parents, and community. Doesn't address school causes for problems.
Detention	Student spends extra hours in the school or classroom as punishment.	Is a nonviolent form of punishment, usually applied the same day. Students can put the time to use by doing homework. Students involved in extracurricular activities have extra incentive to avoid detention.	Staff can see monitoring as noneducational imposition. Often given for trivial offenses. Hours of detention can be a status symbol among peer groups. The detention room can be a dumping ground; students often are not engaged in productive work. School is lengthened as a punishment, implying that school is punishment. Sometimes whole classes are forced to stay as a result of a few students' misbehavior. (Very poor educational practice.) Too many detentions given willynilly destroys effectiveness. Doesn't address school causes for problems. Requires special process for transported students.

Approach	Definition	Advantages	Disadvantages
Sending students to principal's office	The student is told to go to the principal's office to be disciplined by the principal.	Teacher can immediately remove a disruptive student. Teacher is relieved of pressure and responsibility. Principal is informed of problems.	Principal's office is often filled with students. Principal's role is defined as disciplinarian and punisher. Children may learn that teachers can't discipline. Principal has no time for creative administration. Time is taken away from learning activities. Doesn't address school causes for problems.
Transfers	A student who is not working well in a particular classroom or school is transferred to another situation.	A transfer can resolve personality conflicts. A student can be placed in a situation where teaching methods better suit his/her learning style. Student is in a learning situation rather than being suspended or expelled. Student can exercise choice, take responsibility for own program.	Transfers may be used as punishment. Receiving schools may resent or reject new students. Records may label the student in a negative way. Student can be moved around just to get rid of problems rather than trying to solve them. Some "voluntary" transfers are really force-outs. Often used as a step prior to expulsion with little help for the student. Doesn't address school causes for problems.
Loss of privileges	Students who misbehave lose privileges such as assembly, gym, etc. Some systems have a demerit system which results in loss of privileges.	If students want to retain privileges, they are motivated to behave appropriately.	If privileges are not seen as important, the technique will not work. Students may misbehave to get out of some extra-curricular activities. Doesn't address school causes for problems. Special teachers resent loss of student time.
In-house suspension	The student is suspended but stays at school, usually restricted to a certain area such as a study hall or room.	Student is removed from immediate situation. Student can receive counseling and work towards rehabilitation. Parents are pleased that the school is dealing with the problem rather than sending the student home. Suspension and expulsion are reduced. School is not denied to the student. Time can be used productively. Can develop personal relationship between the student and some staff member.	Often such programs are highly regimented. If student is too restricted, experience can build up further dislike for school. Time may not be used productively if proper help is not available. Is expensive in terms of supervision. Students who behave well in the suspension room could often behave well back in the classroom. Students may misbehave again to escape the boredom. Doesn't address school causes for problems.

Approach	Definition	Advantages	Disadvantages
Physical exercise (Doing "laps")	Students who fight or otherwise misbehave engage in physical exercise such as running, doing push-ups, etc.	Excess energy is worked off. Students are distracted from original misbehavior. Permits students to cool-off, regain composure.	Making students tired may in some cases increase the problem. Students may learn that exercise is a punishment rather than a need of the body. Doesn't address school causes for problems. Can be excessive and cruel.
"Fresh air class"	Students who are disruptive spend time in activities as cleaning up the school grounds.	Energies are channeled into productive activities. Needed work is done. Student may gain stature for doing important work.	Students may learn that keeping grounds neat is a punishment rather than a duty as a citizen. Doesn't address school causes for problems.

II. Treatment of Individual Student Needs: Techniques which attempt to fulfill or counteract perceived deficiencies within individual students.

Approach	Definition	Advantages	Disadvantages
Drugs	The student is given tranquilizers or stimulants to modify behavior by increasing attention span or calming activity.	Can be helpful in a small percentage of cases who have been accurately and carefully diagnosed by a physician.	Represents a radical intervention in the student's life. Often misused by being given indescriminately. Are sometimes administered to students who are exhibiting normal behavior in response to rigid teacher expectations. Doesn't address school causes for problems.
Dietary modifications	A change in diet to reduce the intake of certain foods whose chemical content can produce (or is associated with) undesirable behaviors or to increase the intake of certain nutritional elements whose lack is associated with undesirable behaviors.	Works well for students whose behavior is related to dietary intake. Can prevent student from being labeled a "learning disability." Can provide "answer" for otherwise unexplainable behavior. May be substituted for ill-advised drug treatment. Little chance of harming child.	Doesn't work with all children. Can be overused by faddists. Probably should be used after a good medical examination. Doesn't address school causes for problems (unless school food has wrong nutritional balance for student).

Approach	Definition	Advantages	Disadvantages
Special education classes	Students who are having discipline problems are referred to special education professionals for diagnosis and prescription. Sometimes students are put into special classes for "emotionally handicapped or disabled."	Students get professional treatment. Teachers have resources; can get expert advice. Teacher does not have to cope with the disruptive student.	Often used discriminatorily against minority students. Isolates problem students; prevents normal school life. Assumes disruptions are caused by problem students rather than normal frustrations. Stigma attached to special classes. Used instead of suspension or expulsion to avoid due process requirements. Often labels student for entire school career. Tendency to lump together for treatment those who have special problems and those who don't. Doesn't address school causes for problems.
Positive reinforcement (Also called behavior modification, response shaping, success approximation, or contingency management).	The goal is to reward appropriate behavior and not reward those that are not desirable. The technique is built on the theory that we tend to repeat behaviors we find rewarding.	Negative actions and punishment are eliminated. Inappropriate behavior is simply ignored while appropriate behavior is rewarded by praise or other means. The approach is especially effective when the positive reinforcement is inhernt in the consequences of appropriate behavior (such as involvement in work or constructive interaction with other students). Helps teachers understand learning better. Can build emphasis upon the positive throughout the school. Gives teachers an effective tool they can use without additional resources. Helps teachers describe behavior better.	Positive reinforcement is sometimes accomplished by external means only. Can fail to build on intrinsic drives and rewards. When misused, behavior modification programs can destroy initiative and self determination. Some people fear "mind control" over unwitting students. Program can be rigid, inflexible and dull. Doesn't address school causes for problems.
Specialized help for children with special needs	The teacher refers children with suspected physical problems or severe emotional problems to outside resource persons such as psychologists, nurses, therapists, counselors.	Sometimes discipline problems are the result of neglected or unsuspected medical problems. When such problems are relieved, disruptive behavior ceases. Sometimes children's emotional problems or home situations are so severe that professional help is needed. The teacher is relieved of sole responsibility for the student's problems. Consultative help is available to the teacher.	Qualified specialized help is not always available. When resource persons are available, they may not have enough time to devote to individual students. Sometimes professional resource persons diagnose but do little to help the teacher deal with the problems. The danger of "labeling" the child as a learning or emotionally disabled student should be avoided. Doesn't address school causes for problems.

Approach	Definition	Advantages	Disadvantages
Meeting basic needs	The school provides for basic needs which may be missing in the student's life. An example is the breakfast program provided in many city schools or the provision of warm clothing. Also could include programs to provide personal support, "buddies," parent-figures, etc. Could also include activities to help student feel safe and a valued member of the group.	Some of the barriers to learning and involvement are removed. If students lack enough food or warm clothing, they find it difficult to concentrate on school work. Can make student feel secure, valued. Can promote relationship between student and school personnel. Can provide "linkage" with the complex, unresponsive organization.	Extra time is needed to find out about a student's needs and to make provision for them. Money is needed to institute programs such as free hot lunches. Sometimes help is given to children in such a way as to destroy dignity. Staff often resents such activities as "not part of learning." Doesn't address school causes for problems.

III. Interactive Strategies: Techniques which bring the student's world and the school world together.

Approach	Definition	Advantages	Disadvantages
Behavior contracts	A contract is made between the student and the principal or teacher to achieve stated objectives. The contract may be sent to parents.	Can develop personal relationships between student and staff. If worked out cooperatively, the contract puts responsibility on the student to meet his/her own agreements. Parents know what is expected. Expectations are clear. The "official" nature of the contract impresses the student with its seriousness. May be used to address school causes for problems. No extra funding is required.	Extra staff time is needed to make and follow up on the contract. If imposed by authorities, all advantages can be negated. May not address school causes for problems.
Appeal boards or ombudspersons	Appeal boards or ombudspersons constitute a third party to which students can appeal if they feel they have been unfairly treated by school officials. Student ombudspersons may be utilized.	An objective opinion is available. Students learn from the proceedings. Students do not feel helpless in the face of school authority. Some boards are composed of students and community people as well as school people.	Boards take time and effort to organize. Boards and ombudspersons may require extra money. Careful planning is required so that the system will actually work. See "Advocacy."

Approach	Definition	Advantages	Disadvantages
Community involvement in discipline problems	Schools make contact with community agencies which serve as a link with the home.	Community agencies are able to provide resources and make contracts that school people cannot. Agency can serve in a consultative capacity to the teacher. Agencies offer training courses for parents and students and provide counseling services.	Extra time is involved in seeking community involvement. Often not as effective as direct communication with the student's parents. Community agencies may operate under a philosophy which is detrimental to what the teacher is trying to do. May not address school causes for problems.
Community Schools Mott Program Flint Program or other variants of community involvements in the school. Adult education and recreation programs Volunteer or paraprofessional staffing plans	Any practice which involves parents and other citizens in the school as active participants, either as recipients of services, as staff adjuncts, or in problem solving roles. Any practice which makes the school an integral part of community life for persons normally not in school as well as students. Degree of mutual involvement varies widely.	Generally, the more integral the school in community life, the fewer discipline problems will be. Makes it easier to settle discipline problems by focusing more school, home, and community resources. Reduces community opposition to measures taken and support for disrupters. Gives students sense of ownership; greater sense of value and responsibility. Reduces barriers between school/community. Raises respect for and confidence in school personnel. Increases staff self-confidence. Nips problems in the bud. Increases communication and problem-solving. Can address school causes for problems. Reduces cultural barriers, staff fears. Reduces mutual prejudices. Can reduce vandalism. Can improve staff performance. Makes effective use of space freed by lower enrollments. Can facilitate relationships with other agencies involved in educational/recreational services. Makes efficient use of space and people at "down times." Can provide additional employment for staff members. Brings all ages together in school.	Takes time, maybe space and personnel. School personnel may resent feedback. School personnel may fear parental involvement. Sharing space may produce friction. School personnel may dominate groups. Teachers' unions, custodians, or administrators may resist some forms of involvement. Working out working relationships requires a "shakedown" period. Persons or groups currently benefitting from present school practices may oppose new groups' involvement. Can cause staff members to leave (may be an advantage in some cases). Teachers need inservice to develop human relations skills and attitudes (can be advantage to improving total school program). May be inadequately conceptualized or implemented.

Approach	Definition	Advantages	Disadvantages
Advocacy Programs (one variant is ombudsperson)	Each student selects one teacher or administrator to act as an advisor and mediator in the event that he/she has problems or specified members of staff are designated advocate or whole school is trained to protect the rights of others or whole staff acts on behalf of students in preference to other considerations.	Student is able to deal with an adult whom he/she trusts. Provides checks and balances against inappropriate actions. Relationships are built between students and teachers. Possibilities are opened up for ongoing personal counseling. Parents gain confidence that staff works for students. Addresses many school causes for problems. Assures students they are valued.	Mechanism may not allow for changes if relationships fail to achieve purposes. Program must be voluntary on both sides. Students who are in a failure pattern may find it difficult to establish relationship with any school person. Staff may shift responsibility to one or a few persons. Staff (and administration) may resent advocates.
Home visits	Teachers make friendly nonevaluative visits to the students' homes, preferably during the first few months of school. Both friendly and problem-solving visits are made throughout the school year.	Community gains respect for school staff. Students learn that teachers are interested and that their homes are worthwhile places for teachers to visit. Relationships are established with parents before evaluation creates tension. Students know that the teacher has direct contact with the home; therefore, "game playing" and disruptive behavior are lessened. Student self-esteem is increased. The teacher knows the student better. Teacher loses prejudices about parents and vice-versa. Teacher gains confidence.	Sometimes teachers are shy or apprehensive about making home visits. Going in pairs for the first few visits is helpful. Home visits take time. Teacher unions may oppose them. Instructional value isn't recognized. Teachers may go to "study" homes. Teachers may go only to "tattle" to parent. Other teachers resent home visitors.
Parent involvement (various forms)	Parents volunteer in schools or classrooms. Parents are involved and informed about the school situation. If behavior contracts are formed, parents are part of the arrangement. Teachers invite parents into the school for a variety of reasons rather than for discipline or evaluation only. Teachers visit students' homes.	Communication between the home and school gives the student added security and helps in making expectations clear. Added parent contact builds trust on the part of students and parents. Students cannot easily play "games" between home and school. Parents react positively to increased contact.	Sometimes difficult to get parents involved, especially if they work long hours and have economic difficulties. Teachers must be careful not to be judgmental, constantly evaluating or talking about disruptive behavior. Time is needed to build positive teacher/parent relationships.

Approach	Definition	Advantages	Disadvantages
Teacher/student conference	The teacher and student talk together about the violations of rules or discipline problems.	Communication is established on a one-to-one basis; involves student in solving own problems. Both get a chance to talk and to listen to each other; helps get at causes. Student is not given a lecture before peers; can save face; gives student sense of being valued.	Is sometimes not sufficient as a deterrent to misbehavior. As in-depth discussion, especially with a student who has severe problems, takes time and skill. Can turn into a "lecture."
Class meetings and discussion Rap sessions	Class meets as a group to solve problems, to discuss causes of behavior, to specify what behavior is desirable, to improve classroom routines.	Negative reactions are turned into positive interaction. A positive classroom environment is established. Opportunities for choices and decisions are created. Social learning is enhanced. Students have a chance to be heard, feel they belong and are valued. Students have responsibility, learn self-discipline. Students learn ways of interacting positively and working together to solve problems. Can address school causes for problems.	May not yield immediate effects from one rap session. Must be utilized over a period of time. Class time may be limited. Teachers may not see such sessions as "teaching." Staff may resent having students "talk up." Teacher may dominate discussion. Parents may not see the educational value.
Strength bombardment	People in the school begin to focus on the positive attributes each person brings to the school.	Overcomes low moral and negative climate. Fosters creativity in teachers. Raises self-esteem in teachers and students. Fosters pride in the school. Can lift community spirit.	Personnel and students can "go through the motions" but still feel negative. Many school practices depend upon negative evaluations; practices need to change. Uninvolved parents may see it as permissiveness or cover-up of problems. Educators may lack skills.

IV. Support Systems: Techniques which link human resources to help individuals.

Approach	Definition	Advantages	Disadvantages
Proximity	The teacher lets the student work near him/her.	Nearness provides the security and sense of control some students need. The student can receive attention at times when he/she is behaving appropriately.	Is effective only if the student is gradually moved towards independence and self discipline. A teacher cannot always keep one student nearby. Doesn't address school causes for problems.

Approach	Definition	Advantages	Disadvantages
Peer counseling	Students work in groups, receive special training in problem-solving skills, understanding self and their environment, and leadership. Students become co-leaders for other groups of students. They talk and help each other work out problems.	Students, particularly adolescents, are more trusting and likely to discuss problems with peers. Students learn problem-solving skills and working with others. Supportive groups are developed to reinforce positive behavior. Students develop leadership skills. Builds on the fact that peers are the greatest influence on adolescents. May address school-caused problems.	Peer group counseling requires skilled adult guidance. Is most useful at the secondary level.
Adult teams to help students	Teachers, administrators, aides, volunteers (parents and others)—form teams to take students aside when disruptive, talk to them, counsel them, etc.	Student is prevented from becoming more and more disruptive. Energy is channeled into problem solving. Can develop personal relationship between student and staff. Can address school causes for problems. Can help student become self-disciplined.	Adults often need inservice training or some kind of special help to work effectively together. Extra adult help may not be available. Takes time. If one-sided, advantages can be negated. May not address school causes for problems.
Adult teams to relieve teachers	Teachers, administrators, aides, volunteers, etc., form teams to help a teacher solve problems.	Support is provided for teachers. Personality clashes are relieved. Teachers gain perspective. Trains teachers to deal with own problems. Builds confidence as teacher gains ability. Can address school causes for problems. Can give teacher a cooling-off time.	May reinforce teachers' biases. Teachers are often unwilling to talk about their problems to other teachers. Time for group discussion and planning between teachers may not be readily available. Team may not treat teacher as a peer learner. May alienate teachers, cause them to ignore or hide problems.

V. Training Strategies: Techniques which seek to improve discipline problems through increasing the knowledge and skills of the people involved.

Approach	Definition	Advantages	Disadvantages
Case Study	Teacher or other person notices a student who is a source of discipline problems and observes the student, taking careful note of the situations that elicit inappropriate and appropriate behavior, and gathering the relevant information to determine causes of behavior problems and possible solutions. (Child could do a self study)	Teacher works toward discovering causes of behavior problems rather than simply reducing symptoms. The teacher takes active interest in the student; such interest can deter inappropriate behavior. Develops deeper insight into behavior. Can address school causes for problems. Postpones precipitate action.	May encourage amateur psychology or sociology. May not address immediate problems. Time consuming. May treat child as a thing to be studied. May focus too narrowly on child and miss external causes. May reinforce bias that student is deficient. May focus on trivia or irrelevant factors.

Approach	Definition	Advantages	Disadvantages
Courses for students in human relations and psychology	Students are provided courses which help them to understand themselves and others better.	Can teach self-discipline. Students begin to understand the causes for their own behavior and can consciously work to make changes. Students can begin to understand the behavior of others, including teachers, and can learn to deal with it in positive ways. Courses can provide a vehicle for discussion of student behavior. Courses provide an interesting educational alternative. May address school causes for problems.	Often difficult to find money and resources for offering new courses. A teacher who adds the course to his/ her load will have to find time and money for training and preparation. Can be treated too academically; doesn't get acted upon. Instructors may not comprehend, or model the behavior that is taught. May be offered only for "better" students.
Role-playing	Students take the role of another person in conflict situation. They could also play the teacher's role. The technique can be used by teachers to analyze students' problems in inservice sessions.	Increases individual or group sensitivity to underlying causes for behavior problems. Increases ability to see from another persons' perception. Can address school causes for problems.	Students and teachers are often self-conscious in role playing situations. People need to become accustomed to role playing and to discussing it. Can be disturbing to participants; should be carefully used if issues are sensitive. Can be seen as "plays and games."
Behavior chaining	Persons who have been involved in or have observed a situation of conflict make a flow chart or diagram which represents every action, statement, or feeling in sequence. Discussion and analysis accompanies diagraming.	Individuals are allowed to describe actions and their own feelings and perceptions. People involved develop awareness that there are usually several different points of view in any one incident. An incident is described in concrete form so that causes may more easily be inferred. Individuals develop the skills of objective description before leaping to inferences or judgments.	Chaining and describing behavior are skills which take time to develop. Process is time consuming and would not be practical for every discipline incident. Educators often lack skill for accurate description; get frustrated.
Staff development. Inservice training for teachers, administrators, aides, custodians, or any other member of the staff.	Includes teaching skills necessary for creating a school environment which teaches self-discipline. Any attempt, formal or informal, to teach staff members new skills, attitudes, knowledge or functions.	Teaching self-discipline requires knowledge and skill which is seldom adequately developed during undergraduate work and isn't often reinforced in schools. During inservice training sessions, teachers can learn to work together in problem-solving groups. New teachers can profit from the experience of other teachers in the school. The inservice session can provide a time when teachers share their problems and use each other as resources. Skills developed during inservice sessions, such as communication skills or awareness of cultural diversity, can "spill over" into work in other areas of the curriculum. Addresses school causes for problems.	Takes time and money. Sometimes difficult for school officials to recognize the value of such expenditures. Often very poorly done. Parents must be educated to realize the value of released time for teachers to engage in professional development. If teachers are not involved in planning for inservice, they may not respond positively. If all staff are not included, teachers may find their new ideas frustrated by misunderstandings with aides, principals, or custodians. May reinforce every school cause for problems.

Approach	Definition	Advantages	Disadvantages
Social Literacy Training	Helping a group of teachers become aware of shared problems, identify how school rules or organization cause those problems, and work together to improve the system by changing roles, goals, rules, practices, policies and norms.	Improves morale. Increases confidence in self. Improves relationships among staff and with students. Reduces bickering among staff and blaming other people. Addresses school causes for problems. Reduces unfair, unproductive practices. Teaches staff and students to be responsible, to be self-disciplined. Makes people feel valued. Builds a sense of community; improves learning atmosphere. Can have "spin-off" effects such as higher achievement of students and better instructional decisions on part of teachers. Prepares better citizens, both teachers and students.	Takes time. Seems too simple to some staff members. Takes away scapegoats. Will not work if the staff believes the students and their parents to be the only source of problems. Resistance or lack of participation by a few staff member can sabotage the process. Staff members with highly diverse philosophies will find the process difficult (but such a situation makes it even more necessary).

VI. Rule Systems: Techniques which attempt to improve discipline problems by improving the effectiveness of written rules and guidelines.

Approach	Definition	Advantages	Disadvantages
Discipline codes	The school system develops a clearly stated discipline code. Some codes are jointly developed by students, teachers, administrators, and parents. Student rights may be included as well as school rules and procedures.	Development can be used to build a sense of community and agreed upon norms for everyone. Codes which are cooperatively developed are more likely to be understood and supported. Expectations are clearly stated so that they can be understood. Consequences and procedures are outlined so that each student may be assured of equal or fair treatment. A well-developed, fair code can build up trust on the part of students. If a bill of rights is included, the code becomes a social contract and not merely a legal form. (see Bill of Rights) Can address school causes for problems.	The code can be so inflexible that it does not provide for individual personalities or extenuating circumstances. If discipline codes are implemented by administrators alone they may not be supported. Discipline codes must be updated often so that the people following them feel that they have been involved in the creation or interpretation of them. Clearly stating expectations and rights is a difficult process Codes can lead to an emphasis on the form rather than the substance (letter rather than spirit) of the procedures. Often focuses only on student's transgressions. Often treats only procedural "rights" not substantive rights. May not address faculty culpability.
Computerized records on student conduct	Teachers have computer cards listing violations of rules. At each infraction, the teacher sends a card to the computer center. The computer selects the appropriate letter and sends it to the parent.	The computer provides a record of disciplinary action. Parents are informed promptly of rule violations.	May be too expensive for the few advantages. Can be impersonal and sterile. Circumstances of the violation cannot be adequately recorded by computer. Provides only the teacher's view. A phone call to parents for any serious offense is more prompt than going through the computer. Lessens possibilities for communication and cooperative planning between teachers and parents. Doesn't address school causes for problems.

Approach	Definition	Advantages	Disadvantages
Eliminate unnecessary or vague rules	The teacher decides what is and what is not a problem. Rules which are not necessary for facilitation of learning and which may actually cause distraction (such as asking permission every time a student needs to sharpen a pencil) are eliminated.	Students are freed from trivial, oppressive constraints. Can free the teacher from some aspects of disciplinary role. When fewer rules exist, students can follow those necessary rules that do exist more carefully. A less rigid atmosphere causes less frustration and hostility. There is no "fun" in breaking a rule that does not exist. Frees staff for pressing educational duties. Can address school causes for problems.	Individual teachers must decide what rules they consider necessary. When making school rules or eliminating school rules, it may take some time for teachers to reach concensus on what rules are necessary. Staff and some parents may see trivial rules as safeguards against anarchy.
Bill of Rights	Students and school staff work together to develop a Bill of Rights, a set of inviolable freedoms, for all people who work and learn in the school.	Teaches self-discipline. Students learn from the process of developing the Bill of Rights. The Bill of Rights helps students become involved in the governance process of the school and in preventing discipline problems. Students work to keep each other from infringing on rights. Reasons for rules are made more understandable. Both teachers and students get rights protected. Gives students a sense of being valued and responsible. Addresses many school causes for problems.	An effective Bill of Rights takes time to develop. A variety of people with differing perceptions and opinions must find agreement. Teachers or principals may not like granting rights to students. Teachers may not understand how to apply rights in schools. Students have to be taught how a bill of rights is applied to their actions. Deciding about rights violations takes time, requires due process.

VII. Alternative Educational Settings: Strategies which seek to improve discipline problems and help individuals by providing for student and parent choice.

Approach	Definition	Advantages	Disadvantages
Quiet places	Corners, small rooms, or retreats are constructed where students can go to be by themselves without distraction or to "cool off."	Tension is relieved. Student has a chance to calm down before talking about a problem. Escalation of conflict is prevented. No punishment need be involved. Can promote self disciplined behavior.	Teacher may overuse. The "quiet place" may become an "isolation booth" for punishment. If more than one student is sent to the quiet place, it may become a dention area. An entire class cannot be sent to a quiet place. (Seldom need to do so.) Teachers may not accept nonpunitive nature of the alternative.

Approach	Definition	Advantages	Disadvantages
Alternative programs within the school (Voluntary transfers between classrooms)	Any opportunity whereby a student or parent may select an alternative to the assigned class. May be permanent. May be temporary way to withdraw from or avoid an immediately frustrating situation. May be teacher or student initiated for sound educational purposes. Should be nonpunitive.	Recognizes different learning/teaching styles. Individual needs and interests can be considered. Discipline problems are prevented from becoming severe. Students are stimulated and motivated. Students are not simply "dumped" to get rid of problems. Permits nonpunitive way for teachers and students to avoid normal personality conflicts. Can address school causes for problems.	Alternatives are in danger of becoming isolated. Stigma may be attached to students who participate. Can become equivalent to in-school detention. Can become a "dumping ground". Teachers may resent giving students an "escape." Staff may take transfer personally. Violates belief that all classes should be alike.
Alternative Schools (temporary)	The student is removed to an alternative school setting which offers individualized teaching and counseling. The goal is to rehabilitate the student and enable him/her to go back to the regular school situation.	Students can receive needed individual help and counseling. Causes of problems can be more easily determined when individual help is available. Disruptive students are removed from the school and put into situations where they can be productive.	Genuine learning opportunity must be offered; Danger of becoming "dumping grounds" for problem students. Alternative schools are expensive.
Alternative Schools (permanent) (Voluntary transfers to other schools)	Students who do not respond well either academically or behaviorally to assigned school settings may elect to attend an alternative school which may offer a variety of learning options. Difficult to generalize because variety and quality differ so much.	Usually provide more individualized instruction. Programs offer more choice and meet student needs and interests. Teaching methods are selected to fit student learning styles. A new setting offers a "fresh start." Students learn to choose, take responsibility (unless they are sent to school as punishment). Programs can be tailored to interests, learning styles, etc. Staff can be freed to address school causes for problems.	Can be expensive. Require much communication with parents so that programs which differ from "regular" school are understood. Genuine learning opportunities, not just fun, must be offered. Can be punitive and segregatory. Receiving schools may be inhospitable.
Work-study Alternatives	Programs combine school work with on-the-job training. Students spend a portion of the day in classes and work at the job the other part of the day.	Students' self esteem and feeling of responsibility is increased. Boredom and frustration are lessened. Peer norms work to create pride. Motivation is increased as school work seems more relevant. Students have an opportunity to explore careers. Students and coordinators may relate productively.	Staff may view program as a dumping ground. Tracking minority students or poor students into work-study programs may deny them academic excellence of which they are capable. Participation sometimes means a student has less chance of being admitted to college. Teachers sometimes resent students in academic classrooms.

Approach	Definition	Advantages	Disadvantages
Alternative experiences for students (within or among classrooms or schools or community)	A variety of experiences are provided within or outside the classroom. The curriculum is adjusted and methods are organized to provide for choice, exploration, problem solving, and active learning. Examples are special projects, library research, work-study experiences, working with media, art experiences, peer tutoring, etc.	Reduces chance of pushing student into corner. Challenge and a channel for energy are provided. Students become involved, less interested in causing problems, less easily distracted, and less tense and hostile. Self-esteem is increased. Making choices is taught and learned. Meets more interests. Reduces school causes for problems. Puts responsibility on student; teaches self-discipline.	Extra work is required on the part of the teacher. Organization and planning is needed. May reduce teacher contact with student. May let important instruction "slip between cracks."

Notes

1. R. Mukerjii, Japanese University student. "About School," *Colloquy* Magazine, January, 1970 (copyright : United Church Press, 1969).

2. Dr. Thomas Gordon. *Teacher Effectiveness Training*. New York: David McKay Company, Inc., 1974, page 24.

3. Dr. William Wayson and Gay Su Pinnell, "Developing Discipline with Quality Schools," *Citizen Guide to Quality Education*. The Citizens Council for Ohio Schools, 517 The Arcade, Cleveland, Ohio, 44114, copyright 1978.

4. Robert Kaplan, Linda Meeks, and Jay Segal. *Group Strategies in Understanding Human Sexuality: Getting in Touch*. Dubuque, Iowa: William C. Brown Company Publishers, 1978, page 12.

5. Sidney Jourard. *The Transparent Self*. New York: D. Van Nostrand Company, 1971, page 19.

6. John Powell, S.J., *Why Am I Afraid To Tell You Who I Am?* Illinois: Argus Communications, 1969, page 12.

7. Sidney Jourard. *The Transparent Self*. New York: D. Van Nostrand Company, 1971.

8. Robert Kaplan, Linda Meeks, and Jay Segal. *Group Strategies in Understanding Human Sexuality: Getting in Touch*. Dubuque, Iowa: William C. Brown Company Publishers, 1978, page 11.

9. Dr. Thomas Gordon. *Teacher Effectiveness Training*. New York: David McKay Company, Inc., 1974, page 151.

10. Dr. Thomas Gordon. *Teacher Effectiveness Training*. New York: David McKay Company, Inc., 1974, pages 142–4.

11. Dr. Thomas Gordon. *Teacher Effectiveness Training*. New York: David McKay Company, Inc., 1974, pages 66–68.

12. Dr. William Wayson and Gay Su Pinnell, "Developing Discipline with Quality Schools," *Citizen Guide to Quality Education*. The Citizens Council for Ohio Schools, 517 The Arcade, Cleveland, Ohio 44114, Copyright 1978, page 1.

13. Dr. William Wayson and Gay Su Pinnell, "Developing Discipline with Quality Schools," *Citizen Guide to Quality Education*. The Citizens Council for Ohio Schools, 517 The Arcade, Cleveland, Ohio 44114, Copyright 1978, page 1.

14. George Borelli. *Role Simulation*. Copyright © 1975 by George Borelli, Columbus Psychological Services, Inc., 24 East Weber, Columbus, Ohio, page 1.

15. George Borelli. *Role Simulation*. Copyright © 1975 by George Borelli, Columbus Psychological Services, Inc., 24 East Weber, Columbus, Ohio, pages 22–24.

16. George Borelli. *Role Simulation*. Copyright © 1975 by George Borelli, Columbus Psychological Services, Inc., 24 East Weber, Columbus, Ohio, pages 31–32.

17. Larry Cox, "Psycho-social drama is new education approach," *Mental Horizons*. December, 1977.

18. Jim Million, and Dee Mason, "Nine Steps to Prepare Psycho-Social Drama Material," Institute for Human Awareness, 1266 East Broad, Columbus, Ohio.

19. Dr. William Wayson and Gay Su Pinnell, "Developing Discipline with Quality Schools," *Citizen Guide to Quality Education*. The Citizens Council for Ohio Schools, 517 The Arcade, Cleveland, Ohio 44114, copyright 1978, page 9.

20. Dr. William Wayson and Dr. Gay Su Pinnell, "Approaches for Improving School Discipline," copyright 1977 by William W. Wayson, appeared in Citizens Council for Ohio Schools, 517 The Arcade, Cleveland, Ohio 44114, copyright, 1978, pages 13–23.

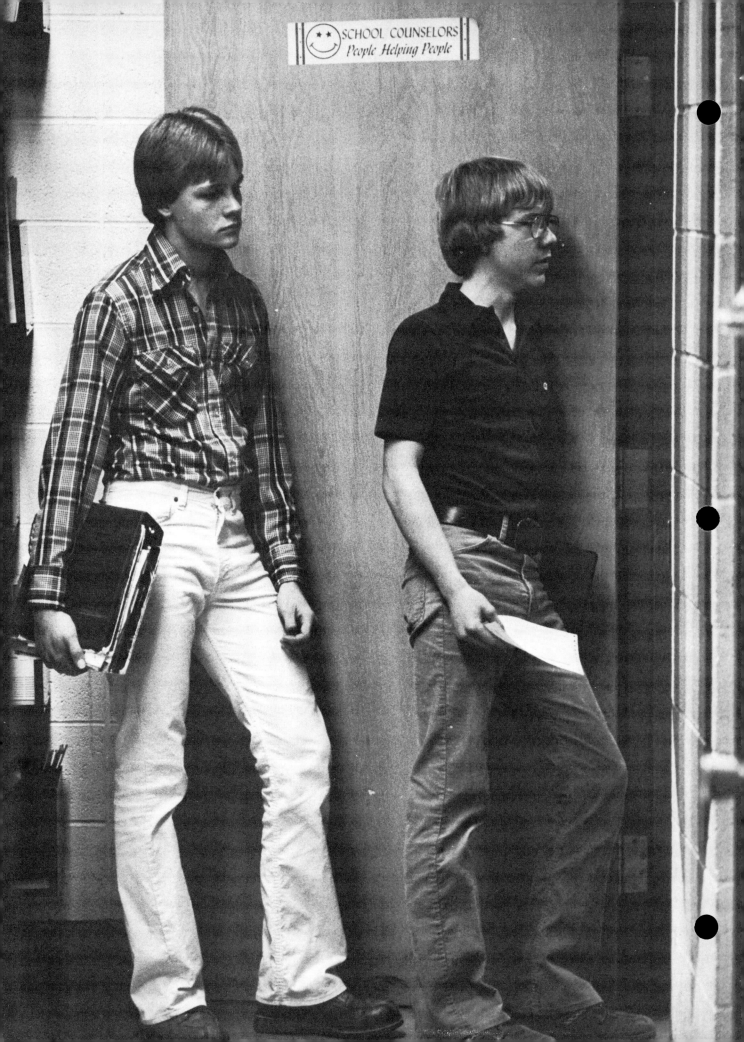

Health Counseling

The Need for Health Counseling

At no time has the need for school health counseling been as great as it is today. With over one-half of today's population under 25 years of age, and one-fourth of those under 18 years of age living at or below the poverty level, the risk for psychological problems has been enhanced.[1] While ten million children in this group will require intervention for mental illnesses, only seven percent will receive it.[2]

Traditional Counseling

If one were to ask a student what role a school counselor plays, the responses most likely to be given would fall within the following areas:

1. academic counseling—many students feel that counselors serve only to help plan academic courses which will help prepare one for college;

2. career counseling—often students feel the school counselor exists to guide them to careers which will lead to satisfying life adjustments;

3. scheduling—many schools use counselors to assist students with course scheduling—i.e., when to include and exclude academic courses.

While each of the roles mentioned is important in the school, by no means do all of them fit into the perspective in which the authors view health counseling.

For the purpose of this chapter, we will view the health counselor as that person in the school setting who possesses the skills necessary to assist students in their quest for achieving positive mental health.

The Health Educator as Counselor

In his professional preparation, the health educator should have been exposed to a course in health counseling. Assuming this as a prerequisite, the authors believe that every health educator is in one way or another a health counselor. The competencies required of a health educator seem to be commensurate with the qualities required to be an effective counselor.

Photo by James L. Shaffer

Having had a wide exposure to the myriad of adolescent health problems, the health educator is often sought out by other school personnel, for advice in dealing with emotional problems in students. Gary S. Belkin[3] in his book "Practical Counseling in the Schools" developed a matrix which can be applied to the competencies needed by a health counselor (Fig. 3.1).

THE COUNSELOR-QUALITIES MATRIX

Quality	Category	Open-mindedness	Sensitivity	Objectivity	Genuineness	Nondominance	Positive regard	Communication skills	Self-knowledge	Respect
Flexibility		●		●		●		●	●	
Warmth			●		●	●	●			●
Acceptance		●	●		●	●	●			●
Empathy			●						●	
Congruence		●		●	●				●	
Honesty				●	●					
Ability to artic.								●	●	
Intelligence		●		●				●		
Interest			●		●	●	●			
Caring			●		●	●	●			
Sincerity			●		●	●	●			
Security				●					●	
Courage									●	●
Trust					●		●		●	
Concreteness		●		●				●	●	
Responsibility									●	
Dedication					●				●	
Commitment					●				●	
Professionalism			●	●	●	●	●	●	●	●
Cognitive flex.		●		●		●				
Perceptiveness		●		●				●		
Nonpossessive		●				●	●			
Self-disclosing					●			●	●	
Nonjudgmental		●	●	●		●	●			●
Awareness of lim.			●						●	

From: Gary S. Belkin, *Health Counseling in the Schools*, Dubuque: Wm. C. Brown Company Publishers, 1975.

Figure 3.1.

The Counselor Qualities Matrix

Included in this matrix are some of the more commonly used adjectives, together with some broader, more inclusive categories of effective functioning. In the nine major categories are twenty-five commonly cited characteristics. Each of the nine category headings can be translated into a broad range of behavioral and perceptual criteria. These criteria will reappear in other categories and break down into more specific behavioral, attitudinal, and perceptual traits.

For example, in the category of openmindedness, we can find nine adjectives that contribute to this characteristic. Then we can look at each of the nine adjectives and see with which of the other categories they have been associated or paired. In this way we can establish a connection between openmindedness and each of these other categories.

Using the above example, a comprehensive picture of the effective health counselor can be constructed by examining the relationships among component parts—a relationship among the terms, among the categories, and between the categories and counselor activities.

The differences between an effective health educator and an effective health counselor are almost minimal. Both professionals need to possess the following qualities:

1. the ability to understand others
2. the ability to understand one's self
3. the ability to relate to others.[4]

Understanding Others

The ability to understand others is determined by *flexibility* and *perceptiveness*. The health counselor must learn to understand and adapt to other frames of references (flexibility) and sense the student's values and feelings (perception).

Sensitivity and *empathy* are two traits which are also needed to understand others. The counselor should be able to respond emotionally—to feel for his student (sensitivity). The empathetic health counselor can feel with students—he can perceive and appreciate his student's feelings in terms of his own frame of reference, so as to *be* the student—with his thoughts and feelings.

Understanding One's Self

A cardinal rule in preparing health educators in the notion that one cannot teach about sensitive topics if the instructor is not comfortable with the subject matter. For example, if the health educator is embarrassed at using the word "penis" during a lesson on anatomy, he should not teach the unit on human sexuality.

The same principle can be applicable to the health counselor. If the health counselor does not have an objective understanding of himself, he cannot be in a position to help others.

The health counselor must be *secure*—he must be free from anxiety and fear. Fear and anxiety can lead the counselor to act more defensively with students than if that student were with a counselor who was secure. The insecure counselor may fear a student's anger and rejection and thus, in order to please this student, he or she may take inappropriate actions.

To understand one's self means to trust and to be trusted. If the health counselor intends to be an effective helper, he must not question a student's every motive. Having trust means to be able to give and receive, to depend on one another.

Previously we mentioned that it is essential for the counselor to understand himself. This section will discuss the significance of this ability of the health counselor to relate to and understand others.

According to Belkin, the following qualities are prerequisites for relating to others:

1. genuineness
2. nondominance
3. positive regard
4. communication skills.[5]

Genuineness

The health counselor who is genuine will not hesitate to give appropriately of himself. He will not create a facade, or, hide behind his role of counselor—i.e., "I am the teacher (health counselor) and you are my student, and don't forget that."

All too often, perhaps due to administrative interference, the counselor uses his position to conceal personal and school imperfections. If this occurs, genuineness is eliminated. As a result, the closeness of the relationship between the counselor and student is impaired.

Nondominance

Perhaps one of the most difficult skills to learn is how to deal with silence. Teachers are often uncomfortable when a class remains silent after a question is asked. The same situation is applicable to the counseling situation. The counselor, in his desire and enthusiasm to elicit responses and help the student, may tend to dominate. This domination can take the form of too much talking, imposition of values, or inappropriate use of techniques.

Often the student can be helped more if the counselor sits back and does not interrupt. In essence, the effective counselor will acquire the ability to listen.

The counselor must learn that acceptance of the student—his ideas, feelings, and responses is prerequisite to a meaningful, helping relationship. The following is an example of a situation experienced by one of the authors:

> While teaching in an inner city high school, the issue of racial discrimination surfaced. A group of black students had met to discuss their feelings and seek change in conditions of the high school. One of the students mentioned that the school should hire ten additional black faculty. Upon hearing that, I shook my head in a manner which reflected a message of "Oh, how ridiculous." After the meeting, a student who had noticed my nonverbal gesture, came up to me and expressed displeasure at my nonacceptance of the feelings expressed by the group.

The implication of this situation for health counseling is significant. As counselors we may be confronted by situations where we may not agree with statements a student may express. It is not our duty to impose values. In the above example, the teacher really said "You're wrong for feeling that way." The effective health counselor will accept what a student feels he must express. While the right to agree or disagree with a statement is the prerogative of the counselor, the labeling of a *feeling* statement as right or wrong is not within the scope of proper counseling techniques.

Communication Skills

Communication between the student and health counselor will take the form of either verbal or nonverbal messages. The counselor must be adept at understanding and using each in the helping interview. The jargon used by students in different parts of the country or for that matter, within different parts of a city, may be similar in meaning, yet opposite in oral expression. For example, black students may indicate approval of an action by a friend by saying "that's bad" when the interpretation was "that's good." In many cases, the counselor may wish to communicate in the student's language provided that language comes naturally. Students often will see through a counselor who tries too hard to be "one of the gang."

Especially in health-related topics, the counselor needs to be a semanticist. The inability to interpret correctly students' comments can mean the difference between adequate and inadequate choices.

Through nonverbal expressions the counselor can determine a student's intent. What the student hears and what he feels the student means can be quite different perceptions. The intent of a counseling situation is to strive for consonance—the student needs to express verbal intentions which are commensurate with his feelings.

The Counseling Techniques

Since the emphasis of this text focuses upon methods and techniques, the remainder of this chapter will concentrate on the "how to's" of counseling.

External and Internal Conditions

Two factors need to be discussed when dealing with communication facilitators—external and internal conditions.

External Conditions

The physical environment in which a counseling situation may occur can be either a positive or negative force in the counselor-student relationship. While the health educator may have to accept the facilities given to him within the school building, he can establish an environment which is conducive to meaningful interchange.

The Room

If the counselor will use his office, certain physical characteristics should be present.

First, privacy must exist. As long as others may be within listening distance, the student may feel inhibited.

Second, the physical arrangement of the room may be an impediment. The counselor may be wise to arrange his desk and chair in a fashion which would enable he and the student to face each other without any barrier (desk) between them. The counselor who converses with a student while behind a desk presents a physical barrier which in turn, may produce a psychological wall.

The counselor should make every attempt to maintain a clear and orderly desk. The student who sees a desk with papers piled up and scattered sloppily, may not view the counselor as an organized and orderly individual. In an orderly environment, the student can feel that he or she is the focus of attention.

Third, the student needs to feel that the counselor, at that moment, is giving one hundred percent of himself to that student. This means that the counselor is to avoid accepting telephone calls, speaking to colleagues, or looking through his day's mail while conversing.

Internal Conditions

According to Alfred Benjamin in his book *The Helping Interview*,[6] desirable internal conditions are more important to the interviews than all the external conditions put together. As a result, Benjamin cites the following two internal conditions as basic to the helping interview:

1. Bringing to the interview just as much of our own selves as we possibly can, stopping, of course, at the point at which this may hamper the interviewer or deny to the student the help he or she needs.
2. Feeling within ourselves that we wish to help him as much as possible and that there is nothing at the moment more important to us. This attitude, communicated nonverbally, will be sensed by the interviewee.

These two internal conditions bring to light a point made previously in this chapter—trust. If the student perceives that the counselor is doing his best, he will gain respect for his efforts. This leads to the development of trust which, in essence, will lead toward a meaningful counselor-student relationship.

How Counseling May Be Initiated

The health educator will be placed in a counseling situation in one of two ways: through a student-initiated action or a teacher-initiated action. In either case, the teacher, soon to be counselor, must know how to deal with each situation.

Student-Initiated

When a student asks to see you, the most sensible thing to do is to let him state why he wants to speak to you. As easy as this may seem, many teachers would want the student to know how perceptive he (the teacher) is. For example, when the student comes to the teacher with a request to speak about a concern, the teacher may say, "I bet you want to speak with me about your involvement with drugs." The student, if he is timid may feel very dominated and as a result may not wish to pursue his concerns.

While there is no set method according to which a counselor can pursue a student-initiated interview, the authors feel that the counselor who allows the student to state in his own words his reasons for wanting to see him will have a greater chance of meaningful interaction.

Another mistake often made in a counseling situation occurs when the teacher uses the word "problem." "What is your problem?" This word may lead to a communication barrier since:

1. the student may not have a problem;

2. the student may not have thought of his concern as a problem;

3. the student may think the word "problem" is too intense and loaded.

These three interpretations can serve as a barrier to communication.

The teacher who wishes to initiate an interview will proceed in a manner different from the student who initiates the approach. As was mentioned previously, through classroom observation the teacher will often notice changes in student behavior. Upon noting this, the teacher may decide he would like to help the student. The following are some "do's" and "don'ts" for teacher-initiated conferences."

Don't:

1. highlight your observation or concern during a classroom session;

2. *confront* the student on a one-to-one basis with a blatant statement as opening;

3. act alarmed over a particular observation.

Do:

1. start a conversation with the student at the end of a class period and use this situation as an icebreaker for further conversation;

2. show concern but without acting nervous or feeling panicky.

When the teacher has "broken the ice," it is desirable at the outset to share with the student the reason for your concern. For example, "I wanted to speak to you because I have noticed you were acting nervous about something." This comment indicates an intention to assist the student; it also shows him that you are open and honest. Sometimes the teacher, although well intentioned, may open a counseling session with a comment such as, "I guess you know why I've asked to see you." This type of statement can be threatening to the student. In addition, the student may not know why he has been approached by the teacher, and as a result may become confused.

Defining Your Role

The teacher may wish to share with the student his role in the helping relationship. A statement such as, "My experience as a health educator has made me well aware of some of the issues and concerns of youth your age. We can talk about your concern and take steps to work effectively to deal with it."

There is no need to involve the student in the details of your role as a health counselor. You do not need to describe your professional training and your experiences, since these aspects are of little importance to your troubled students.

Individual Values Versus School Rules

At times the teacher may be placed in a situation where student well-being and school policy may conflict. The following case study can help clarify this point:

> While Mr. Rogers is teaching a lesson, he notices a student who is rolling a joint (making a marijuana cigarette) secretively at his desk.

> Mr. Rogers has several options; among them are:

1. He could abruptly stop his lesson and report the student to the principal;

2. Ignore the situation and pretend nothing has happened;

3. Speak to the student after class and determine what action he will take.

If the teacher decides to forego the first two steps, the final option places him in a one-to-one situation where counseling skills must be utilized. In a confrontation such as this, the teacher must choose between going against school policy and not reporting the student, or playing by the rules. The teacher may decide to ignore the school rules because he may feel the punishment for possession of marijuana is not proportionate to the offense. Yet the teacher must protect himself. To deal with this and similar occurrences, the instructor may wish to place the student in a *limit* situation—that is, give the student a warning and take action should the same thing happen. Thus, the teacher can call the student up to the front of the room *after* the class and tell him that he hopes the student will not be in possession of any illegal drug in the future, since this would then be reported. In this situation the teacher has acted responsibly in that:

1. (s)he never admitted to the student or other class members that he actually saw him with marijuana

2. (s)he never accused the student of anything illegal.

Had the teacher not taken either of the steps mentioned, he would have no choice but to report the student.

This example does not endorse this practice. However, it does illustrate a situation which contrasts school policy with the teacher's inner feeling. While the student-counselor relationship must maintain confidentiality, the counselor needs to discriminate between reporting or not reporting school infractions.

Student Records

The teacher who does health counseling in the school should be familiar with the rules governing access to students' records. Any notes that the teacher may place in a student's file can be subpoenaed by the courts. The only person in the school who is not required to provide student records is the school psychologist. Therefore, the teacher or counselor may need to consider carefully before maintaining formal files or placing information in a student's permanent file.

Chapter Summary

Innumerable health problems confront middle and secondary school students. To help students cope effectively with their concerns, teachers should have some knowledge of counseling skills which can help students in their quest to attain a higher level of wellness. Often, the health educator, because of his/her knowledge about health, is called upon to offer assistance in this area.

The health educator in his/her role as counselor should have the following skills in order to serve effectively: the ability to understand others, ability to understand one's self, skill in relating to others, communication skills, and freedom from pretense or affectation.

There are many counseling techniques which one must master if one is to be effective. Establishing an internal and external atmosphere conducive to positive communication is essential, whether a counseling session is counselor- or student-initiated.

The teacher in the role as counselor should be aware of the legal ramifications within which he or she operates. A good working knowledge of school rules is a prerequisite, if such advice will be sought after and eventually given.

Notes

1. Sandra Dale, "School Mental Health Programs: A Challenge to the Health Professional," *The Journal of School Health,* 48:9, November, 1978, 526.
2. T. Langner, J. Gersten, E. Green, et al.: "Treatment of Psychological Disorders Among Urban Children," *Journal of Consultant Clinical Psychology,* 5, 1976, 26–32.
3. Gary S. Belkin, *Health Counseling in the Schools,* Dubuque: Wm. C. Brown Company Publishers, 1975.
4. *Ibid.,* 108–110.
5. *Ibid.,* 112–116.
6. Alfred Benjamin, *The Helping Interview,* Boston: Houghton Mifflin Company, 1969, 4–8.

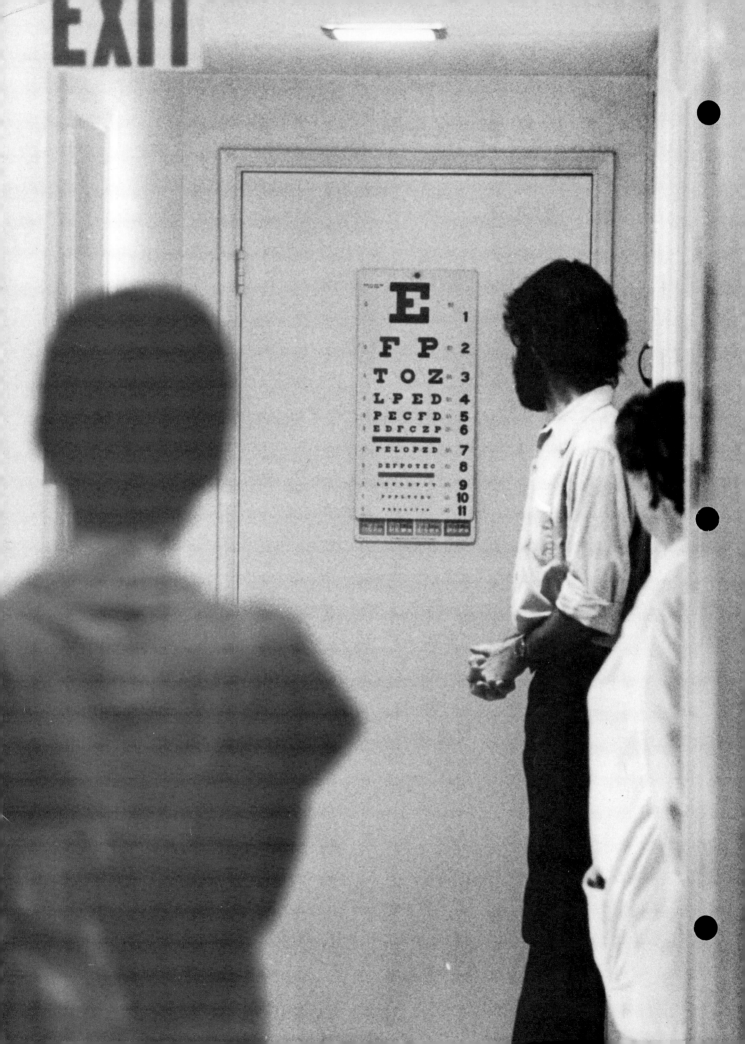

The School Health Program

Today's Middle and Secondary school students are confronted with social, psychological and physiological health-related issues which differ from those of previous years. This in turn requires greater judgement and maturity for satisfactory health decision-making. The secondary school teacher can play a vital role in the prevention and treatment of these problems by integrating related aspects of the school health program throughout the school day. Essentially, the teacher can make use of all activities within the school that have been developed to promote and preserve the health of the student. These activities and resources—school health services, health instruction and healthful school environment—are the components of the school health program.

School Health Services

School health services include those school activities directly concerned with the present status of school youth. These services are designed to appraise, promote, protect, and maintain the health of students. The justification for the importance of school health services is based upon the fact that the schools have a captive audience of 50 million children. Thus, many in the health related areas feel that schools are the logical place where suspicion—sometimes identification—of illness is made.[1]

Following are the major components of school health services.

Health Appraisal

Since the middle and secondary school health educator often sees his students one period per day, five times per week, he or she is in a position to notice physical and psychological changes which may occur. The health educator's professional preparation in health-related issues places him in a position where other faculty and administrators will seek his help.

Observation

The middle and secondary school health educator is one of the more qualified individuals in the school, able to detect problems related to drug abuse, sexually transmitted diseases, and alcohol, to name a few. Therefore, the health educator, through continuous attention to students in his classes, as well as observing his colleagues' students, can make more valid determinations of actual and potential problems. Among the signs that may indicate problems exist are: withdrawal from peers and teachers; sudden acting out; a sharp dip in grades; a decrease in participating in extra curricular activities; and engaging in disruptive classroom behavior.

Cumulative Health Record

In many middle and secondary schools, students' cumulative health records are maintained in the health education office. The health educator, through his knowledge of school health services, is usually in a better position than most other school personnel, to interpret the materials within the health folder.

The cumulative health record should always be updated with information about height, weight, and vision, with the results of physical exams added yearly.

The guidance counselor or school nurse should be aware of the patterns on the health record. For example, the health record may indicate that a particular student becomes ill at least two Fridays per month and is either sent home from school or absent for the day. This pattern may indicate several things. One, the student desires long weekends and therefore uses illness as an excuse for absence. Two, a certain teacher may give written examinations on Fridays. Some students become ill due to the pressures of exams, and therefore they often seek to leave school. Three, the student's parents may keep their child out of school because of family commitments to outside activities. A host of other examples can be given.

Suspect, Detect and Refer

In all of the above mentioned cases, the secondary school teacher is limited in the types of action that he can take. The teacher may *suspect* that a particular condition exists; *detect* any clues that will help identify that condition; and *refer* the student to an appropriate person in the school or community.

Diagnosis and Treatment

Diagnosis and treatment are two areas which are outside the realm of the legal and moral responsibility of the middle and secondary school teacher. Participation in either area (except for the immediate and temporary care of a student in an emergency situation) opens the door for negligence and liability suits. Licensed professionals in the medical and psychological fields are the ones who ought make judgements related to these areas.

Screening

By the time a student enters the middle or secondary school, many screening examinations have been administered. These examinations, which are preliminary evaluations of the growth and development of various body organs, are often discontinued in the middle and secondary school screening program. Among these screening tests may be vision, hearing, and dental health. However, much data concerning these areas can be obtained from a regular physical check-up by the student's family physician or the school doctor. Most states require a general physical examination at least once during middle or secondary school.

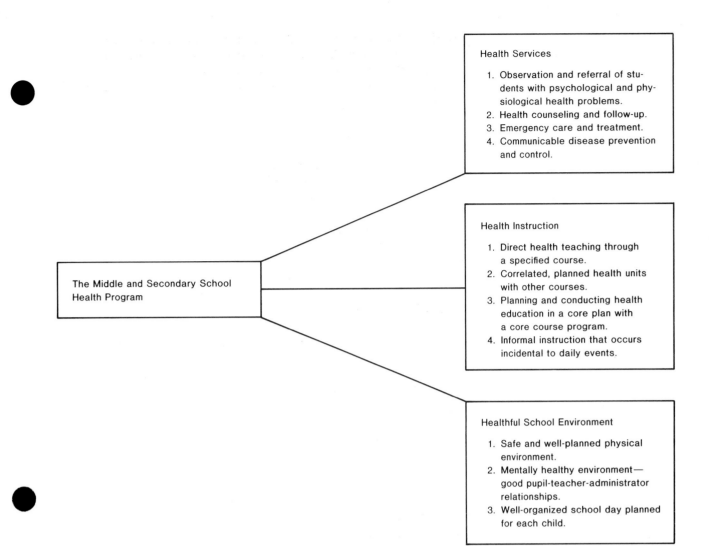

The Middle and Secondary School Health Program

Health Services

1. Observation and referral of students with psychological and physiological health problems.
2. Health counseling and follow-up.
3. Emergency care and treatment.
4. Communicable disease prevention and control.

Health Instruction

1. Direct health teaching through a specified course.
2. Correlated, planned health units with other courses.
3. Planning and conducting health education in a core plan with a core course program.
4. Informal instruction that occurs incidental to daily events.

Healthful School Environment

1. Safe and well-planned physical environment.
2. Mentally healthy environment— good pupil-teacher-administrator relationships.
3. Well-organized school day planned for each child.

Figure 4.1. The total middle and secondary school health program

Characteristics of Screening Tests

According to the Joint Committee on Health Problems in Education of the National Education Association and the American Medical Association,[2] certain factors must be weighed in determining the feasibility of administering screening tests.

1. Is the test applicable to the health problems of children of school age? The incidence of some conditions should be detectable in sufficient instances by means of the screening process.

2. Is the test medically sound? The screening procedures used should provide information that is specific in regard to health status. It should not lead to over—or under—referrals, and follow-up should be feasible.

3. Is the test educationally sound? Screening tests incorporated in the school setting should be able to provide useful health practices to students in post-school life, should be incorporated in the school teaching program, and should provide teachers with the tools needed to prepare students for the test.

4. Is the test economically feasible? Can the tests be conducted within the schools budget allocation? Costs for personnel and equipment need to be considered.

5. Is the test acceptable public relations? The implementation of screening tests should promote good relations between the school, the child and his family, physicians, and community health agencies.

Health Counseling

At one time or another all school personnel are placed in a health counseling situation. Chapter Three covers theory and practice of health counseling. This section will deal with the role of counseling within the scope of school health services.

The Parent's Role

The school should report its assessments of pupil health and needs to parents, so that the family can be informed concerning proper care, treatment, and referral procedures.

Assessment can be shared during parent's visitations to school, by telephone or by home visits. The latter, although used sparingly today, is a good school-family endeavor.

Schools and parents should help the student assume responsibility for his or her conduct. This may be achieved by allowing the student to understand the cumulative health record, including student input about health-related decisions, making students aware of the rationale for health practices and policies, and allowing one's self to listen effectively, providing immediate, specific, and worthwhile feedback.

The Teacher's Role

For teachers to counsel effectively in health-related areas, they need to be informed of the health status of each student. In the secondary school setting, each student may be exposed to as many as eight different teachers per day, one per class period. Each teacher may teach five periods per day—each period involving thirty students. With 150 students per day, the teacher is limited in the number of health problems that he can detect. However, there can be a considerable degree of effectiveness.

Informing the Teacher of Health Problems

The school nurse or health services coordinator can distribute to each child's teacher, a note or form which indicates a health problem or condition. After the teacher is made aware of the student's condition, the note is maintained on permanent file in the students permanent health folder. The health educator or school nurse should be consulted about questions concerning treatment, emergency care, or special precautions to be observed in the classroom.

Community Resources

Today more than ever before, voluntary and public health agencies are receiving referrals from schools. Venereal disease, pregnancy, abortion, alcoholism, drug use and abuse, cigarette smoking, weight control, suicide, and depression are just a few of the many health problem areas for which referrals are made.

The schools must discriminate among the agencies to which its students are referred. Although not possessing the skills needed to evaluate community health agencies, schools can ascertain to some degree the extent to which these agencies assist the students referred to them. Table 4.1 provides a framework for evaluating a community health agency. Assessments can be made by school personnel—teachers, counselors, school nurses, school psychologists, and administrators.

Table 4.1
Evaluating a Health Agency

I. Policies and Practices
   1. What age groups does the agency service?
   2. What is the fee structure?
   3. How many hours and days per week is the agency open?
   4. Can personnel be reached in an emergency?
   5. How are records maintained?
   6. Are names released indiscriminately?
   7. What precautions are taken to assure confidentiality?
   8. What are the follow-up procedures for clients?
   9. What evaluation efforts have been taken to assess effectiveness?
   10. Must clients wait for long periods of time before seen?

II. Personnel
   1. What kind of training and/or professional degrees do employees possess?
   2. What kinds of experience do personnel have?
   3. Did the students referred find agency personnel easy to talk to and helpful?
   4. Did the agency personnel appear knowledgable?
   5. Do they take the time to talk at length?
   6. Were agency personnel easy to talk to?
   7. Are they professionals?

III. Physical Facilities
   1. Are the waiting rooms and offices well kept?
   2. Is the agency easily accessible by public transportation or motor vehicle?
   3. Is the agency situated in a community in which one feels safe traveling?

Follow-up after Counseling

One of the more significant aspects of health counseling is follow-up. Every school has a moral and legal responsibility to insure that this is done after every referral.

The policy in most schools is that a student must provide a teacher with a note from home if an absence has occurred. Usually a physician's statement will suffice if the student has been to see him. In either case, the reason for absence should be stated.

The classroom teacher is sometimes responsible for checking admittance papers when a student has not been in his class for several days. This serves two purposes. One, the student who may have had a communicable disease will be "cleared" so that contact with other students will be safe. Two, in the middle or secondary school setting, students often "cut" class. Knowing that (s)he may be referred to the attendance officer for admittance to class, the "cutter" may think twice before attempting a similar move.

What is done after follow-up is important. Concerns such as a reduction in the number of courses a student is taking, on-going counseling, administering daily medication, and tutoring need to be taken into account.

Prompt and detailed follow-up policies enable the school to ascertain the effectiveness of referral agencies. In cases where the school sends a student to a community health agency, especially one with which the school has not dealt previously, feedback is needed.

Referring a student to an agency which mistreats its clientel can serve to alienate the student from the teacher or counselor who made the referral. Although the school may not have been aware of the inadequacies of the agency, a loss of client-counselor trust may occur.

Emergency Care

The school is responsible for providing immediate and temporary care in case of sudden illness or accident.

Ideally, every teacher in the school building should be qualified to perform first aid. Since this is not the case, health educators, school nurses, or school administrators are often the ones called upon for this task.

In his role, the health educator can teach in-service courses (health educators are, in most cases, certified first aid instructors) and certify other staff in first aid and cardio-pulmonary resuscitation (CPR).

Liability in Emergency Care

Sometimes the question of liability may surface. The outcome of such an issue may be based upon the question of what a person of reasonable prudence would have done. Therefore, the following should serve as guidelines in an emergency first aid situation:

1. Assume the worst. If you come across a student who is lying on the floor unconscious, do not move him and assume he may have had a serious injury which could be aggravated by a sudden shift;

2. Use common sense. Most first aid procedures are simple;

3. Be calm and do not unnecessarily rush to administer first aid;

4. Only perform those first aid procedures which you know are appropriate and correct.

In most states, teachers are automatically covered by liability insurance. However, some states have a policy by which boards of education cannot be sued and it is the teacher against whom a claim is made. In such cases, teachers may be encouraged to purchase liability insurance.

Student Records

Every student should have a card on file in the school which has the following information:

1. Where his or her parents or guardian can be reached during the day—work and home addresses and phone numbers.

2. Name and phone number of the family physician.

3. Any health conditions that the student may have.

4. Name and phone number of someone close to the family if family members cannot be reached.

Sending Students Home

Often a student needs to be sent home because he may feel ill. The above mentioned card can be used to contact parents. Generally, students should not be sent home from school unless a parent or another adult can come to school to take the student home. In rare cases, the teacher or administrator, after speaking to the parent may allow the student to go home by him or herself.

Informing Parents

In any emergency, the parents should be notified of all actions the school is taking. The school should avoid making a diagnosis and administering medication.

In addition to informing parents, the school should guide them toward community facilities at which the injured child may be treated. The family should also contact its physician about the emergency. The family physician is the one usually best acquainted with the student's health history and status; he may therefore be in position to offer valuable assistance and information regarding care and treatment of the injured child.

The Accident Report

The school has the responsibility for completing an accident report for any injury occurring on school grounds. According to the National Safety Council, the following should be recorded on an accident report:

1. Name
2. Address
3. School
4. Sex
5. Age
6. Grade/special program
7. Date and time of accident; day of week
8. Nature of the injury
9. Part of the body injured
10. Degree of the injury
11. Number of days lost
12. Cause of the injury
13. Jurisdictional classification of the accident
14. Location of the accident
15. Activity of the victim
16. Status of the activity
17. Supervision
18. Agency involved (apparatus, equipment, etc.)
19. Unsafe acts
20. Unsafe mechanical-physical conditions
21. Unsafe personal factors
22. Corrective action taken or recommended
23. Property damage
24. Description (paragraph form)
25. Date of report
26. Report prepared by (signature)
27. Witness's signature
28. Principal's signature[3]

Almost all schools have a room which is designated as an emergency or sick care room. This provides students and teachers with a facility for emergency treatment, a bed upon which to rest, a first aid kit, health records, guidelines and procedures concerning first aid and temporary care.

Communicable Disease Prevention and Control

The health department is legally responsible for communicable disease control. It reports symptoms of diseases, as well as regulations about exclusion from school.

Other than the common cold, students showing symptoms of a communicable disease should be referred for proper diagnosis and/or treatment.

Teachers should not emphasize the need for perfect attendance, since this may encourage ill students to come to school. Pupils should be commended for staying home when they have a contagious condition.

In cases of actual or potential epidemics, the school, with assistance from the health department, may wish to initiate an immunization program. Typical might be a mass inoculation campaign for a measles outbreak.

Health Instruction

Health instruction is "the process of providing a sequence of planned and spontaneously originated learning opportunities comprising the organized aspects of health education in the school or community."[4]

In the middle and secondary school, health is taught as a separate subject. A health educator should be responsible for health instruction, whether this instruction is for students or teachers (in-service).

By means of the health instruction program, the school health educator's major responsibility is to provide classroom instruction that assures students the opportunity to receive accurate factual information, clarify values, and promote sound health practices that will prepare them for future health needs.[5] This can be accomplished by direct teaching approaches or by integrating instruction with other disciplines.

Cognitive and Affective Instruction

The health educator is responsible for providing students with accurate information which will enable them to attain such skills as knowing, analyzing, comprehending, and applying information.

The middle and secondary school teacher must promote affective behavior through activities which assist students in clarifying their attitudes and values as these relate to health areas.

Promoting Healthy Practices

The health educator has as his ultimate goal a responsibility for promoting positive behavior change in students. As a result, externally demonstrated practices will indicate to some extent, how effective we are. These behaviors can include:

1. those that are observable in the classroom—i.e.,—good grooming, social interaction with peers, motivation and enthusiasm in classroom activities;

2. conduct patterns that are observable due to behavior outside the classroom—i.e.,—visits to the dentist, participation in physical fitness and diet program;

3. those that are to be practiced in the future—i.e.,—yearly physical check-ups, involvement in community health policies, and participation in smoking-cessation programs.[6]

Healthful School Environment

A healthful school environment is the promotion, maintenance, and utilization of wholesome surroundings, organization of day-by-day experiences, and planned learning procedures which contribute to favorable emotional, physical and social health.[7]

Physical Environment

The physical layout of a room can set the tone in a health education class. Some characteristics which the health educator may wish to examine are:

1. Is my classroom cheerful and bright?

2. Do students have to sit in straight rows or can I have them seated in a circle?

3. Is it necessary for me to sit behind my desk each period and therefore create a "barrier," or can I sit on my desk or have it moved behind me?

4. Are there health-related messages posted in my room that are appealing to the students' eye and imagination?

5. Even with energy problems, is the physical environment warm—both emotionally and physically?

6. Do students feel comfortable about using the school bathrooms without worry of being "ripped off" by others who are "hanging out."

7. Does the school provide ample and safe facilities?

8. Is the school a good role model? For example, how does one teach good nutritional habits, and yet try to rationalize the existence of candy machines in the school?

Custodian

One of the key people in the school building is the custodial engineer. Since this person is responsible for reporting to superiors other than the school principal, he is in a position to act independently. Therefore, the teacher often needs to work through this person directly in order to obtain certain favors, such as having classroom furniture arranged and facilities cleaned up for special events. A rule of thumb is to remain on the good side of the custodial engineer.

Social-Emotional Environment

Student learning can be affected by the social and emotional climate in the school setting.

Teachers and program coordinators must be attuned to the day-to-day schedule of students. Issues to be considered are:

1. Is the student carrying too many courses?

2. Are lunch periods built into the student's program?

3. Is the student too involved in extra-curricular activities?

4. Does the student have ample free time during the school day?

5. Are undue pressures concerning performance placed on students?

The Teacher

Teachers need to be in an environment which is conducive to effectiveness. The following considerations should be noted:

1. Is the teacher teaching too many classes? In the secondary school setting, teachers should not teach more than five, forty-five minute class period per day nor more than three consecutive periods without a break.

2. Does the teacher feel insecure about job stability? With declining enrollments and budget restrictions, many teachers are concerned about forced early retirement or tenure denial. While these problems have no immediate answers that will satisfy personnel, they do create emotional strains which may affect classroom teaching. Administrators need to be supportive of their faculty and provide positive feedback when applicable.

3. Is the teacher able to handle stressful situations? Teaching today is considered a significantly stressful occupation.[8] Psychological stress placed upon teachers by parents, school administrators, and students can have a negative impact on a teacher's performance. Because of the many stressors which confront teachers, the "burn-out" rate in the profession has reached the thousands.[9] To deal effectively with this problem, one must be able to identify the sources and consequences of stressors and in turn, develop effective coping strategies.

Chapter Summary

The middle and secondary school health educator has a major responsibility to his students, colleagues, and the community, for promoting health and well-being. Knowledge and application of principles and practices of the school health program can help meet these needs in this area. As a result, the teacher needs to understand those factors in the school which can influence students' health and safety.

The teacher has a moral and legal obligation to his students, their families, and to any other person connected to the school. The teacher must understand the scope of emergency care, plan safety measures, and be aware of the responsibilities essential to providing an optimum environmental facility commensurate with student wellness.

School personnel should have a good working knowledge of the health related agencies within the community, since referrals are often made to these agencies. For the most part, these referrals are made by counselors, principals, or school nurses. Because of his professional preparation, specifically insights regarding community facilities, the health educator is found often in the position of recommending an agency to assist with particular student health problems. Some of these may be drug treatment facilities, family planning agencies, or suicide-prevention clinics. It is important to note that agencies vary in the kinds of services provided, therefore student needs should be identified as closely as possible with agencies which have services that match these needs.

Notes

1. Dorster, Mildred, "The Role of Schools in Primary Health Care," *The Journal of School Health,* February, 1979, 49:2, p. 113.
2. Joint Committee on Health Problems in Education of The National Education Association and The American Medical Association, *"Health Appraisal of School Children,"* Washington, D.C., 1969, 8–9.
3. *Student Accident Reporting Guidebook,* Chicago: National Safety Council, 1966, 29.
4. Green, Lawrence W. (Ed.), "New Definitions: Report of the 1972–1973 Joint Committee on Health Education Terminology," Health Education Monographs, No. 33, 1973, 63–70.
5. Galli, Nicholas, *Foundations and Principles of Health Education,* New York: John Wiley and Sons, Inc., 1978, 277.
6. Fodor, John T. and Dalis, Gus T., *Health Instruction: Theory and Application,* Philadelphia: Lea and Febiger, 1974, 6–7.
7. Green, Lawrence W. (Ed.), 63–70.
8. Needle, Richard H.; Griffin, Tom; Svendsen, Roger; Berney, Coleen. "Teacher Stress: Sources and Consequences," *The Journal of School Health,* February, 1980, 50:2, p. 96.
9. *Ibid;* 96.

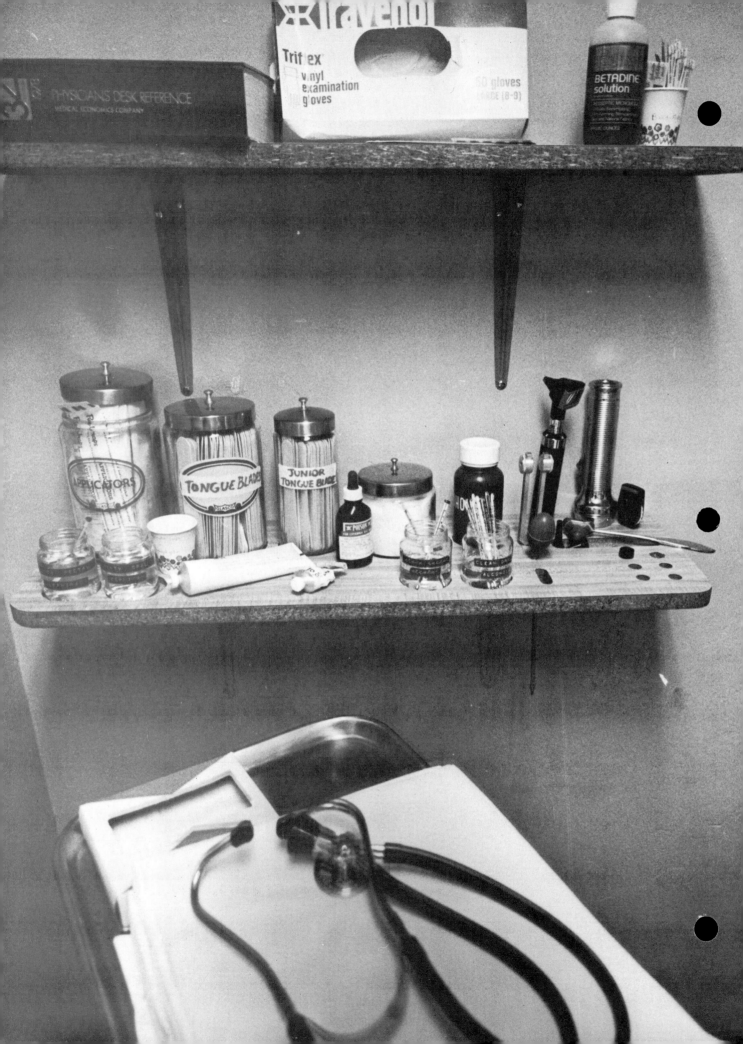

5

The Health Education Curriculum

The Contents of the Curriculum

A curriculum is an orderly plan for implementing health instruction that includes a framework for organizing health instruction to meet the needs of the learner, to convey subject matter in a meaningful way, and to evaluate the effects of instruction.

A curriculum and a related curriculum guide may depict a complete program, or it may only be a rough outline of a program plan for a community. The most successful curriculums include the following as a *minimum:*

1. Philosophy of Education.
2. Philosophy of Health Education.
3. Statement of Need.
4. Overall Objectives or Goals of the Curriculum.
5. Plan for Instruction to meet the objectives and goals:
   Units
   Topics
   Objectives
   Sources
   Content and Procedures
   Materials
   Evaluation Items
6. Plan for Evaluation of Curriculum Goals and Objectives.

Developing the Curriculum

There are several different ways to develop curriculum and curriculum guides for your middle and secondary school students. According to Goodlad[1] curriculums have traditionally been developed or centered around one of the following concerns:

1. a concern for subject matter;
2. a concern for the learner's total education;
3. a concern for the individual as a human being.

It is our belief that a successful curriculum is developed or centered with reference to all three of these concerns.

We further believe that a curriculum serves to raise a series of questions about a specific discipline, in our case a series of questions about health science. Relating this curriculum function to the concerns mentioned previously, we might ask ourselves the following questions:

1. What questions about health science do we want to ask?

2. How does the teaching of health science relate to the learner's total education in the middle and secondary school?

3. What questions will we raise in our health science class that will relate to our learner as a human being?

When we examine alternative approaches to solutions to these questions, we have a basis for the health science curriculum. But who begins this search?

The Curriculum Advisory Council

After the selection of a health science curriculum project co-ordinator who will oversee the development of the curriculum, a health education curriculum advisory council is formed.

Keogh Rash and Morgan Pigg in their excellent book, *The Health Education Curriculum,*[2] identify the three important broad functions of the health education curriculum advisory council:

1. to provide resources from which to draw in determining the health education needs and interests of pupils, as well as the community health needs;

2. to provide opportunity for increasing the understanding and appreciation of the community as they relate to health and the school health program;

3. to secure support for the conduct and growth of the program and for meeting unfair or unjustified criticism.

Rash and Pigg further specify the responsibilities of the health education advisory council[3]:

1. Developing statements of philosophy concerning the nature of the health program.

2. Determining the principal health and health education needs of the community.

3. Determining the principal health education needs of the pupils.

4. Deciding some areas of health education outcomes to be stressed in schools.

5. Determining general policies concerning development and application of the health education curriculum.

6. Acquainting the public with the needs and progress of the school health curriculum project.

7. Surveying the opportunities for coordination of efforts of all health workers.

8. Stimulating a keen interest in the project.

9. Acting as a consultant group for the health education curriculum committee.

Rash and Pigg suggest that membership on the advisory council should be representative of the following agencies and organizations[4]:

Official Agencies
Health Department
Public Welfare
Fire Department
Police Department
Schools

Government
City
County

Professional Associations
Dental
Medical
Nursing
Ministerial

Labor and Management
Unions
Manufacturers association

Parent-Teacher-Student Associations

Voluntary Agencies
Cancer Society
Society for the Crippled
Heart Association
The National Foundation, Inc.
Red Cross
Lung Association
Mental Health Association
Social Health Association
Council on Family Relations

Civic and Service Clubs
American Legion
Chamber of Commerce
Women's Club
Fraternities and Sororities
with health interests
Service clubs
Senior citizen clubs

The Health Education Curriculum Committee

The Health Education Curriculum Committee has the responsibility of supervising the development of all aspects of the health education curriculum.[5]

According to Rash and Pigg "The personnel of the health education curriculum committee will consist of representatives from all aspects of the school health program, a few key community representatives, selected teachers who are not directly concerned with health education, students, representatives of the administration, and representatives of the parent-teacher-student association. It is important that some members of this committee also be on the advisory council, and some on the central course of study committee.

Membership on the health education curriculum committee should be representative of the following[6]:

School Health Program
Health education teachers
Custodians
School nurse
School physician
Nutritionist
Supervisor of health education
Health coordinator

Administration
Curriculum director
Elementary school principal
Secondary school principal

Nonhealth Teachers
Biology
Social studies
Physical education
Elementary school
Secondary school

P.T.S.A./O.
Chairman of health commission
Interested parents
Students

Community representatives
Health department
Voluntary agencies
Medical society
Dental society

The Available Health Education Curriculum Plans

There are a variety of curriculum guides available from which to choose and develop a framework that will meet the needs of a given locality. In keeping with our philosophy of personal responsibility for choice, we believe that it is our task to assist you in the evaluation and intelligent selection among the various alternative curriculum designs available.

We will identify and discuss several alternative curriculum designs in the following pages. Keep in mind as you examine each, that curricula and curriculum guides are not mutually exclusive. There is no need to select one and use it by itself. Evaluate and select the best, choosing from the many different alternative guides and plans available the one which is most adapted to your needs.

The Life Style Curriculum

We will begin with the Life Style Approach to curriculum design as it is compatible with our approach.

The Life Style Approach is based on the premise that the we are responsible for our health. This approach recognizes the advances that have been made through medical science and holds that future advances in the improvement of health will come from the individual's behavior.

The Life Style Approach to health education developed by Dr. John Burt[7] identifies a clear purpose for health education in the schools: To assist in the evaluation and intelligent selection of the alternatives in life style.

According to Burt, the life style approach involves three steps:

1. Identifying the alternatives in life style.

2. Evaluating these alternatives (or reevaluating in the case of old habits).

3. Intelligent selection of personal alternatives (or change in life style in the case of old habits).

The life style approach to health education provides a framework within which a meaningful curriculum can be developed. The life style curriculum is based on the premise that much of health behavior is determined by our life style patterns. The differing patterns of behavior are organized by Burt into a *Taxonomy of Life Styles*.[8] This *Taxonomy* is shown in Table 5–1.

Burt's *Taxonomy of Life Styles* could be briefly summarized to include:[9]

1. *Coping style*—each individual develops a style whereby he attempts to cope with a variety of life stressors.

2. *Relating style*—To overcome our aloneness, each of us develops a style of relating to others. The style might be heterosexual, homosexual, bisexual, or purely psychic.

3. *Risk-taking style*—Each of us develops a style for risk-taking, engaging in trade offs between present goals and long range health risks.

4. *Decision-making style*—Each of us has the power to focus the direction and intensity of our consciousness or to suspend our thinking and let the mind drift passively. Thus, some of us make our own decisions, some of us make no decisions, and others leave decision-making to someone else.

5. *Working-creating-producing-style*—It is characteristic of some to be productive but not creative, others are both creative and productive, and some may be neither, or even destructive.

6. *Self conservation style*—A self-conservation style is one where life style components are altered to conserve the heart, arteries, pancreas, gall bladder, teeth, eyes, etc. The opposite style, where no regard is given, is termed self-dissipation.

Table 5.1 Taxonomy of Life Styles

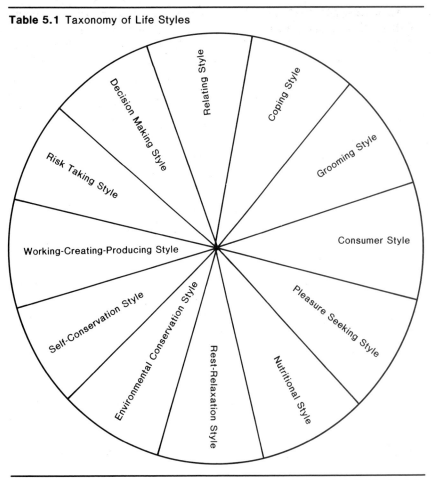

John J. Burt, Linda Meeks, and Sharon Pottebaum. *Toward A Healthy Life Style Through Health Education in the Elementary School.* (Belmont, California: Wadsworth Publishing Company, 1980).

7. *Environmental conservation style*—The style that is selected to deal with conserving our natural resources such as land, water and air.

8. *Rest-relaxation style*—Transcendental meditation, yoga, biofeedback, sleeping pills, etc. are among the possible styles to select for rest-relaxation.

9. *Nutritional style*—A style of food and fluid intake including such choices as what to eat, when to eat, where to eat, and how much to eat, to list only a few.

10. *Pleasure-seeking style*—Pleasure-seeking is one of the most difficult tasks that man has ever undertaken. Deciding between the alternative styles of pleasure seeking certainly is related to one's health.

11. *Consumer style*—The consumer may develop a style that includes careful evaluation of the health and safety risks of the products and services that he purchases, or he may ignore these risks.

12. *Grooming style*—Many of the alternatives to grooming style have major implications for health; others are of little significance.

From a developmental view, the twelve components of life style must be considered concurrently. A student must deal with each of these components at each grade level—evaluating and revising as he moves from grade to grade.

The Conceptual Approach to Curriculum

The conceptual approach to curriculum design stresses key concepts as "basic central ideas, an understanding of which opens the door to an entire field of knowledge. The concepts serve as the major organizing elements of the curriculum.[10]

The School Health Education Study

The School Health Education Study, often referred to as SHES, pioneered the way for a conceptual model by accumulating information about health experiences and understandings in several school systems, and organizing the findings. The result was a publication titled *Health Education: A Conceptual Approach to Curriculum Design, Grades Kindergarten Through Twelve.* Three key concepts were used as unifying threads to hold the curriculum together.[11]

> *Growing and developing:* a dynamic life process in which the individual is in some ways like all other individuals, in some ways like some other individuals, and in some ways like no other individuals.
> *Interacting:* an ongoing process in which the individual is affected by and in turn affects certain biological, social, psychological, economic, cultural, and physical forces in the environment.
> *Decision-making:* a process, unique to man, of consciously deciding to take an action, or of choosing one alternative rather than another.

After the identification of these three key concepts, ten concepts were identified which reflect the scope of the health education curriculum. These ten concepts are[12]

1. Growth and development influences and is influenced by the structure and functioning of the individual.

2. Growing and developing follows a predictable sequence, yet is unique for each individual.

3. Protection and promotion of health is an individual, community, and international responsibility.

4. The potential for hazards and accidents exists, whatever the environment.

5. There are reciprocal relationships involving man, disease, and environment.

6. The family serves to perpetuate man and to fulfill certain health needs.

7. Personal health practices are affected by a complex of forces, often conflicting.

8. Utilization of health information, products, and services is guided by values and perceptions.

9. Use of substances that modify mood and behavior arises from a variety of motivations.

10. Food selection and eating patterns are determined by physical, social, mental, economic, and cultural forces.

With these ten concepts as a framework, behavioral objectives or long range goals were identified for health teaching. The strength of this type of conceptual model is that rapidly changing factual data does not outdate the framework.

New York State Health Strands Program

The State of New York has also developed a comprehensive health education program utilizing the conceptual approach. The New York State Health Strands Program[13] is set up in five strands, with substrands as follows:

I. Physical Health
   Health Status
   Nutrition
   Sensory Perception
   Dental Health
   Disease Prevention and Control

II. Sociological Health Problems
   Smoking and Health
   Alcohol Education
   Drugs and Narcotic Education

III. Mental Health
   Personality Development
   Sexuality
   Family Life Education

IV. Environmental and Community Health
   Environmental and Public Health
   World Health
   Ecology and Epidemiology of Health
   Consumer Health

V. Education for Survival Safety
   First Aid and Survival Education

This program is easy for the teacher with little background to use. There are teaching guides available for the different substrands. They employ a cookbook approach by including detailed lesson plans with an outline of content, fundamental concepts, teaching aids and suggested learning activities, as well as supplementary information for the teacher.

The Health Instruction Framework for California Public Schools

The Health Instruction Framework for California Public Schools is another example of a curriculum guide organized by concepts. There are ten content areas and three multidisciplinary goals. They are: to grow in self awareness, to develop skills for effective decision making, and to grow in coping action.[14] Each objective is related directly to one or more of the multidisciplinary goals.

Pennsylvania Department of Education

The Pennsylvania Department of Education also has a curriculum guide[15] that is organized by concepts. In addition there are 17 units identified for grades 7–9 and 10–12, with learning activities for each. These units are:

1. Alcohol
2. Anatomy
3. Community Health
4. Consumer Health
5. Dental Health
6. Disease Control
7. Drugs and Narcotics
8. Family Relationships
9. Health Careers
10. Heredity and Environment
11. Human Sexuality
12. Mental Health
13. Nutrition
14. Physical Fitness
15. Physiology
16. Safety
17. Smoking

Body Systems Approach to Curriculum

Another means of developing curricula, is the formulation of teaching concepts, activities, etc. organized by body system. The School Health Curriculum Project[16] undertaken in 1969 by the National Clearinghouse for Smoking and Health, A Division of the Center for Disease Control of the Federal Department of Health Education and Welfare, developed a highly successful curriculum using this approach.

The goals of The School Health Curriculum Project (SHCP), previously known as the "Berkeley model," are to impart knowledge, develop healthy attitudes, and change behavior. The curriculum is organized by body system (4th grade-digestive, 5th grade-respiratory, 6th grade-circulatory, and 7th grade-nervous). Each body system is a unit of study requiring about eight to ten weeks for completion.

The model has objectives, using teaching activities and materials to facilitate lesson planning. Books, filmstrips, pamphlets, transparencies, casette tapes, anatomical models, and slides are the components of the eight to ten week learning session.

The current program is developed for the elementary school, although there is the 7th grade curriculum on the nervous system. Thus, it appears that this curriculum will have major impact on school health programs throughout the country. Already many school districts are using the program in the United States, as well as school districts in Saudi Arabia and England.

Competency Based Approach to Curriculum

A competency-based approach to curriculum design specifies minimum performance levels for students to complete at the various grade levels. When discussing the competency-based approach to instruction, it is important to understand three terms:[17]

1. *Program goal*—where the teacher hopes the student will be by the end of the course; a long range target for success.

2. *Competency*—possession of skills, knowledge, and understandings to the degree they can be demonstrated.

3. *Performance indicator*—a description of a student behavior which takes place within a prescribed setting (when a student is able to perform in certain specified ways the teacher may assume that the student has reached the desired competency).

The WOW Health Education Curriculum Guide

The WOW Health Education Curriculum Guide[18] is an excellent example of a competency-based curriculum. The guide identifies four content areas: mental health, physical health, safety, and community health. Although at the time of printing this text, we are uncertain as to the adoption of this guide, we liked many of the ideas.

Competencies are developed for primary, intermediate, junior high, and senior high school instruction. A decision-making model is used, in which knowledge is combined with the exploration of attitudes, beliefs, and values. Specific ideas and directions for these competencies are identified.

One of the significant facts about the WOW Guide (and unique) is that it was developed by teachers in Washington, Oregon, and Wisconsin. In addition, the directions and suggestions were field tested.

The Unit Approach to Curriculum

Another approach to health education curriculum involves the unit approach. In this approach health is considered in terms of several units or areas. Once these units have been identified, a time allotment is assigned. Often, the same time allotment is used for each unit. Thus, areas are grouped together to become units with approximately equal value to the curriculum.

The unit approach is traditional and has features which render it easy to use. This approach facilitates organizing the school year into blocks of time. The unit approach can be easily combined with a textbook approach. Units can be ordered to fit the sequence and philosophy of a text.

In addition, the unit approach is flexible enough to meet teacher needs. Since all of the units usually have the same weight they can be ordered and used at a time of the year that is most convenient for the teacher. If a teacher is very busy when school begins, the unit that he or she is most familiar with can be used.

The unit approach is readily combined with a competency-based approach, a life style approach, a conceptual approach, etc.

The Theme Approach to Curriculum

The theme approach to curriculum design utilizes a central idea or philosophy to give perspective to the development of health instruction.[19]

One of the important health educators in theme development has been Howard Hoyman, Professor Emeritus at the University of Illinois. Some of the themes[20] that Dr. Hoyman was described:

Human life cycle approach—This relates health behavior to the major transitional stages: prenatal, infancy, childhood, adolescence, early adulthood, middle age, old age, senility, impending death.

Personality-lifestyle approach—This approach studies the lifestyle and personality of youth related to: drug abuse, drinking, accidental injury, death, premarital sex, venereal disease, abortion, environmental pollution, suicide, obesity, violence and crime, psychosomatic stress, and disease.

Human potentialities approach—This enables the student to examine the full range of health: optimal health, minor disease, major illness, critical illness, impending death, and death.

Ethical approach—This focuses on students learning to make value judgements without the influence of parents and peers.

Ecological approach—This approach plans health instruction from an ecological perspective, including the evolution of ecology of man as a unified organism in the earth's ecosystem.

Preventive-constructive approach—This approach emphasizes the preventative aspects of health care such as the value of periodic medical examinations, the dangers of quackery and self diagnosis, and personal health care.

Community experience approach—This is based on the saying "It is better to see once than to hear a hundred times over." Field experience is the principal source of learning.

Another example of a theme approach is The Risk-Taking Curriculum[21] developed by Janet Shirreffs. Her curriculum integrated subject matter with a focus on behavior that threatens the well being and or life of the individual.

Chapter Summary

In summary, a curriculum is an orderly plan for implementing health instruction that includes a framework for health instruction to meet the needs of the learner, to convey subject matter in a meaningful way, and to evaluate the effects of instruction. A curriculum serves to pose a series of questions and to identify probable alternative solutions.

To develop curricula, a project co-ordinator, a health education advisory council, and a health education curriculum committee is needed. The project co-ordinator co-ordinates efforts. The health education advisory council provides resources from the community, provides increased understanding and appreciation, and secures support for the conduct and growth of the program.

The health education curriculum committee is responsible for supervising the development of all aspects of the curriculum. There are many possible alternatives available from which to evaluate and select the best possible learning situations for a given locality. A brief summary of these approaches:

1. *The life style approach* involves three steps: (1) Identifying the alternatives in life style, (2) Evaluating these alternatives (or reevaluating in the case of old habits), (3) Intelligent selection of personal alternatives (or change in life style in the case of old habits).

2. *The conceptual approach* stresses key concepts as basic or central ideas around which the curriculum is designed. The School Health Education Study is a well known conceptual approach to curriculum design.

3. *The body systems approach* focuses on units of study by body system. The School Health Curriculum Project is an example of the body systems approach.

4. *The competency based approach* specifies minimum performance levels for students to complete. The WOW Guide is an example of competency based education.

5. *The unit approach* breaks down health instruction into equal time allotments for grouped areas of study. The unit approach is compatible with the organizations of many health books.

6. *The theme approach* selects a central idea or philosophy to give perspective to the development of health instruction.

Notes

1. John Goodlad. *School Curriculum and the Individual.* (New York: Blaisdell Publishing Company, 1967).
2. J. Keogh Rash and R. Morgan Pigg. *The Health Education Curriculum: A Guide for Curriculum Development in Health Education.* (New York: John Wiley and Sons, 1979), pages 88–9.
3. *Ibid.* 89–90.
4. *Ibid.* 90–91.
5. *Ibid.* 91.
6. *Ibid.* 92.
7. John Burt, Linda Meeks, Sharon Pottebaum. *Toward A Healthy Lifestyle Through Health Education in the Elementary School.* (Belmont, California: Wadsworth Publishing Company, 1980). pg. 10–12.
8. *Ibid.* pg. 14.
9. *Ibid.* pg. 12–17.
10. School Health Education Study. *Health Education: A Conceptual Approach to Curriculum Design.* (St. Paul, Minnesota: 3M Education Press, 1967), page 15.

11. *Ibid.* 15.

12. *Ibid.* 20.

13. The State Education Department, *Suggested Guidelines for the Development of Courses of Study in Health Education for Junior and Senior High Schools.* (Albany, New York: The State Education Department, 1970).

14. State of California, *Health Instruction Framework for California Public Schools.* (Sacramento: The California State Board of Education, 1970).

15. Pennsylvania Department of Education. *Conceptual Guidelines for School Health Programs in Pennsylvania.* (Harrisburg: Pennsylvania, Department of Education, 1970).

16. Phil Heit, "The Berkeley Model," *Health Education.* Vol. 8, No. 1, January-February, 1977, page 2.

17. Robert E. Kime, Richard G. Schlaadt, and Leonard E. Tritsch. *Health Instruction: An Action Approach.* (Englewood Cliffs, New Jersey: Prentice Hall, 1977), pg. 82.

18. *WOW Health Education Guide* (Salem, Oregon: Oregon State Department of Education; Olympia, Washington: Washington State Department of Public Instruction; Madison, Wisconsin: Wisconsin State Department of Public Instruction, 1975).

19. John Burt, Linda Meeks, and Sharon Pottebaum. *Toward A Healthy Lifestyle Through Health Education in the Elementary School.* (Belmont, California: Wadsworth Publishing Company, 1979).

20. Howard S. Hoyman, Ed. D. "New Frontiers in Health Education," *The Journal of School Health.* Vol. XLIII, September, 1973, No. 7.

21. Janet Shirreffs, "A Risk-Taking Curriculum," *School Health Review.* July/August, 1973.

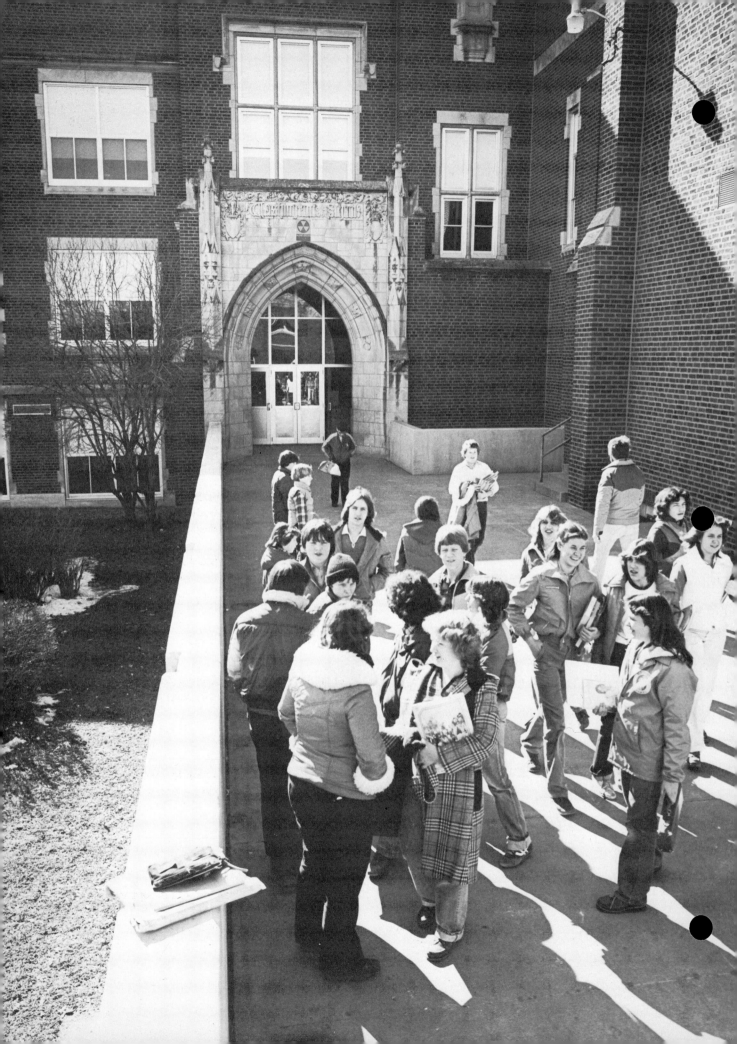

6

Health Instruction
Implementing the Curriculum

An Organized Plan to Implement the Curriculum

Lack of focus, direction, and planning in implementing the curriculum jeopardizes our efforts to establish effective instruction in the middle and secondary school. It can be said that "Planning without action is futile, and action without planning is fatal."[1]

Thus, after our curriculum is developed an organized plan is needed to provide effective instruction.

The next step is the development of lesson plans that carry out the intent of the curriculum. A lesson plan is an individualized format used by the teacher to state clearly how his or her health education classes will be conducted.

The health education lesson plan is individualized in at least two important ways:

1. The lesson plan takes into account the individual needs, interests, and abilities of the students.

2. The lesson plan is designed with the goals, needs, and style of the individual teacher.

The teacher who designs lesson plans for effective classroom instruction, answers the following questions *before* health instruction takes place:

1. Where am I going?
2. How will I get there?
3. How will I know that I have arrived?

The teacher who has thought out the answers to these questions has established direction and purpose. A systematized approach to managing classroom instruction exists.

Lesson Plan Format

A lesson plan should contain each of the following:

1. Unit title
2. Topic
3. Objectives
4. Sources
5. Content and Procedures
6. Materials
7. Evaluation

Each of these seven aspects of a carefully designed lesson plan will be discussed in detail below. These seven aspects are also utilized in Section 2 of this text, Creative Lessons for Teaching Health Science in Middle and Secondary Schools.

The Unit Title

The selection of a curriculum model will assist the teacher in identifying the major units to be considered during the school year. We have identified the following units for the middle and secondary school:

1. Mental Health and Self Concept
2. The Human Body
3. Cardiovascular Fitness and Health
4. Nutrition and Weight Control
5. Drugs: Use and Abuse
6. Tobacco and Health
7. Diseases and Disorders
8. Communicable Diseases
9. First Aid and Safety
10. Human Sexuality and Family Life
11. Consumer Health and Medical Care
12. Environment
13. Aging, Dying, and Death

The Topic

After the selection of a curriculum and the designation of units, the teacher selects the most appropriate topics to be covered in the middle and secondary schools.

The selection of vital topics in a given area is very important. With the limitations on time for health instruction in the middle and secondary school, it is usually necessary to spend time on vital issues only.

There are two pitfalls experienced by teachers who do not establish priorities among topics for each unit:

1. They try to cover too much, and the learning experience lacks focus.

2. They run out of time, and several important units are still not covered by the time the school year ends.

There are different ways to go about selecting the most important topics. Our method of topic selection might work well for you.

We made a comprehensive list of curriculum areas and gave the list to the following groups associated with secondary schools:

1. principals and assistant principals
2. health education teachers
3. teachers of other subject areas
4. counselors
5. school nurses
6. parents of students in the school
7. students

We asked each group to identify what they considered to be the most important topics in each curriculum area. The results of this survey, are found in Table 6–1.[2] A careful look at the topics identified and the discrepancies between the two groups will show the importance of assessing needs when developing health education lessons.

Table 6.1

Students' and Teachers', School Administrators' and Parents' Priorities of Areas of Importance Within Secondary School Health Curriculum Topics

Topics	Students N = 1,673	Number of Times Selected	Teachers, Administrators, Parents N = 479	Number of Times Selected
1) Mental Health	1. causes of emotional problems	1,253	1. developing a healthy self-concept	387
	2. care and treatment of emotional problems	997	2. interpersonal and family relationships	362
	3. developing a healthy self concept	956	3. stress	301
	4. suicide	844	4. care and treatment of emotional problems	297
	5. peer pressure	787	5. peer pressure	270
2) Body Systems	1. circulatory system	1,483	1. circulatory system	452
	2. nervous system	1,368	2. nervous system	440
	3. respiratory system	1,352	3. reproductive system	411
	4. muscular-skeletal system	1,073	4. respiratory system	408
	5. digestive system	976	5. digestive system	399
3) Fitness and Health	1. the best exercises for health improvement and maintenance	1,428	1. the best exercises for health improvement and maintenance	429
	2. effects of jogging on health	1,179	2. exercise and weight control	425
	3. how to stay in shape	1,034	3. how to stay in shape	414
	4. exercise and weight control	983	4. effects of jogging on health	379
	5. reasons for exercise	955	5. fitness facilities	314
4) Nutrition and Weight Control	1. what constitutes a balanced meal	1,314	1. facts and fallacies of diets	455
	2. facts and fallacies of diets	1,308	2. what constitutes a balanced meal	426
	3. how to deal with the psychological and physiological aspects of overweight	1,241	3. how to deal with the psychological and physiological aspects of overweight	411
	4. how to deal with the psychological and physiological aspects of underweight	1,073	4. junk food	390
	5. junk food	904	5. vitamins	236
5) Drug Use and Abuse	1. marihuana	,260	1. decision-making and drugs	396
	2. psychological and physiological effects of drugs	1,258	2. reasons for drug use	350
	3. reasons for drug use	1,176	3. treatment for drug abuse	341
	4. the "positives" of drugs	1,077	4. alcohol	338
	5. alcohol	943	5. psychological and physiological effects of drugs	319
6) Tobacco and Health	1. physiological effects of smoking	1,521	1. physiological effects of smoking	463
	2. smoking-related diseases	1,430	2. smoking-related diseases	448
	3. reasons for smoking	1,164	3. how to stop smoking	412
	4. how to stop smoking	1,139	4. reasons for smoking	396
	5. effects of smoking on nonsmokers	949	5. decision-making and smoking	362
7) Communicable Diseases	1. types and signs and symptoms of diseases	1,574	1. venereal diseases	428
	2. venereal diseases	1,251	2. physiological effects of diseases	415
	3. physiological effects of diseases	1,121	3. treatment and prevention of disease	409
	4. treatment and prevention of diseases	1,063	4. types and signs and symptoms of diseases	405
	5. causes of diseases	1,002	5. the role of the health care system in disease control	321
8) Noncommunicable Diseases	1. types and signs and symptoms of diseases	1,396	1. physiological effects of diseases	407
	2. cancer/leukemia	1,117	2. treatment and prevention of diseases	393
	3. physiological effects of diseases	1,108	3. types and signs and symptoms of diseases	360
	4. causes of diseases	1,033	4. cancer	357
	5. treatment and prevention of diseases	995	5. causes of diseases	351

Table 6.1—*Continued*

Topics	Students N = 1,673		Number of Times Selected	Teachers, Administrators, Parents N = 479	Number of Times Selected
9) *First Aid and Safety*	1. accident prevention		1,132	1. CPR	380
	2. CPR		1,081	2. accident prevention	350
	3. first aid for bleeding		983	3. automobile safety	337
	4. first aid for fractures		975	4. first aid for bleeding	326
	5. first aid for heart attacks		968	5. first aid for fractures	309
10) *Human Sexuality*	1. birth control		1,373	1. venereal diseases	459
	2. venereal diseases		1,266	2. anatomy	455
	3. dating		1,142	3. dating	372
	4. childbirth		1,136	4. decision-making skills	321
	5. anatomy		992	5. birth control	320
11) *Consumer Health and Medical Care*	1. community health care services		1,079	1. health insurance	391
	2. how to select a doctor		1,055	2. consumer rights	377
	3. consumer rights		921	3. community health care services	372
	4. consumer product safety		817	4. quackery	366
	5. health care costs		815	5. OTC and prescription drugs	341
12) *Environment (Ecology)*	1. air pollution		1,442	1. air pollution	449
	2. pesticides		1,324	2. water pollution	434
	3. water pollution		1,303	3. energy	384
	4. energy		947	4. pesticides	370
	5. how to maintain a clean environment		934	5. how to maintain a clean environment	368
13) *Aging, Death and Dying*	1. how to deal with a dying friend or relative		1,479	1. how to deal with a dying friend or relative	446
	2. causes of death		1,398	2. psychological and physiological changes occurring with aging	430
	3. physiological and psychological changes occurring with aging		1,284	3. dealing with grief	429
	4. preparing for ones own death		1,245	4. preparing for ones own death	418
	5. funeral arrangements		1,128	5. preparing for old age	402

Behavioral Objectives

After an important topic is identified, the teacher constructs behavioral objectives which describe the desired outcomes to be expected at the completion of the lesson plan.

Rules for Constructing Objectives

There are four important rules to remember when constructing behavioral objectives.[3]

The first rule states that behavioral objectives are expressed in terms of student behavior. It would be correct to say "The student will be able to" while it would be incorrect to say "This lesson describes" or "The teacher will."

The second rule states that behavioral objectives specify the kind of behavior that will be accepted as evidence that the learner has achieved the objective. Some words which specify evidence of student behavior are to list, to compare, to identify, to differentiate, to solve, to write, and to recite. Words which are incorrect because there is no evidence of behavior are to know, to have faith in, to believe, to really understand, to understand, and to appreciate.

The third rule states that behavioral objectives describe the important conditions under which the behavior will be expected to occur. Some examples of conditions are:

With his textbook open . . .
After seeing the film . . .
Using a model of the heart . . .
Given a fifty minute time period . . .

The fourth rule states that behavioral objectives specify the criteria of acceptable performance by describing how well the learner must perform to be considered acceptable. Thus, the objective "The student will write an essay on the danger signals of heart disease," would not be an example of an objective with an acceptable criteria. Correctly stated the objective would read "The student will write an essay on heart disease which includes at least two danger signals."

Examine the following objective to see if all four rules for constructing objectives are satisfied: The student will be able to identify in writing the correct food group for at least 90 out of 100 foods appearing on a grocery list.

1. Is the preceeding objective stated in terms of student behavior? (The student will . . .)

2. Is a measurable behavior identified by name? (identify in writing)

3. Are conditions stated? (foods appearing on a grocery list)

4. Is a criteria of acceptable performance identified? (90 out of 100)

The four rules are satisfied so that we know this objective is correctly written.

Categories of Behavior

In addition to correctly constructing behavioral objectives, the teacher needs to differentiate between desirable student behaviors. Student behaviors can generally be described as thinking behavior, feeling or attitudinal behavior, or action behavior.

These three different categories of behavior make it necessary to classify objectives into three domains: the Cognitive Domain, the Affective Domain, and the Psychomotor Domain.

The Cognitive Domain
The Cognitive Domain is a category dealing with thinking behavior. Objectives in the Cognitive Domain emphasize learning and problem solving tasks. Cognitive objectives are divided into six classifications:[4]

1. Knowledge objectives which require students to reproduce or recall something that they have experienced previously in the same or similar form.

2. Comprehension objectives require students to reproduce or recall something previously experienced in a new form.

3. Application objectives require students to use previously experienced procedures or knowledge in new situations.

4. Analysis objectives require students to break down into its component elements something which they have not broken down previously.

5. Synthesis objectives require students to put something together which they have not put together previously.

6. Evaluation objectives require students to render judgements regarding something for which they have not rendered judgement previously.

The Affective Domain

The Affective Domain is a category of behavior dealing with feelings and attitudes. The objectives in the Affective Domain contain behaviors which have emotional overtones and encompass likes and dislikes, attitudes, values, and beliefs. Affective objectives are divided into five classifications[5]:

1. Receiving objectives require students to recognize and receive certain phenomenon and stimuli.

2. Responding objectives require students to demonstrate a wide variety of reactions to stimuli.

3. Valuing objectives require students to display a behavior with sufficient consistency.

4. Organization objectives require students to organize values into a system, determine the interrelationship among them, and establish dominant and pervasive ones.

5. Characterization by a value or value complex objectives requires students to act consistently in accordance with the values they have internalized at this level.

The Psychomotor Domain

The Psychomotor Domain deals with action behavior. The objectives in the Psychomotor Domain emphasize some muscular or motor skill, some manipulation of materials and objects, or some act which requires neuromuscular coordination. Psychomotor Objectives are divided into four classifications[6]:

1. Gross bodily movement objectives which require students to move entire limbs.

2. Finely coordinated movements which require students to coordinate movements of the extremities, usually with the eye and ear.

3. Nonverbal communication objectives require students to convey a message to a receiver without the use of words.

4. Speech objectives require students to communicate through speech, such as public speaking.

In a classroom designed to promote the selection of healthy behavior, each type of behavior is important. Thus, when constructing behavioral objectives careful attention should be centered on including objectives that measure thinking, feeling, and acting.

Sources

Thus far the teacher has: (1) selected a curriculum, (2) identified pertinent topics to be covered, and (3) constructed behavioral objectives which describe desirable student performance at the completion of the lesson.

It is now essential to obtain and examine appropriate sources of information relative to the topic and to the behavioral objectives constructed. Select a variety of sources and obtain information that is as current as possible. Identify the sources that you plan to utilize in detailed bibliographical form such as the following example:

Meeks, Linda Brower and John Burt. *Education for Sexuality: Concepts and Programs for Teaching.* (Philadelphia: W.B. Saunders Company), 1975.

A list of the names of names and addresses of appropriate health resources can be found in Chapter 9.

Content and Procedures

The teacher examines reliable sources to find the content to which to expose the students to so that they can achieve the behavioral objectives. There are five cardinal rules in the collection and arrangement of content:

1. The material should be organized in detailed outline form.

2. It should contain appropriate information to achieve the behavioral objectives.

3. The outline should avoid information which is unnecessary.

4. The content should be appropriate for the designated grade level.

5. When material in the outline is quoted directly from a source, that source to be clearly identified.

There are numerous styles for outlining content. We have used a specific style in the lesson plans found in chapters 11 to 23. You will notice that the detailed content outline contains sufficient information to reach the objectives, avoids unnecessary information, is appropriate for the grade level, and the source of information is clearly marked.

Interspersed among the provisions of the content outline are procedural directions explaining how the content will be covered. For example, you might want to discuss the seven danger signals of cancer in your lesson on cancer. Rather than reciting them orally to the class, you might select a film from The American Cancer Society which shows the seven danger signals.

You would still list the seven danger signals in your content outline but you would indicate in your procedural directions that the method of conveying this information would be to use a film. You would state the name of the film and the length of the film, as well as a brief summary of the contents.

Thus, by procedures we mean methods. Methods of instruction are crucial in a classroom which focuses on healthy behavior development. The methods should be varied, in order to stimulate and motivate the student to positive health behavior.

The methods which can be employed to this end are innumerable, and careful examination of each is of utmost importance. Chapter 8 will focus on identifying numerous methods that could be utilized with the different content areas.

Materials

There are many materials that can enhance health instruction in the classroom. These materials are available upon request from different voluntary and official or commercial agencies; they can be made by the teacher or by the student.

Once again using the example of a unit on cancer, you might want to show the students how much tar collects in the lungs when cigarettes are smoked. You might borrow a smoking machine from your local Cancer Society.

In Chapter 9 we have presented a list of the names and addresses where health education materials can be obtained.

Evaluation is the means by which we assess whether or not we have reached the desired behavior that we stated at the beginning prior to the lesson.

Exactly what behavior do we want to measure? With regard to the lesson plan, we will want the teacher to evaluate the performance of each student in terms of the designated behavioral objectives.

We will want each student to examine his or her own performance. Thus, student self evaluation is important.

In addition to student self-evaluation, students can also benefit by evaluating other students. Although student evaluation of other students should be designed with care by the teacher, it is highly beneficial.

The teacher will also want to evaluate his or her own performance. The teacher should evaluate himself/herself, allow student evaluation, and be evaluated at intervals by peers.

There are at least six types of evaluation utilized in the classroom to examine the effectiveness of instruction:

1. Students by the teacher.
2. Students by other students.
3. Student self-evaluation.
4. Teacher by students.
5. Teacher by peers (other teachers, administrators).
6. Teacher self-evaluation.

The following chapter will examine evaluation in greater depth.

Chapter Summary

We have just completed a discussion focusing on implementing the curriculum through the development of lesson plans which clearly state how the health education class will be conducted. A lesson plan which answers the questions "Where am I going?" "How will I get there?" and "How will I know that I've arrived?" includes the following:

1. A *unit title* determined from the curriculum selected.

2. A *topic* which is vital to the needs of the students.

3. *Behavioral objectives* which measure thinking (cognitive), feeling and attitudinal (affective), and action (psychomotor) behaviors.

4. A variety of appropriate and current *sources,* identified in detailed bibliographical form.

5. A detailed *outline of content* needed to achieve the objectives, interspersed with *procedural directions (methods)* which explain how the content will be covered.

6. A description of the *materials* needed to implement the lesson.

7. *Evaluation* techniques to determine the effectiveness of classroom instruction.

Notes

1. Mary E. Hawthorne and J. Warren Perry, *Community Colleges and Primary Health Care: SAHE Report* (Washington D.C.: American Association of Community and Junior Colleges), 1974, p. v.
2. Phil Heit and Linda Meeks, "A Comparison of Students' and Teachers', School Administrators' and Parents' Perceptions of Major Areas of Importance in the Secondary School Health Education Curriculum," presented at the 52nd Annual Convention of The American School Health Association, October 15, 1978.

3. Robert F. Mager, *Preparing Instructional Objectives* (Belmont, California: Fearon Publishers, 1975 (Second Edition), pg. 21.
4. Robert J. Kibler, Larry L. Barker, and David T. Miles, *Behavioral Objectives and Instruction.* (Boston: Allyn and Bacon, Inc.), 1970, pg. 93–4.
5. Benjamin S. Bloom et. al., *Taxonomy of Educational Objectives—The Classification of Educational Goals, Handbook II: Affective Domain.* (New York: David McKay Company, Inc., 1956).
6. Kibler. *Behavioral Objectives,* p. 68–74.

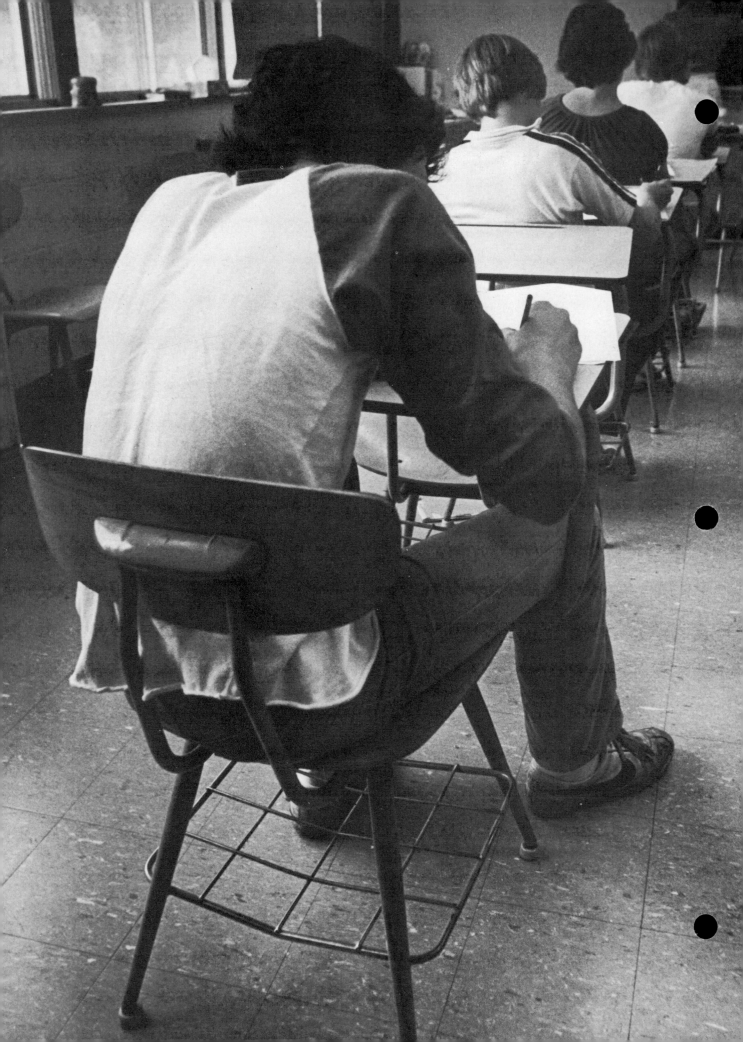

Evaluating Health Instruction

Evaluation is perhaps one of the least emphasized areas in health instruction. Most classroom teachers believe paper and pencil tests are all that is needed to ascertain student achievement. A situation which occurred recently, can shed some light on the concern school administrators and communities have in the area of accountability. The following is a description of the interaction between a principal and a recent health education graduate who was responding to an advertisement for a health education position opening:

> Principal: Mr. Smith, I see you are interested in the health education position we have open in our school.
>
> Mr. Smith: Yes I am. I was just graduated from Southeastern Northern State University with a B.S. in Health Education and I am anxious to share my knowledge of health along with the teaching skills that were provided me by my professors.
>
> Principal: Well, Mr. Smith. I have had full-time health educators in my high school for the past ten years. During that time period, I have seen an increase in the number of students who begin to smoke cigarettes, an increase in the number of young girls who become pregnant out-of-wedlock, an increase in the number of youngsters who become alcoholics and an increase in the number of young people who attempt and commit suicide, to name a few. With these facts in mind, why should I hire you? Are health educators making a positive impact upon influencing health behavior? Could I not use the position for a reading specialist so that I can appease the community when they complain about poor reading scores?

As expected, our young health educator was placed in a difficult position. In an age of accountability, parents, administrators and *students* are demanding results. As has begun to happen today and will occur increasingly in the near future, students are suing teachers for incompetence. With increasing costs and stabilized budgets, decisions must be made concerning discriminate expenditures of funds. Health education as a profession must begin to demonstrate its qualitative and quantitative worth. Now more than ever before, the secondary school teacher must begin to objectify the results of his classroom endeavors. The purpose of this chapter is to examine the components of evaluation and place them in perspective as they relate to middle and secondary school health education programs.

Photo by Allen Ruid

What Is Evaluation?

Evaluation in health education is a process whereby health related data are gathered and assigned a worth so that a judgement can be rendered concerning degree of change or maintenance of status.

In a lesson on sexually transmissible diseases the health educator had the following behavioral objective: On an examination, the student will be able to list the ten signs and symptoms of gonorrhea listed in the textbook.

Testing—The teacher gave the class an examination about the signs and symptoms of gonorrhea. Students were required to enumerate the ten signs and symptoms of gonorrhea which were listed in the text.

Measurement—With a maximum score being 100%, the following was the breakdown of scores and grades on the exam for 30 students:

# of students	Score Range	Grade
3	90–100	A
5	80–89	B
15	70–79	C
4	60–69	D
3	below 60	F

Evaluation—According to the interpretation of the teacher's grading standards, few of the students performed in the excellent (A) range. As a result, the objectives were, for the most part, not attained. Several interpretations may be made:

1. The teacher was not effective in communicating material.

2. Students did not study for the exam.

3. The test did not cover the material that students received in lectures and from the textbook.

4. Students did not know what was expected of them.

5. All, a combination, or none of the above may be correct.

In essence, after we collect and collate responses to an instrument (test) and assign a score (measure), we can assess a worth (evaluate).

Purposes of Evaluation

The most common reason for evaluation, at least in the mind of many, is to determine student knowledge. While this may be a necessity, it is not the only purpose.

One of the problems facing health education is the lack of research which indicates the long term effect of health instruction. The literature is replete with statements concerning the need to evaluate the outcomes of health education.[1-6] While numerous studies have been conducted which indicate behavior and attitude change before taking a course and immediately after, the need exists for follow-up one, two and three and more years later. It is reasonable to expect that if one is given a treatment, immediate effects should take place, especially in the cognitive domain. We need fewer "The cognitive effects of . . . on eighth grade students" studies and more "The long term effects of . . . on health behavior" studies.

Assessing Knowledge, Attitudes, and Practices in the Learner

Teachers need to ascertain changes in students' knowledge about health-related topics as well as changes related to attitudes and practices, so that they can determine whether or not sound health education is taking place.

Hopefully, if the health educator can influence positive attitudes, the appropriate behavior will result. The ultimate goals of health education are to promote the maintenance of healthy behaviors and to alter the patterns of unhealthy life style selections.

Determining Teacher and Program Strengths and Weaknesses

In addition to using evaluation to arrive at a grade for students, the teacher can assess his own strengths and weaknesses as well as the strengths and weaknesses of the health education curriculum. Evaluation also indicates the specific needs of students and health programs based upon these strengths and weaknesses. With proper evaluation, the health teacher and health program can be provided guidance toward greater effectiveness.

What Do We Evaluate?

Assuming the aforementioned goals of health education are valid, our next step is to assess component parts that lead to a successful end product. To evaluate successfully the outcome of health education, we must know what components are integrated in the learning process. Although these components are numerous, we selected those which are of major importance. Without measurable objectives, evaluative endeavors would be an impossibility.

Evaluating Objectives

Thus, Hilda Taba[7] in her book *Curriculum Development: Theory and Practice* succinctly states the following as principles needed in the formulation of objectives:

1. Objectives should describe the kind of behavior expected as well as the content to which that behavior applies.

2. Objectives should be stated specifically enough so that there is no doubt as to the kind of behavior expected or what that behavior applies to.

3. Objectives should state clear distinctions among learning experiences required to attain different behaviors.

4. Objectives should be stated in a developmental nature as opposed to a terminal outcome.

5. Objectives should be realistic.

6. Objectives should be broad enough so as to encompass all types of outcomes.

Evaluating Health Content

Since health education is a discipline whose content is always changing, the health educator must keep informed of the rapid changes in student's behavioral trends. The health problems that existed ten years ago may not be significant to today's middle and secondary school students. For example, if one were to examine the drugs used and abused ten years ago, it would be apparent that many are no longer in vogue—i.e., there has been sharp decreases in the use of LSD, heroin and uppers and downers and an upsurge in the use of PCP and alcohol. Regardless of the health area, one can notice principal shifts in emphases. Therefore, the content incorporated in the health curriculum needs to be continuously assessed. The teacher needs to ask of himself the following questions:

1. Am I maintaining a current knowledge of the popular and professional literature concerning student health problems?

2. Is the content in my lesson plans reviewed for accuracy?

3. Is the proper content presented at the appropriate age?

4. Is the content related to the needs and interests of my students?

5. Are the materials I selected appropriate for the reading skills my students possess?

The teacher who does not frequently review his lesson plans will deny his students the current and future information needed toward the proper guidance of healthy behavior.

Evaluating the Physical and Emotional Setting

The health educator must examine those factors which may have an effect on student learning. A healthful school environment is conducive toward the attainment of teacher and student objectives. Among the questions the health instructor can examine with regard to evaluating the role he plays in the physical environment are:

1. Is my classroom neat, cheerful and large enough to accommodate the number of students in my class?

2. Is the fiscal situation in my school district sound enough so that adequate materials and equipment are at my use?

3. Does my classroom have moveable chairs so I can incorporate the many classroom methodologies necessary for health instruction?

The teacher must also evaluate his role in establishing a sound emotional environment. Specifically he must ascertain:

1. his rapport with students, faculty, administrators, and community;

2. his position as role model for students;

3. his methods of providing feedback to students;

4. his student's perceptions of how he is viewed.

Evaluating School and Community Needs

There is a continual need to evaluate the relative concerns of the school and community. A community may have values indigenous to only that community. For example, one school in a district may have a large number of blacks while another school in that district may have few, if any blacks. While a health education curriculum may have been developed for an entire school district, the fact may remain that sickle cell anemia needs be discussed more thoroughly in the school with the large black population. The health educator must be cognizant of the values of the community and assess the worthiness of these values in the health education curriculum.

In the same respect, the health educator must assess community values to ascertain whether or not he will disagree with community wishes. A sex education unit may evoke outcries of antagonism from a small number of community residents. Does the health educator then include this unit in the curriculum, or does he eliminate it, thereby siding with a small group of dissidents who may not reflect the values? Evaluation of community values can assist the health educator in developing a sound health education program.

Evaluating Evaluation

Every evaluation effort itself needs to be evaluated to ascertain the relative validity and reliability of the strategies employed. Assuming that the outcomes of evaluation attempts will be used to improve health curricula, it is evident that improper evaluative endeavors will lead to invalid recommendations concerning curriculum development and revisions.

Every health educator must understand the evaluation process. He must answer the following questions:

1. Why did I choose to evaluate my efforts?

2. Did the instruments I used succeed in measuring my objectives?

3. Will the results of my evaluation provide me with specific directions?

4. Are the results of my evaluation based upon sound evaluation practices?

5. Was the curriculum based upon theory related to child development and learning?

Who Do We Evaluate?

Any facet of the population that may have a direct or indirect impact on the health and well-being of students should be evaluated. Among those may be students, teachers, school administrators and parents.

Students

The student is the focus for behavior change. The health educator needs to ascertain whether or not:

1. he has made an impact on student health knowledge;

2. he has provided students with the opportunity to examine the health-related attitudes and values of the peer group;

3. changes in student behavior are observable.

Teachers

The teacher needs to ascertain how effective he has been. He must evaluate his knowledge of subject matter, rapport with students, techniques of delivering health information and overall, whether or not he achieves his daily objectives, as well as the objectives of the curriculum at its culmination.

Every teacher knows when he or she is "on" as well as "off." At the end of each lesson, the teacher should ask himself such questions as:

1. What things did I do well in class today?

2. Where could I have changed my lesson so as to facilitate communication between student-to-student and teacher-to-student?

3. What activity, exercise or strategy can I use if I teach this lesson to another class?

4. If my supervisor were observing my lesson, what would he or she have said about my teaching?

The concerned teacher will evaluate daily activities and seek to improve upon shortcomings. Reactions from students and administrators will serve to provide more meaningful classroom experiences, provided the feedback is valid, specific, and constructive.

Administrators

The key toward successful health education programs is the degree of support provided by administrators. An administrator can help make health education an important subject in the academic curriculum or a "rainy day" fill in.

One of the reasons for the success in implementing the School Health Curriculum Project is the prerequisite that teams, consisting of two teachers and an administrator be trained prior to having the program placed in a school.[8] The reasoning behind this requirement is that an administrator will be supportive if he becomes involved and thus understands first hand, the potential value of a program. In essence, the administrator is continually evaluating the content and process of health instruction.

The Proper Time for Evaluation

Evaluation is a process which should take place before a program is implemented, throughout the program, and after the program. Unfortunately, most evaluation efforts continue to take place at the last stage, and at that point, only immediately after the program. What were the existing conditions before the program was implemented? If we showed that students possess a wealth of knowledge, could this not be due to the fact they entered the course with knowledge gained from previous health education experiences? Will this knowledge be retained one or more years after the course? Or more important, will this knowledge effectuate behavior change? If behavior change did occur, was it necessarily due to the health education course?

Questions like these are very difficult to answer. The multiplicity of intervening variables makes it difficult to evaluate the outcomes of health instruction. However, if data can be collected before a program is developed (i.e.—needs assessments), during the program (assessments of knowledge and observations of behavior), and after a program (longitudinal studies that examine health knowledge, attitudes, and behaviors), then assessments of the value of health instruction may be made.

Evaluation Processes

Since the objectives of any health instruction program fall within the cognitive, affective, or psychomotor domain, it is essential that evaluative endeavors should measure change within these areas.

Evaluations of attitudes, practices, and knowledge need to be objectified so as to ascertain program worthiness. The following are some general methods and techniques that may be used to accomplish this task.

Evaluating Health Attitudes and Behaviors

Perhaps the easiest method of ascertaining attitudes and behaviors is through observation, since the middle and secondary school health educator has a familiarity with adolescent health problems. Although this teacher sees his students as little as once per day, he is in a position to observe the effects of his health instruction. Through watching his students during classroom activities such as role play, or by reading homework assignments, like reaction papers, the health instructor can determine behaviors and attitudes. While observation can be a subjective form of evaluating attitudes and behavior, it is the easiest method to employ.

Techniques for Acquiring Feedback about Health Behavior and Activities

Through conferences as well as classroom question and answer periods, the teacher can acquire direct information concerning health behavior and attitudes. If the student is embarrassed to speak during class, the teacher can confer with him individually and thus make judgments.

Self-reporting data can be used to help evaluate student attitudes and behaviors. If topics may appear threatening, the teacher can ask students not to sign their names on any papers submitted. However, the teacher may be able to ascertain the class position relative to significant health topic areas. Instruments such as checklists, attitudinal surveys and questionnaires, both standardized and teacher-made, can provide the instructor with effective information. These types of instruments can provide specific feedback concerning student attitudes and behaviors. This in turn can assist the teacher in quantifying his effectiveness. If conducted in *pre* and *post* stages, the teacher may see clearly the effects of his course and instruction. Unfortunately, most evaluation is often *ex post facto*.

Among the different methods that the teacher can use for evaluating attitudes are Likert-type items and the semantic differential. The following are examples of each:

Likert Scale:

Directions: Please give your reactions to the following statements regarding cigarette smoking. Record your first impression.

Draw a circle around *AA* if you completely agree with the item.

Draw a circle around *A* if you are in partial agreement.

Draw a circle around *N* if you are neutral.

Draw a circle around *D* if you partially disagree.

Draw a circle around *DD* if you totally disagree.

AA A N D DD 1. Smoking in restaurants should be banned.

AA A N D DD 2. The cigarette manufacturers have too much influence in the U.S. government.

AA A N D DD 3. People who smoke cigarettes do not care about their own health.

Semantic Differential:

Directions: In this study, I would like to find out how you describe different things. There are no "right" or "wrong" answers. The rest of this page has pairs of words that you will use to describe your image of the heading at the top of the page. Place a circle around the letter that best indicates the image you have about the heading.

	Cigarette Smoking	
Healthy	A B C D E	Unhealthy
Legal	A B C D E	Illegal
Enjoyable	A B C D E	Unenjoyable
Sophisticated	A B C D E	Unsophisticated

Dull	A B C D E	Exciting
Enjoyable	A B C D E	Unenjoyable
Bad	A B C D E	Good
Informative	A B C D E	Uninformative

Assessing Student Health Knowledge

While great emphasis has been placed recently on the need for bringing the affective domain to light in the health education field, the cognitive may appear to be overshadowed. The authors believe that knowledge is an essential vehicle for creating behavior change and as a result, stress the importance of assessing skills in the cognitive area.

Assessment of student knowledge can take place through the use of teacher-constructed tests—either in the form of short answers (objective) or essay. In developing essay or short answer tests, the teacher needs to examine his course objectives to identify the kinds of behavior that need to be assessed. For example, if a teacher established as one of his objectives, "The student will identify the signs and symptoms of sickle cell anemia," he will need to ask questions that will provide feedback in the cognitive domain.

According to Norman Gronlund,[9] the teacher should keep the following principles in mind when constructing an examination:

1. Test construction must take into account the use to be served by the test.

2. The types of test items used should be determined by the specific outcomes to be measured.

3. Test items should be based on a representative sample of the course content and the specific learning outcomes to be measured.

4. Test items should be of the proper level of difficulty.

5. Test items should be so constructed that extraneous factors do not prevent the pupil from responding.

6. Test items should be so constructed that the pupil obtains the correct answer only if he has attained the desired learning outcome.

7. The test should be so constructed that it contributes to improved teacher-learning practices.

Keeping these principles in mind, we will examine the common types of tests used to evaluate students and provide information on the valid construction of these exams.

Essay Examinations

Essay examinations have several advantages. Among these are:

1. It may be easy to construct since few questions need be asked.

2. It allows students the opportunity to be creative and organizational.

3. It can be used for any topic in health education.

4. It allows the student to apply knowledge.

Disadvantages of essay examinations may be:

1. Difficult to grade.

2. Sometimes difficult to find the proper wording for the question.

3. Possesses low reliability.

4. Promote what is known in student language (and often teacher language) as baloney.

5. Can be time consuming.

Hints in the Construction of Essay Examinations

1. In writing an essay exam, the teacher should be specific.
   item (poor)
   Discuss the marijuana controversy.
   item (somewhat better)
   Do you feel marijuana should be legalized? If a student answered the above question with only a "Yes" or "No" response, the teacher would be hard pressed to fail a student since a response was provided for the question as stated.
   item (good)
   Select a position, pro or con on whether marijuana should be legalized. List and describe five reasons for your position.

2. The teacher should take the exam before giving it to his students. Since time is an important consideration, the teacher can ascertain the reasonable limit with which an exam can be completed.

3. Assign a value (points) to each essay question. This will enable the student to set priorities in allocating time to be spent writing for each question.

Hints for Grading Essay Exams

1. Since one of the shortcomings of essay exams is the subjectivity in grading, the teacher can read through each question and place checkmarks next to each pertinent statement or group of statements. This can assist the teacher in objectifying his scoring.

2. The teacher should read only several papers during a time period. During the reading of essay examinations, especially those requiring many pages of writing, the instructor may begin to grade objectively, but soon the remainder of the papers begin to take on a "middle of the road," monotonous consistency. As a result, all responses as well as grades may appear the same. Short breaks between sets of papers—i.e., every five papers, will minimize this effect.

True-False Examinations

Among the advantages of true-false exams may be:

1. easy to construct, since each question consists of only one statement;

2. graded objectively;

3. easy to score;

4. easy to distinguish right from wrong.

Disadvantages of true-false exams may be:

1. the student has a 50–50 chance at a correct guess;

2. greater chance than essays for developing ambiguous questions;

3. higher thought processes may not be measured;

4. a great deal of time required to prepare the exam.

Hints in the Construction of True-false Examinations

1. Keep away from value judgments in the wording of questions. i.e.—Children under the age of twelve should not drink alcohol.

2. Avoid questions which use the words "always," "never," "all" or "none." Many students know by now that an answer of "false" will most likely be the proper answer to this type of question, since one exception breaks the rule.

3. Avoid double negatives and long and confusing sentences, since often the tasks become one of the student trying to understand sentence structure, as opposed to formulative answer.

4. Do not use sentences with more than one idea (i.e., compound sentences)

Hints for Grading True-false Examinations

1. Use a separate answer sheet, as opposed to having students write on the question paper. Thus exams can be used repeatedly for different classes during different semesters.

2. Avoid having students write "t" for true and "f" for false on their answer sheets since often, the two may be confused. Instead, the student should write a "t" or "T" for a true answer and an "O" for a false answer. Another technique is to have the student *circle* T or F on an answer sheet.

3. The teacher can use a system which can expedite the grading of true-false exams. Figures 6.1 and 6.2 are examples of how true-false responses can be arranged on a 50 item answer sheet. The use of this system permits the teacher to grade each student's paper without the use of a master comparison sheet.

1	O	11	O	21	O	31	O	41	O
2	O	12	O	22	O	32	O	42	O
3	O	13	O	23	O	33	O	43	O
4	O	14	O	24	O	34	O	44	O
5	O	15	O	25	O	35	O	45	O
6	+	16	+	26	+	36	+	46	+
7	+	17	+	27	+	37	+	47	+
8	+	18	+	28	+	38	+	48	+
9	+	19	+	29	+	39	+	49	+
10	+	20	+	30	+	40	+	50	+

Figure 7.1. Example of a systematic answer sheet in which the top-half of all questions on the answer sheet are designed to be false and the bottom-half true.

1	+	11	+	21	+	31	+	41	+
2	O	12	O	22	O	32	O	42	O
3	+	13	+	23	+	33	+	43	+
4	O	14	O	24	O	34	O	44	O
5	+	15	+	25	+	35	+	45	+
6	O	16	O	26	O	36	O	46	O
7	+	17	+	27	+	37	+	47	+
8	O	18	O	28	O	38	O	48	O
9	+	19	+	29	+	39	+	49	+
10	O	20	O	30	O	40	O	50	O

Figure 7.2. Example of a systematized answer sheet in which true and false answers are alternated.

One may be inclined to look at this arrangement and conclude that students will discover a pattern. After exams conducted with hundreds of students, this system has proven reliable. If a test is designed that is valid and reliable, must students will naturally get some answers wrong. When this occurs, the pattern is broken. The rare student who will guess the pattern is required to answer almost all or all the questions correctly.

Multiple Choice Examinations

Advantages of multiple choice exams may be:

1. a lowered chance of guessing correctly, as when compared to true-false exams;
2. ease of grading;
3. adaptability to item analysis, and thus to further refinement;
4. forcing students to critically analyze the implications of several alternatives

Disadvantages may be:

1. time consuming to prepare;
2. more than one answer listed;
3. guessing encouraged;
4. encouragement of rote memorization

Hints in the Construction of Multiple Choice Examinations

1. In the directions, the teacher should state "Select the *best* answer." This may protect the teacher from student complaints which state that "Choice C can also be the correct answer."

2. Make each choice a worthy choice.
   Example (poor)
   Which of the following has a primary, secondary and tertiary stage?
   A. syphilis
   B. gonorrhea
   C. Salt Lake City   (wasted choice)
   D. herpes simplex II

3. Do not make multiple choice examinations a puzzle for the student to complete.
   i.e. (poor)
   Which of the following is a communicable disease?
   A. syphilis
   B. lung cancer
   C. ringworm
   D. the common cold
   E. none of the above
   F. all of the above
   G. choices A and B only
   H. choices A, C and D
   I. choices A, C and E

Use no more or less than four or five choices. More than five becomes too confusing, and fewer than four increases the chances of a correct guess.

Hints for Grading Multiple Choice Examinations

Have students write answers in capital letters. This minimizes errors in interpreting script.

The teacher can also distribute an answer sheet upon which the student can circle the correct choice.

Matching Examinations

Advantages of matching exams are:

1. scoring is easy and reliable;
2. students are required to discriminate in a manner more rigorous than other exams; students guessing is minimized;
3. can be made highly valid for specific health-related topics.

Disadvantages of matching exams are:

1. can be difficult to construct;
2. may take too long a period to complete;
3. answers may be correct or wrong in pairs;
4. may have several answers for one question.

Hints for Constructing Matching Examinations
1. Do not include more than ten nor less than five or six items. Too many choices may lead to confusion and too few items may lead to "correct guessing."
2. The alternatives from which to choose on a matching examination should exceed the number of items by one or two. In this manner, the student cannot automatically match the remaining item if he has but one alternative.

Completion Examinations

A completion test requires the student to add missing information to a sentence fragment.

Advantages of this type of exam are:

1. requires the student to know all aspects of a subject;
2. minimizes the ability to guess correctly;
3. allows the student to organize information;
4. easy for the teacher to prepare.

Disadvantages of completion exams are:

1. several answers may be correct;
2. may be difficult to grade;
3. student is required to select an answer he feels the teacher is seeking even though he may have several alternatives from which to choose;
4. questions may be ambiguous.

Hints for Constructing Completion Examinations
1. Word questions so that only one answer can be correct.
   item (poor)
   Hashish is more potent than marijuana.
   item (good)
   Hashish which is made from the resin of the hemp plant, is more potent than marijuana.

2. Have students write answers on a separate answer sheet. Since completion items may fall any place on the question paper, (the beginning, middle, or end of a sentence) grading can be time consuming. In addition the teacher would have trouble tallying the incorrect answers.

1. When grading short answer exams, place a line through the incorrect answer (example 1) and not through the question number (example 2).

   Example 1   *Example 2*
   1. A   1. A
   2. C   2. C
   3. D   3. D

   In example 2, the student can cross out his original answer (choice C) and substitute the correct answer. This cannot occur in example 1 since the teacher placed a line through the original answer.

2. If an answer is left blank by the student, place a line through the space as well as through the question number.

   Example

   1. A
   2. - - - - -
   3. C

This will prevent the student from filling in the blank when he gets his paper back. Your line through the space indicates an answer was never entered.

Using a Variety of Exams

We do not know what is the best type of exam. Student performances vary, depending on the type of test administered. Therefore, the teacher may wish to use a variety of different tests throughout the semester.

A Word about Cheating

Some students may try to "slide through" a course through illegal maneuvers. If you suspect a student is cheating on an exam, make sure you have *proof* before making an accusation. If you suspect a student is looking at another student's paper, several options may be examined:

1. Make an announcement to the class that you have noticed some people looking at other's papers and the next time action will be taken.

2. Stare at the student, since most cheaters will frequently look at the teacher to see when its "clear" to let the eyes wander. As soon as the student knows you are suspicious, his actions will often cease.

3. Move the students to another seat in the class.

4. Stand next to the student. He will usually know you are "on to" him.

Student Evaluation of Teachers

While much has been said about teacher evaluation of students, by no means should this comprise the entire evaluative process. Often students can enlighten teachers as to the strong and weak points of his instruction as well as the course.

The arguments for and against student evaluation of teachers are multifaceted. The teacher who is insecure may not take kindly to students assessing his abilities. On the other hand, some schools hold student evaluations of teachers as an integral part of the rehiring process—especially in cases of tenure.

As is often the case, an efficient administrator knows whether or not a teacher's performance is up to par. Conversations with and comments from other students enable an administrator to make fairly accurate assessments.

On the other hand, teachers are often rated "good" or "bad" by students based upon criteria such as: "He's a nice guy," "She is good looking," "Mr. Jones is a lousy teacher. He gives difficult exams." "Mrs. Johnson is a great teacher. I got an "A" in her course."

Valid and reliable instruments can assist in developing meaningful evaluations of teacher performances as well as ascertaining whether or not the health education course met student expectations.

Table 6.1 is an example of a modified instrument which is used at The Ohio State University. Called the "Student Evaluation of Teacher" (SET) instrument, students can evaluate their instructor and course strengths and weaknesses in the following categories: I General (the first five questions must be answered), II Course Goals, Objectives and Expectations, III Lectures, Seminars, Sections—Instructor and Course, IV Assignments and Media, V Special (Team Teaching, Guest Lectures, Field Trips, etc.), VI Exams, Grades, Feedback, VII Evaluation of Forms.

Using a Likert Scale (strongly agree, agree, undecided, disagree, strongly disagree) students can respond to questions from each category. These questions are selected by the instructor and consist of approximately 25 items. Included in these items must be the core questions (1–5). For each category, the teacher is free to add statements he feels are applicable to assessing his skills.

Interpretation of SET

The teacher should look at the SET results as only a part of the evaluation process. Depending upon the statements selected as well as those added, the teacher may wish to revise this instrument each semester.

By means of this instrument, not only does the teacher receive feedback about his performance, but the course he teaches is also evaluated in terms of its organization, content, and relevance.

Student Evaluation of Student

While evaluation is usually the sole responsibility of the teacher, student input cannot be ignored. Since health educators are concerned about promoting sharing and interacting in the classroom, it follows that students ought have the opportunity to assess the qualitative and quantitative worth of peer performance.

Student evaluations of students can become a popularity contest. The teacher can minimize this occurrence by providing specific criteria with which students can evaluate each other.

The following is a list of criteria the teacher can provide students for peer evaluation:

1. accuracy of factual material;
2. meaningfulness of responses;
3. creativity;
4. ability to share;
5. dependability;
6. concern toward classmates;
7. amount of preparation for class projects;
8. flexibility toward receiving feedback;
9. ability to think independently;
10. cares about subject.

Each of these items can be stated in sentence form in a unified structure.

To promote honesty in completing evaluations, the teacher can tell his students that all responses will remain confidential.

Checklist

He/she provided
factual material
which was accurate

SA	A	U	D	SD

SA = Strongly Agree
A = Agree
U = Undecided
D = Disagree
SD = Strongly Disagree

Continuum

The accuracy of the
factual material
he/she provided
in class

1	2	3	4	5

worthwhile   not
worthwhile

Agree-Disagree

The factual material
was accurate

Agree	Disagree

Often-Sometimes-Never

The factual material
was accurate

Often	Sometimes	Never

Table 7.1
SET Question List
Student Evaluation of Teacher Form*

For each statement, you are to select the code which best represents your feelings.
Code
SA = Strongly Agree
A = Agree
U = Undecided
D = Disagree
SD = Strongly Disagree

Category I: General (High Inference Level)

core 1. The instructor was well prepared for class.

core 2. The instructor had a thorough knowledge of the subject.

core 3. The instructor communicated his/her subject matter well.

core 4. The instructor stimulated interest in the course subject(s).

core 5. The instructor is one of the best OSU teachers I have known.

6. The overall teaching ability of the instructor was high.

7. I would be pleased to have another course with this instructor.

8. I would recommend this course to other students.

9. I would recommend this instructor to other students.

10. This is one of the better courses I have taken.

11. I learned a great deal from this instructor.

12. I learned more in this course than in most other courses.

13. ---

14. ---

Category II: Course Goals, Objectives, Expectations

15. Course goals or objectives were clearly presented.

16. Important objectives of the course were met.

17. Objectives were helpful in developing understanding.

18. Course objectives helped me to appraise my progress.

Table 7.1—*Continued*

19. Lectures and discussion were relevant to course objectives.
20. Objectives encouraged independent work.
21. Objectives encouraged development of analytic ability.
22. Class size was consistent with course objectives.
23. Class composition was consistent with course objectives.
24. Course content was consistent with prior expectation.
25. Course was accurately described in catalog.
26. Prerequisites provided adequate preparation for this course.
27. ---
28. ---
29. ---

Category III: Lectures, Seminars, Sections
A. Instructor (See also Category I)

30. Presentations were well organized.
31. Instructor spoke clearly and audibly.
32. Instructor's command of English was adequate.
33. Instructor followed course outline closely.
34. Teaching methods used were appropriate for this course.
35. Instructor presented material at an appropriate pace.
36. Instructor presented material at an appropriate level.
37. Presentations were largely free of distracting mannerisms.
38. Instructor seemed interested in course material.
39. Instructor's explanations were clear and concise.
40. Instructor answered questions carefully and clearly.
41. Instructor adequately summarized material to aid retention.
42. Instructor raised stimulating and challenging questions.
43. Instructor stimulated independent thinking.
44. Instructor used good examples and illustrations.
45. Instructor seemed up to date and included recent developments.
46. Instructor emphasized particularly important course material.
47. Instructor discussed topics in sufficient depth.
48. Writing and drawing at board were legible.
49. Instructor encouraged questions/discussion in class.
50. Instructor led class discussion skillfully.
51. Instructor encouraged differing points of view.
52. Instructor helped students to learn from each other.
53. Instructor helped clarify difficult materials.
54. Instructor seemed able to anticipate student problems.
55. Instructor seemed able to recognize student problems.
56. Instructor's relationship with students was good.
57. Instructor motivated me to work effectively.
58. Instructor helped open new areas of knowledge to me.
59. Instructor seemed to treat students impartially.
60. Instructor seemed to respect constructive criticism.
61. Instructor demonstrated importance/significance of course topics.
62. Instructor related course material to practical situations.
63. Instructor distinguished clearly among fact/theory/opinion.
64. Instructor helped apply theory to solve problems.
65. Instructor helped me to read the language.

Table 7.1—*Continued*

66. Instructor helped me to write the language.
67. Instructor helped me to speak the language.
68. Instructor stimulated interest in further courses in area.
69. Instructor effectively held class attention.
70. Instructor provided an effective range of challenges.
71. Instructor seemed able to help many kinds of students.
72. Instructor was sensitive to individual interests and abilities.
73. Instructor was reasonably available for personal help.
74. Instructor's office hours were adequate.
75. Instructor incorporated views of women and minorities.
76. ---
77. ---

Category III: Lectures, Seminars, Sections
B. Course (See also Category I)

78. Separate parts of this course were well integrated.
79. Separate topics of this course were well coordinated.
80. I learned a great deal from this course.
81. Course provided useful factual knowledge.
82. Course helped develop rational thinking.
83. Course helped develop problem-solving ability.
84. Course helped develop skills/techniques/views needed in field.
85. Course broadened student views.
86. Course provided a healthy challenge to former attitudes.
87. Course helped develop creative capacity.
88. Course fostered respect for diverse points of view.
89. Course sensitized students to views or feelings of others.
90. Course helped develop rational decision-making abilities.
91. Course developed appreciation of intellectual activity.
92. Course developed appreciation of cultural activity.
93. Course developed writing ability.
94. Course developed skills in expressing myself.
95. Course helped develop responsibility and self-discipline.
96. Course helped develop effective work habits.
97. Course developed more positive feelings toward this subject.
98. Course developed awareness of process used to gain new knowledge.
99. Knowledge gained in course will be useful in the future.
100. Course developed understanding of concepts and principles.
101. Balance of basic and applied material was appropriate.
102. Background assumed for this course was realistic.
103. Course was important to my academic program.
104. Course contributed significantly to professional growth.
105. Course was up to date.
106. ---
107. ---

Category IV: Assignments and Media

108. Course assignments contributed to my learning.
109. Course assignments were of reasonable length.
110. Course assignments were at an appropriate level.
111. Course assignments were clear.

Table 7.1—*Continued*

112. Number of course assignments was reasonable.
113. Lectures were adequately supplemented by other work.
114. Work required was appropriate for credit given.
115. Work required was appropriate for amount learned.
116. Assignments helped achieve course objectives.
117. Textbook was a good choice for this course.
118. Textbook was clear and readable.
119. Supplemental reading was well chosen.
120. Assigned reading was important for understanding course material.
121. Assigned reading appreciably aided learning in this course.
122. Assigned reading complemented instructor's presentation.
123. Assigned reading was readily available.
124. Assigned reading was interesting and of high quality.
125. Amount of required reading was reasonable.
126. Number of problems was reasonable.
127. Level of difficulty of problems was reasonable.
128. Types of assigned problems were appropriate.
129. Assigned problems were important for understanding material.
130. Assignments involved application of concepts discussed in class.
131. Assignments were largely free of "busy-work".
132. Number and length of assigned papers were reasonable.
133. Suggested or assigned topics of papers were appropriate.
134. Time allowed for papers was reasonable.
135. Handouts were valuable supplements to course.
136. Assignments included useful examples of course concepts.
137. Assignments reinforced course concepts.
138. Group projects were appropriate for this course.
139. Group projects were well organized.
140. Group projects were stimulating.
141. Group projects provided good experience in applying course ideas.
142. Instructor made effective use of visual aids.
143. The models/samples/demonstrations were helpful for learning.
144. Films/filmstrips used in course aided learning.
145. TV was used effectively in this course.
146. Televised portions of course aided learning.
147. Audio and video TV reception was of good quality.
148. Programmed learning modules were well organized.
149. Programmed learning modules aided learning.
150. Instructor corrected racist or sexist bias in assigned materials.

Category V: Special (Team Teaching, Guest Lectures, Field Trips, etc.)
151. Team teaching was appropriate for this course.
152. Course was more effective because of team teaching.
153. Instruction was well coordinated among team teachers.
154. The size of the teaching team was appropriate.
155. The composition of the teaching team was appropriate.
156. Guest speakers were appropriate and effective for this course.
157. There was an appropriate number of guest speakers.
158. Guest speakers communicated effectively.
159. The topics of the guest speakers were appropriate.
160. Field trips were appropriate and effective for this course.

Table 7.1—*Continued*

161. There was an appropriate number of field trips.
162. Field trips were useful supplements to other course work.
163. ---
164. ---
165.

Category VI: Exams, Grades, Feedback

166. Exam questions fairly reflected course content.
167. Exam questions were clear.
168. Exams avoided unnecessary detail.
169. Exams emphasized understanding rather than memorizing.
170. Instructor clearly indicated material to be covered on exams.
171. Exams tested well my learning/understanding of course material.
172. Exams covered a reasonable amount of course material.
173. Sufficient time was allowed for exams.
174. Exams had instructional value.
175. Exams required creative or original thought.
176. Exams required synthesis of course concepts and information.
177. Exams emphasized important or major topics.
178. Exams were of appropriate level of difficulty.
179. Exams seemed carefully prepared.
180. Exams were compatible with course objectives.
181. Exams were graded fairly.
182. Exams were returned promptly.
183. Exams were useful for gauging strengths and weaknesses.
184. An appropriate number of exams was given.
185. Written comments on returned exams were helpful.
186. Written comments on returned assignments were helpful.
187. The grading system was clearly explained.
188. Grading was consistent with stated objectives.
189. The instructor's expectations for good performance were realistic.
190. Mix of concepts and applications on exams was appropriate.
191. Information on my relative standing in class was available.
192. Instructor offered suggestions for improvement.
193. Instructor regularly reviewed exams in class.
194. Instructor regularly reviewed assignments in class.
195. Closed-book exams were appropriate for this course.
196. Open-book exams were appropriate for this course.
197. Take-home exams were appropriate for this course.
198. Quizzes were appropriate for this course.
199. ---
200. ---
201. ---

Category VII: Evaluation of Forms

202. This type of questionnaire is useful for course evaluation.
203. This type of questionnaire is useful for instructor evaluation.
204. These are good questions for evaluation of this course.
205. These are good questions for evaluation of this instructor.
206. This questionnaire is an appropriate length for this course.
207. These items let me evaluate this course fully and fairly.

*This instrument was adapted from The Ohio State University Student Evaluation of Teacher Instrument.

Chapter Summary

In the age of accountability, health educators need to justify their existence. Not only do they need to prove they are performing well in the classroom; they also need to demonstrate to their administrators as well as to the public that they are promoting healthy behavior among students. Due to the number of intervening variables, the latter is almost impossible to determine. Only through sophisticated evaluation endeavors may we be able to prove our worthiness as a profession. Evaluating one aspect, health instruction, is one step in the accountability process.

The purpose of this chapter was to help the prospective teacher examine one aspect of evaluation in health education—instruction. With more refined skills in assessing student health status, health educators will take one step toward responding to the public outcry for accountability. This chapter outlines those classroom evaluation-related skills needed by every health educator. Hopefully these skills will be applied.

Notes

1. Madeline Hurster, "Critical Issues in Health Education," *The Journal of School Health,* 47:1, January, 1977, 42.
2. Darrell Crase and Michael H. Hamrick, "Health Education: A Reexamination of Purpose," *The Journal of School Health,* 47:8, October, 1977, 470–474.
3. John A. Conley and Clarence George Jackson, "Is a Mandated Comprehensive Health Education Program A Guarantee of Successful Health Education?," *The Journal of School Health,* 48:6, June, 1978, 337–340.
4. Marshall W. Kreuter and Lawrence W. Green, "Evaluation of School Health Health Education: Identifying Purpose, Keeping Perspective," *The Journal of School Health,* 48:4, April, 1978, 228–235.
5. John T. Fodor and Gus T. Dalis, *Health Instruction: Theory and Application,* Philadelphia: Lea and Febiger, 1974.
6. Robert E. Kime, Richard G. Schlaadt and Leonard E. Tritsch, *Health Instruction: An Action Approach,* New Jersey: Prentice-Hall Inc., 1977.
7. Hilda Taba, *Curriculum Development: Theory and Practice,* New York: Harcourt, Brace and World, Inc., 1962.
8. Phil Heit, "The Berkeley Model," *Health Education,* January-February, 1977, 1–2.
9. Norman E. Grunlund, *Measurement and Evaluation in Teaching,* New York: Macmillan, 1971, 8.

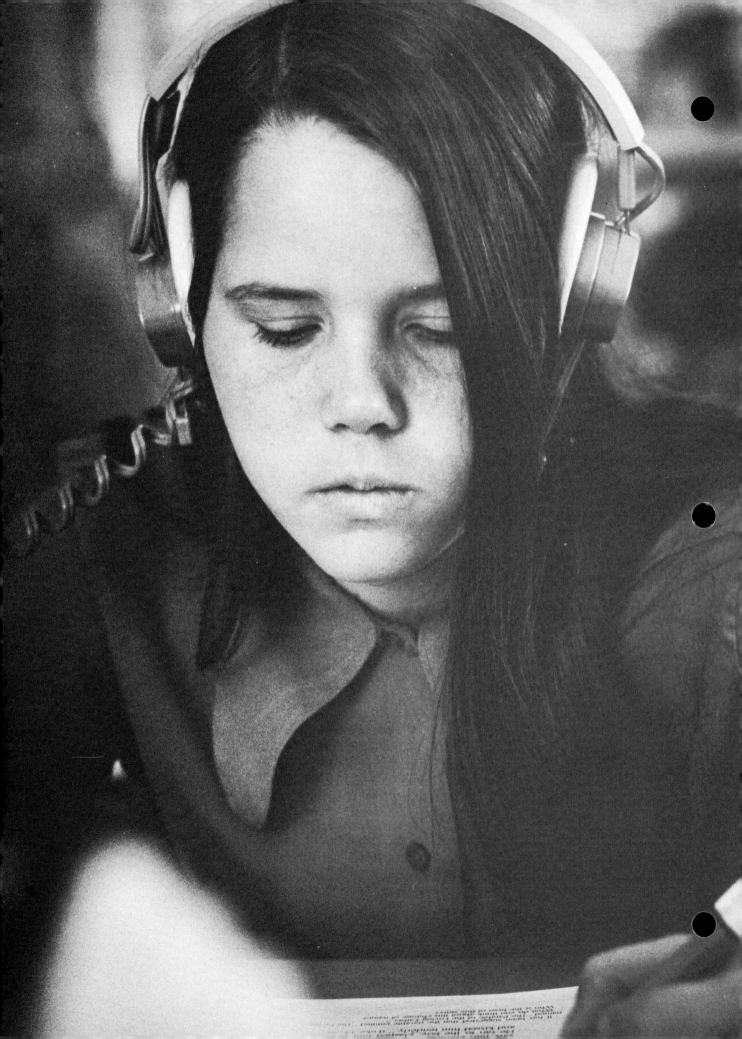

8

Methods of Instruction for
a Creative Classroom

No teacher can teach long with enthusiasm and energy without sensing an intellectual exhaustion unless there is an opportunity for recharging his intellectual vitality.

—Dean Brown, Princeton

The Self-Renewing Teacher

How can we combat the mental staleness which comes from over-familiarity with well-worn subject matter? How can learners be motivated to learn and then communicated with in ways that keep their motivation from dwindling?

Good teachers systematically seek to recharge their intellectual vitality by reading, exchanging ideas, attending seminars and workshops. They recognize the importance of self-renewal and agree with John W. Gardner that "apathy and lowered motivation are the most widely noted characteristics of a civilization on the downward path. Apathetic men (teachers) accomplish nothing. Men (teachers) who believe in nothing change nothing for the better."[1]

The self-renewing teacher explores the full range of his or her potentialities and encourages his or her students to do likewise. Utilizing a wide variety of methods, materials, and media, the teacher aids in developing the student's capacity for sensing, wondering, learning, understanding, loving, and aspiring.

Motivation

Although learning occurs within the individual it is influenced by the teacher and is often considered to be the BASIC purpose of schools. Jack Frymier, in his booklet, *Motivation and Learning in Schools,* defines the ultimate objective of education as helping students learn to "behave according to the best knowledge that is available at any given time."[2] Motivation to learn should aim students in this direction.

Many teachers have a very narrow view of motivation. They may simply view it as "applying incentives and arousing interest for the purpose of causing a student to perform in a desired way." But experts who have studied motivation say it is "related to man's inner impulses and is closely associated with his values. Motivation gives direction and intensity to man's behavior. It significantly affects his abilities and his achievement. . . ."[3]

Thus, self-renewal and motivation are very important in a classroom that deals with healthy life style. After all, we are quite interested in the "direction and intensity" of behavior. One of our primary goals was for each of our students to demonstrate self-direction, self-responsibility, self-control, and self-evaluation.

Methods, Materials, and Media

The teacher assists the student in the development of these skills by creatively using a variety of methods, materials, and media. In a classroom dedicated to the selection of healthy behaviors, we feel that teachers need to understand and utilize the following:

1. Changeable display graphics;
2. Graphic visual materials;
3. Art projects;
4. Common audio-visual materials that require special equipment;
5. Activities requiring writing, thinking, and discussion;
6. Activities involving feelings and values;
7. Games, dramatizations, and simulations;
8. Real things, models, and demonstrations;
9. Community resources.

Let us examine each of these types of methods, materials, and media so that you will be better equipped to make them a regular part of your health education classroom.

Changeable Display Graphics

Changeable display graphics serve a variety of purposes and are among the least expensive instructional resources.

Bulletin Boards

Bulletin boards can be planned and designed by the students; used for instruction and for evaluation. Display single copy materials, jackets from health books, biological specimens, and items of current interest. Materials can be displayed for identification and for comparing and contrasting. Although bulletin boards are usually thought of as horizontal wall space or vertical panels, they may also be supported by an easel.

Buzz Boards

Buzz boards can be easily constructed by the teacher and used by the student for independent review and evaluation. The following design, illustrates one simple construction method:

Purchase the following materials:

1—18″ x 24″ piece of plywood, masonite, or particle board ⅜″ thick
1—6 volt lantern battery with screw terminal
1—6 volt buzzer or bell
20—#8—32 machine screws 1″ long
40—#8 flat washers
40—#8—32 hex nuts
1 radiator hose clamp, large enough to go around the battery
2 telephone plugs
25 feet of 18 AWG stranded wire
Heavy duty staples
Question and answer cards

The procedure: Drill 20 holes on Buzz Board. Insert machine screws from the front, and screw a nut on the back of each screw and tighten it. Loosely add two washers and another nut for each screw. Staple hose clamp to the back of the board (to hold battery). Connect bell to battery and phone plugs. Questions and answers may be connected in various patterns.

Chalkboard Displays

Chalkboards are more than something to scribble on! Not only can lessons be effectively outlined and certain points emphasized, but material can be written on the board ahead of time and then uncovered at the appropriate moment. Use an opaque projector to project original drawings and book illustrations in enlarged form onto the chalkboard. Trace major lines. Pictures from slides and transparencies can also be transferred to the chalkboard. When writing on the chalkboard, keep sentences brief and to the point. Make sure that your writing is legible and can be seen from the back of the room.

Cloth Boards

An old time teaching device that is merely a board covered with material and used to display visuals or tell a story is still in use today. These boards are usually called by the name of materials used in their construction, i.e., "flannel boards," "felt boards," or "velcro (hook and loop) boards."

Flannel boards have the advantage of being inexpensive and easily available. Coarse sandpaper, fuzzy yarns, and flannel attached to pictures that are glued to light-weight cardboard can be gently pressed against the flannel board. The imagination of the teacher often determines how effective this device will be.

Felt boards are more expensive, but felt has the advantage of being durable and available in rich colors. A disadvantage to both flannel and felt boards is that attachment is often minimal. Through manipulation, items will often fall off the boards.

Velcro boards have several advantages. Velcro is the name of a sturdy nylon material that is available in a variety of colors. The surface of Velcro yard goods materials is covered with a very fine, fuzzy-like surface made of tiny nylon hooks; the companion material, used for attaching things to the surface of the board, usually comes in rolls or strips of tape-like cloth which has a surface of coarse, loop-like texture. When the loop material is pressed onto the hook-like surface of the Velcro cloth, the two surfaces stick firmly together with strong holding power and will not let objects change positions until they are firmly pulled away.

Magnetic Boards

Magnetic boards. Some chalkboards have a backing made of steel which will permit magnets to cling to the board. Not only do you retain the value and convenience of the chalkboard, but you have many additional display techniques. Essays, pictures, etc. may be mounted on cardboard that has small magnets either temporarily or permanently attached (use masking tape or glue). The materials can be easily moved, and chalk drawings or lettering can be added when necessary. A variety of commercially available materials for use on magnetic chalkboards (magnetic letters, symbols, arrows, etc.) can be purchased. You may extend the versatility of magnetic boards by mounting flannel or Velcro on the back of portable magnetic chalkboards.

Peg Boards

Peg boards. Excellent display boards can be made by purchasing peg board at lumber or discount stores and using commercial hooks to fasten materials such as plastic body organs, food boxes and cans, or first aid materials to the panel.

Graphic Visual Materials

Graphic visual materials present ideas or concepts which are sometimes difficult to understand if presented in oral or written form.

Cartoons

Cartoons are a major form of graphic communication with the power to capture attention and influence attitudes and behavior. Ask your students to collect cartoons related to some aspect of health and share them with the class. Display the cartoons on a bulletin board—"To Tickle Your Funnybone." Let students draw and label their own health cartoons. In doing this, they are compelled to define ideas and attempt to communicate them accurately.

Charts and Diagrams

The main criticism leveled at wallcharts is that they usually contain far too much information, thereby making them confusing and difficult to read. However, there is something useful about being able to summarize a great deal of material for semi-permanent display. Wallcharts are useful as a reference tool. They may be composed of several different types of graphics—pictures, graphs, diagrams, verbal materials, etc. Consider the purpose of the chart—is it an introductory overview or a summary?

Experience charts describe a group experience. The chart can be made up of one large picture accompanied by a brief narrated story about it. (verbal). Standards of health behavior or health principles may be illustrated. Use words that the students understand.

Graphs can sometimes make material easier to understand. Let students practice making circle, line and bar graphs to illustrate population levels, rise and fall of communicable diseases, amount of sugar in various foods, etc.

Strip charts and flip charts are used to present data in sequence. The strip chart is actually a single chart with sequential parts covered by strips of paper which can be removed to disclose various points during a discussion. Flip charts can be made from several sheets of newsprint or from commercially available 18″ x 24″ all-purpose sketch pads. Place appropriate pictures, cartoons, graphs, or written materials on each page, then turn sheets over as needed.

Commercially prepared charts are usually accurate and well drawn. Anatomy, biology, health and safety education topics are available from dependable, established companies.

Flat Pictures and Photographs

Experienced teachers usually have a file of pictures that are good enough to mount, preserve, and file. The pictures should be interesting, accurate, well reproduced and capable of providing a good basis for discussion.

Ask students to look for contrasts—differences among the people, objects or conditions depicted. Develop the skill of continuity by using two or more pictures, each showing a different stage of development, i.e., growth of a baby.

Pictures can trigger the writing of poems, short stories, and essays. Compile pictures and photographs in scrapbooks—nonalcoholic beverages; families; can you name the body part?

Mount pictures on fairly stiff mounting board, using either rubber cement, liquid adhesive, dry mount tissue and hand iron or press, or between plastic sheet laminations.

Study prints are commercially available in a large number of health related areas, as well as photo study discussion kits.

Posters and Signs

Wall posters and signs usually attempt to convey only a limited piece of information. They are usually attractive, forceful and clear in their message. The colors are bold and vivid to focus attention on their topic, and large enough to be easily seen and understood in a brief glance.

Posters can be made by students and judged. Prize winning posters can be donated to health organizations in the community. Posters may range in content from how to prevent accidents, how to protect your vision, good grooming hints, or proper use of drugs.

Art Projects

Art projects can be used to develop drawing, painting, and lettering skills. They may require observing, imagining and visualizing, as well as psychomotor skills.

Collages

A *collage* is an artistic display where various materials such as paper, cloth, or wood are glued onto a surface. A collage could be made of life styles or of self concept using magazine pictures, and/or real objects.

Construction Activities

Health instruction offers many opportunities for creativity and manipulation of materials.

Building a puppet theater is simple. At the front of the classroom arrange a screen that is large enough to hide all the operators. Use a cardboard box to form the stage itself; make it open to the front and closed on the top and at both sides. It should be at least partially open at the bottom to permit puppets to be moved from underneath. String a curtain across the front, then run pull cords to each side to permit opening and closing from one position. While one group of students is constructing the actual theater, let another group of students paint scenic backgrounds on pieces of paper or cardboard that can be tacked to the stage or quickly shoved into position. Other students may like to construct simple furniture or three dimensional objects like rocks, trees, and safety hazards. Special effects may include background music, tape recorded sounds, and light from a flashlight.

Drawing and Painting

Students can develop their *drawing and painting* skills as they produce displays, bulletin boards and transparencies. Again, a variety can be utilized—pencils, colored chalk, India ink, watercolor paints, finger paints, and felttip pens.

Mobile Construction

A *mobile* can be made of health articles (i.e., comb, toothbrush, toothpaste) or pictures. To make a mobile of pictures, paste the pictures on construction paper and trim off any parts showing around the edges. Cut strings into various lengths. Punch a hole in the top of each picture and tie one of the strings to the picture. Insert one hanger inside the other so that they are at right angles. They can be secured with tape or with rubber bands. Tie the remaining ends of the string to the hangers. The pictures should hang at different lengths. Besides grooming articles, different empty containers of food from the four food groups or prescription and over-the-counter drug containers may be used.

Mosaic Pictures

Mosaic pictures or decorations can be made from small glazed ceramic tiles, soft floor tile, and seeds, as well as from colored glass. The pieces are arranged to form a design. A design made with various macaroni pieces, dried fruits and cereals could be surrounded with pictures illustrating the food habits of people around the world.

Murals

Murals are pictures painted on long sheets of paper and placed at one side of a classroom to illustrate events that happened over a period of time, i.e. development of medicines; landmarks in medical treatment; important people in the health fields, epidemics of major diseases. Usually scale is not strictly followed in illustrated time-line murals, and human figures may be portrayed symbolically rather than realistically.

Puppets

Puppets have been used to entertain and inform people for thousands of years. They are usually divided into five different types:

1. *Glove and finger puppets.* To make this type of puppet, you will need old gloves that have been discarded. Cut off the first and second glove finger. These will be used as the puppet legs and operated with the index and middle fingers. The puppet body can be flat cutouts of figures that are painted and glued to cardboard for extra strength. Cut two holes at the bottom of the figure large enough to slip gloved fingers through for legs.

2. *Hand puppets.* These puppets usually consist of a head and a loose garment or dress that covers the operator's hand. The puppet's head is supported with the index finger and the arms are moved with the thumb and middle finger.

3. *Marionettes* are flexible, jointed puppets operated by strings attached to a crossbar and maneuvered from above the stage. They are usually between 16 and 24 inches in length and considerably more complicated to operate than puppets.

4. *Rod puppets* are cutouts of figures that are usually jointed and have stiff wire or thin wooden sticks attached to the arms, legs, and head so they can be moved.

5. *Shadow puppets* may be easily constructed by cutting various shapes from cardboard or thin wood and attaching handles to the back to permit manipulation. The puppets are seen as moving shadows when they are held close to a rear-lighted white cloth.

Scroll Theaters

A scroll theater is an interesting art project that can be used to simulate television programs, movies, and filmstrips. Materials needed are often in the form of scrap (wooden boxes from the grocery store or simply a cardboard box, or cardboard for the front). Pictures are mounted or drawn on a long, continuous roll of paper, such as butcher paper, and may be arranged like separate frames of a filmstrip or shown as a continuous, interrelated, moving panorama.

Let each student work on individual pictures that help tell a story, then label their particular picture according to the plan of the narrative. The pictures may be taped together or pasted on a continuous roll of paper that is attached to spindles (rods) of the rod theater. By turning the cranks, the pictures will slowly move across a screen which can be illuminated with the light from a slide or filmstrip projector to heighten the dramatic effect. Students can tape record music and sound effects to embellish the presentation. They may want to read or describe the various events as they pass by.

After the production has been completed, the students may want to share it with another class. Video-tape the performance, or display the continuous strip as a mural.

Sculpture

Sculpture is the fine art of forming figures or designs in relief or in the round by carving wood, soap, or wax; modeling clay; twisted wires together; and making molds for casting purposes. Students enjoy carving likenesses of teeth and other objects out of soap, using a blunt knife. Use your imagination to form items out of clay, wax, molds, etc.

Common Audiovisual Materials that Require Special Equipment

Although instructional equipment may not be as easily available as the materials previously mentioned, these resources can make the abstract more concrete, provide indirect learning experiences, and focus class attention on important topics.

Filmstrips

Filmstrips have the advantage of providing a means of presenting information that is inexpensive, convenient, and suitable for effective viewing by groups of almost any size. A filmstrip is useful because it can be stopped at an appropriate time for class discussion. Filmstrips which are purchased are not as expensive as a film. They take up little space and are easily stored.[4]

With the foregoing and other instructional activities, you should help the class develop a readiness for what they are about to view, encourage their participation during the showing, and follow the filmstrip with appropriate activities. Advance previewing on your part will enable you to adapt the filmstrip to your purposes, to make a list of important terms and concepts in the presentation, and to determine student activities to clarify unclear points.

Sound filmstrips are accompanied by records or cassette tapes. They are becoming increasingly popular since they add the dimension of sound; however, problems arise when the filmstrip and recording are not synchronized. The use of automatically synchronized cassette-filmstrip projectors, when available, will provide you with the greatest convenience and dependability.

Motion Picture Films

Sixteen millimeter films are widely available. They can communicate effectively, incorporate special techniques (microphotography, photomicrography, animation, etc.), provide continuity of action (including action that is speeded up, slowed down, and "frozen"). Finally, such films enable us to see events that may never occur in real life. Like filmstrips, they are both convenient and suitable for groups of almost any size.

Health films may be obtained from your school district media resources center, city and state health departments, local mental health agencies, libraries, some universities, industry (i.e., Eli Lilly and Company) commercial associations and your local voluntary health agencies (Cancer, Diabetes, Heart, Red Cross, etc.).

Teachers can use films to impart health information, to change or strengthen attitudes, develop skills (i.e., safety and first aid) to arouse interest, to promote discussion and decision-making, or to summarize a unit. Increased learning results when viewers are told in advance what they are expected to learn from it, view films dealing with complex subject matter a second time, and participate in related learning activities after the film is over. Note taking during film showings is usually not a good idea since it interferes with attention and learning, however, it is sometimes suitable to stop the film occasionally and permit students to ask questions or to clear up misconceptions. Open-ended films may be discussed in small groups after the presentation.

No matter what type of activities your students engage in after the film is viewed, they should also be asked to write down comments and evaluate the films they see. This will help you decide whether or not to use the film in the future.

Trigger Films

A *trigger film* is a short, open-ended film which stimulates and generates discussion. It may simulate a familiar situation and is followed by extensive classroom exchange of views and conclusions. Actions alternative to the situation are discussed. The student thus has the experience to view a situation, consider alternatives, and make a decision. If the student comes upon a similar situation in life, he will already have had some experience in making such a decision.[5]

Guidelines for the evaluation of a trigger film[6]:

1. The film should be short and to the point. It should probably occupy no more than five minutes.

2. The information presented should be limited in amount. It is better to have too little information given than too much.

3. The objective of each film should be clearly delineated in advance, then pursued diligently through classroom discussion. Side issues will detract from the desired outcome.

4. The situations should be realistic in terms of the viewer's frame of reference and likelihood of his encountering similar situations in the future.

5. Points and issues should be presented simply and not belabored.

6. The situations should be open-ended, with many alternative sequels possible. There should be no sermon or moral. Complete stories and closure are to be avoided, as well as situations with obvious or clear cut solutions. The purpose is for the viewer to generate feelings and ideas, to work through them, rather than to discover or arrive at any predetermined answers.

7. The termination point for the film should be the point for optimal triggering of reactions and discussion.

Opaque Projection

Flat, printed, or drawn health pictures that are only available in one book can be successfully shown to both small and large groups if an *opaque projector* is available. Some three-dimensional objects, such as first aid materials can also be projected as part of a game to see whether the student can identify the object and knows how it is used. Since projection by reflected light is much less efficient than by transmitted light (as with filmstrips and slides), the projection must take place in almost total darkness. Do not show objects which may be damaged by heat. The opaque projector is especially convenient when you want to enlarge a picture—simply trace the projected picture on butcher paper, poster-board, or some other material and cut it out, color it, or mount it.

Overhead Projection and Transparencies

The overhead projector is one of the simplest visual communication devices available. It is easy to maintain and use, and can be designed for large-group instruction or for conventional classrooms and smaller groups. Since light is being transmitted through translucent material to a nearby screen, the projected image can be seen in a lighted room.

Many teachers are regular users of overhead projectors because they can completely control their presentation, encourage the participation of every student in the class, disclose ideas in sequence and prepare their materials ahead of time. You can hold student attention by writing, pointing, underlining with color, and using overlays as part of your presentation.

Commercially prepared transparencies range from simple printed materials on clear film to elaborate color presentations with multiple overlays. Transparency masters can be purchased in printed form in packages, in loose-leaf binders, or taken from books, (such as our teaching chapters). With these master sheets, you can prepare transparencies in your own school by using a Thermo-Fax copy machine, a Masterfax unit, or any similar thermographic (heat-process) machine having an infrared light source to expose the film to original material. It takes only a few seconds to produce a transparency ready for projection when you use this method. Depending on the film you select, your image may be black on a clear background, black on any one of a number of colors, or clear lines on a black background.

Transparencies made with the heat process method require that the original drawing be done in India ink, soft lead pencil, or black printing ink, since these marks absorb heat. Drawings done with ball-point pens, colored printing ink, or spirit-duplicator copies, will not be reproduced.

Spirit-duplicator masters that have been used to prepare student handout materials can produce transparencies if a sheet of frosted or matte acetate plastic (with etched side up) is fed into the spirit-duplicator after first running several sheets of paper.

Transparencies can also be made through the diazo or ammonia process; drawing directly on a sheet of clear acetate with colored felt pens or grease pencils; and lifting pictures printed on clay-coated paper to adhesive backed acetate placed on the face of a picture and pressing with a laminating machine. The latter method can only be used with expendable pictures since the process destroys the original.

Transparencies may be colored by using translucent inks, cellophanes and foils, and adhesive-backed films and translucent letters and lines purchased from an art supply house. Colored liquids can be mixed on glass trays to produce psychedelic effects. Movement can be suggested by employing patented Technamation materials to polarize light. When projected, the image from the transparency passes through a rotating "spinner" of polarized glass, and wheels seem to turn and fluids to flow.

Transparent dishes can be placed on the projector stage when you are performing chemical reactions or color-mixing experiments. Colored plastic cutout pieces can be moved around on the stage to tell a story instead of using a felt board.

By adding additional acetate sheets, each containing more information, directly over the base sheet, sequence can be shown. Accurate registration is especially important with such overlays, but the final results are well worth the increased effort. Progressive disclosure is a related technique. Cover your transparency with a piece of paper (temporary use) or hinged pieces of light cardboard (permanent use) and reveal information step-by-step.

Some final hints when teaching with transparencies:

1. Direct attention to details in a diagram by placing a pointer or sharpened pencil directly on the transparency.

2. Add details to transparencies with felt pen or wax-based pencil, before or during projection, but make sure they can be removed—unless you intend for them to be permanent.

3. Create your own overlays to add new material to commercial transparencies.

4. When you use prepared masters, such as the printed materials in the teaching chapters of this book, you can adapt them to the needs of your class in several ways;
   a. Change vocabulary that is too advanced for your students.
   b. Add underlines, arrows, etc. to the master with a soft lead pencil or carbon ink.
   c. Cut up the master to eliminate certain parts, to rearrange the material, or to make two transparencies from one master. If you do not wish to deface the original, use a copying machine to make a paper duplicate and do your editing work on that.

Photography

Photography helps students to understand subjects by making them focus on something and look at familiar objects in new ways. Let students take photographs during field trips and then write a description about what they saw. Develop self worth in your students by taking photographs of each student working on a special project and create a bulletin board display. Assign students to photograph people of various ages during a unit on aging. Use a camera to explore your environment—inner city, rural, suburban . . . show the good things and the bad things. Discuss various forms of pollution. Search out and photograph safety hazards. Document recreational services in your community and forms of physical activity.

Radio Programs

Educational radio is a useful and convenient means of providing learning experiences, especially for remote, isolated schools. One disadvantage to radio use is that many programs are not available when needed, but this can now be remedied by taping the program for later use.

Records and Tapes

Records and prerecorded tapes are available in school media centers (including college and university media centers), from commercial producers, health agencies, government agencies and business organizations. They come in teaching kits and from the National Center for Audio Tapes.

Make a tape recording of sounds heard during a neighborhood walk and ask your students to identify the sounds. Use records or tape record sound effects in conjunction with puppet shows, skits, and other presentations. Let students tape their oral presentations and prepare a simulated radio broadcast concerning a current health topic. A broadcast will involve choosing a topic; writing a script as a class or letting each student write a story outline and combining three or four or the best ones; casting the play and assigning responsibilities for sound effects, musical excerpts, and editing; practicing and revising the script; and making a final tape recording.

Have students listen to problem situations that you have prerecorded, then write down how they would react. Use pre-recorded tapes for individual or group review. Tape record special health documentaries on television, as well as people who speak to your class. Exchange tape recordings with students in other countries.

Television and Videotaping

Television occupies a substantial amount of the free time of both students and adults and consequently exercises significant influence upon all of our lives.

As teachers, our chief purpose here is to briefly discuss recent television developments which promise to improve teaching and learning—both in and out of school. Obviously, the effectiveness of television in education rests upon the quality of programs available and the skills of the teachers who use them.

National Educational Television (NET), which is a national program production organization, provides a major portion of the evening programming seen on public television channels. The National Instructional Television Center (NIT) "seeks to strengthen education by developing, acquiring, or adapting television and related materials for wide use as major learning resources." These two agencies prove that entertainment and education can be combined to teach basic skills and that television programs and have student participation activities built into them.

Teaching through television should only be used after the teacher is thoroughly informed about the content and objectives of the programs; physical arrangements for optimum viewing have been made; and the students are prepared for what they are to see. Learning activities may lead into the televised lesson as well as clarify what the students have learned.

By becoming a discriminating television viewer yourself and discovering the numerous fine programs that are available, you can occasionally suggest home television viewing assignments for your students. These assignments should be optional, since some students may not be able to complete them.

Portable television camera/recorder systems are becoming available in many school systems and present the possibility of valuable classroom television production activities. Video tape recorders are used to tape programs that appear at night and to eliminate dependance upon a fixed schedule of broadcast programming.

Low-cost, portable television camera/tape recorder systems allow teachers to record dissections and other demonstrations from the best point of view and for use at the most convenient time.

Student and instructor performance can be recorded, and later reviewed and evaluated. You may wish to video-tape a speaker who is available to speak with only one of your classes. Details observed on a field trip can be filmed for follow-up class study.

Video-tape recorders have an advantage over motion picture cameras, in that the tape can be erased and rerecorded, thus providing economy and increased freedom to experiment. Since immediate results can be evaluated, interest is maintained.

Besides learning how to operate simple portable television cameras and recorder systems, you may be asked to teach before a television camera. Television teachers are usually selected because they are good teachers, have pleasant voices and good personalities. They are willing to work hard to prepare effective presentations, and easily adapt to the special requirements of television.

Activities Requiring Writing, Thinking, and Discussion

Activities requiring *writing, thinking and discussion* encourage middle and secondary school students to organize their thoughts, define ideas and develop basic communication skills.

Analysis

Analyze, discuss, and evaluate health news clippings.

Brainstorming

The students identify as many solutions as possible to a problem in a given time limit. After each idea is recorded, the students rank the solutions from the most acceptable to the least acceptable.

Computing

The students determine by calculation the solution to various problems such: as if you ate three meals a day plus one snack, and lived exactly 72 years and 20 days, how many meals and snacks would you have eaten? The students may compare costs of toothpaste, toothbrushes, and dental floss, and be asked to compute the cost per use of toothpaste and dental floss.

Current Events Newsletter

The students prepare a newsletter containing information on ten health topics of current interest. The newsletter is mimeographed for students in another classroom. This activity could also be coordinated with another school.

Dear Helper

The students write letters to Dear Helper about specific health concerns—or the teacher can write letters structuring them to include questions for introducing or examining health information. The students research the questions and prepare written answers.

Debates

A debate can be used in which each student or team presents a detailed, well-documented viewpoint on a health issue:

Example: Students should have a smoking room somewhere in the school.

Detective

In the "Detective" activity, one student is appointed to scrutinize a particular health habit. The detective may be given a clever badge. Examples of detective activities include: to see if students select well balanced meals at lunch; to observe eating habits at fast food places after school; to observe the use of seat belts.

Diary of Events

Each student records special events in a diary to learn about himself. A diary of events could contain descriptions of emotions felt during a day, new experiences for a week, and/or physical activities engaged in.

Famous People Notebook

Students can gather bits of health information or habits about famous people to share with the class and be compiled in a notebook.

Example: Who was the first President to wear dentures? What famous people have epilepsy?

Jingles and Poetry Writing

The students write short jingles or poems that discuss various health practices.

Problem Solving

The students use the problem-solving approach discussed in Chapter Two in order to work out problems presented. This approach might be used with an open-ended story or an open-ended film where the students write the ending.

Research and Reporting

The students use books, pamphlets, and magazine articles to research health reports.

Activities Involving Feelings and Values

Activities involving *feelings and values* encourage decision making and are useful when teaching about controversial issues.

Values Clarification

The *values clarification* approach tries to assist young people to answer questions and build their own value system. The focus is on how people come to hold certain beliefs and establish certain behavior patterns.[7]

A person selects the process of choosing, prizing, and acting in order to arrive at a value. Completing all seven of the following criteria is essential in defining a value:[8]

Choosing	1. Freely
	2. From alternatives
	3. After consideration of the consequences of each alternative
Prizing	4. Cherishing, being happy with the choice
	5. Willing to affirm the choice publicly
Acting	6. Doing something with the choice
	7. Acting with a pattern, consistency, and repetition.

To successfully implement the values-clarification approach, the teacher should:[9]

1. Encourage a classroom atmosphere which is conducive to open and honest communication;

2. Provide practical value activities for individuals, small groups, or the class;

3. Allow for mutual respect by permitting the student to say "I pass," whenever he does not wish to participate;

4. Carefully select activities to accomplish a definite purpose;

5. Select activities that will stimulate considerable student involvement and group interaction.

Values clarification does not aim to instill any particular set of values. The goal is to help students utilize the seven processes of valuing in their own lives, to apply the processes to already formed beliefs and behavior patterns and to those still emerging. Students are given options. The evaluation is almost a self evaluation since the process, rather than the product, will be evaluated by the learner.[10]

Belonging to a Club

The student can express a value he holds and publicly affirm it by joining a club designed by the teacher, the class, or a health agency. An example is the "I'll Never Smoke" Club developed by the Franklin County Cancer Society of central Ohio. The student signs a membership card in class and carries the card in a wallet or keeps it in his desk. The club meets occasionally to reaffirm its position.

Brown Bag

The student expresses something about himself by placing an object in a paper sack. The teacher opens the sack and asks the class to give reasons why the item might be valued by someone. After each item has been discussed, have the students claim their items and explain why they cherish it. This activity can be modified to promote discussion of a variety of health topics.

Example: Ask the students to bring one object in a brown bag that typifies their family.

Color the Behavior

The teacher gives the student a list of health behaviors at the completion of a unit. A symbol depicting the unit appears in front of the statement. If the student demonstrates the behavior, he colors the symbol.

Example: After a heart unit:

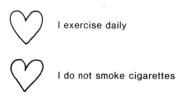

As an alternative, the teacher can draw a face in front of the statement. If the student is proud of his behavior, he draws a smile on the face. If the student is not proud, he draws a frown.

"Happiness" Is

The students complete "happiness" statements to express the attitudes they hold after a unit of study.

1. "Happiness" is using *I* messages.
2. "Happiness" is eating the four basic food groups.
3. "Happiness" is wearing a seat belt.

Happy Faces

Give each student a happy face. Ask him or her to write a few words on the face to describe themselves when he or she is happy. Have all the students turn the faces over and draw a picture of how they feel today. Let them share the faces with each other. Repeat this activity throughout the school year, saving the faces in individual envelopes. How do the faces change? Why?

Hidden Treasure

In this strategy, the students decide what items they would put in a metal box for the next generation or civilization. The items could be health products (toothpaste, syringes, etc.), or health facts printed on index cards. Each student adds one idea to a list. Then the class decides on half of the number of items on the list.

I Learned

"The teacher prepares a chart with the following (or similar) sentence stems. The chart may be posted permanently in the room or it may be posted just when it is to be used. I learned that I . . . I realized that I . . . I relearned that I . . . I was surprised that I . . . I noticed that I . . . I was pleased that I . . . I discovered that I . . . I was displeased that I. . . . Right after a values activity or discussion, the teacher asks the students to think for a minute about themselves or their values. They are to use any of the sentence stems to share with the group one or more of their feelings. Students are not called on, but volunteer to speak whenever they feel comfortable about it."

From Simon, Howe, and Kirschenbaum. *Values Clarification,* p. 163.

I Urge Telegrams

"The teacher gives each student a 4 × 6 card or, better yet, a Western Union telegram form. He asks the students to choose a real person and write a telegram to that person beginning with these words— 'I urge you to. . . .' The message is to consist of 15 words or less (or 50 words for a night letter). The student is to sign his name to the telegram."

From Simon, Howe, and Kirschenbaum. *Values Clarification,* p. 264.

Life Style Autobiography

The student is asked to draw a picture which pictorally represents his philosophy of life style. Then the student is asked to write an autobiography which describes how he has arrived at his current life style.

Likert Scales

A Likert scale may be used to measure the strength of the student's feelings on a particular issue. The scale can be constructed as follows:

strongly agree	agree	disagree	strongly disagree

The teacher makes a statement and the students express themselves by putting a check on the line that describes their feelings.

From Renis Likert, "A Technique of Measuring Attitudes," Archives of Psychology, No. 140, 1932.

Proud Postcard

The student designs a clever postcard out of cardboard. He prints on the badge a description of health behavior that he is proud of. One morning is designated as "Proud" morning. The students share their feelings with each other.

Unfinished Sentences

The teacher provides students with a list of unfinished sentences.
Example:

1. When I exercise . . .
2. My friend with epilepsy . . .
3. If I had a venereal disease I would . . .

The teacher then moves around the room, calling on students to complete aloud any one of the sentences with whatever comes to mind. As an alternative, the students can complete the sentences in writing, then break into groups of three to discuss their finished sentences.

From Simon, Howe, and Kirschenbaum. *Values Clarification,* p. 241.

Values Voting

"The teacher reads aloud one by one questions which begin with the words, 'How many of you? . . .' Example: 'How many of you smoke marijuana?' After each question is read the students take a position by a show of hands. Those who wish to answer in the affirmative, raise their hands. Those who choose to answer negatively, point their thumbs down. Those who are undecided, fold their arms. And those who want to pass, simply take no action at all. Discussion is tabled until after the teacher has completed the entire list."

From Simon, Howe, and Kirschenbaum. *Values Clarification,* p. 38.

Winner-Loser Continuum

In this strategy, a continuum is drawn with one end labelled "winner" and the other "loser." Although the original authors of this article used the strategy with mental health, any topic can be examined. When it comes to making friends, which are you? Regarding your daily exercise program, are you a winner or a loser?

Winner	Loser

From James, M., and D. Jongeward. *Born to Win.* Reading, Massachusetts: Addison Wesley, 1971.

Games, Dramatizations, and Simulations

Middle and secondary school students enjoy and learn through *games, dramatizations, and simulations.* They offer the opportunity for active participation, wholesome competition and pleasant instruction.

Instructional Games

Instructional games are structured activities with set rules. Two or more students interact to reach clearly designated instructional objectives. Games may be purchased, found in this textbook and educational magazines, or created by you and your students.

Experienced teachers suggest that you decide whether a particular game will suit your purposes and help your students. Try it out with a few friends or students and discover any problems that may arise. Decide whether the game will involve the entire class or only a few students at any one time. Briefly and simply explain to the class how to play the game, but then restrict your own intervention. Since games and simulations usually create an atmosphere of enthusiasm, be prepared for increased "noise." After the game is over, reserve time for discussion and evaluation. Discussion is needed to help students recognize what they have learned during their game playing.

The *bowling game* can be used as a tool to reinforce factual information. The student is given a bowling sheet. A perfect score is 120. Each frame on the sheet represents a different category within a health unit. For example, if the unit is on communicable diseases, each frame is a different disease; if the unit is about drugs, each frame is a different drug. There are spaces for 10 pins in each frame. The student writes a fact on as many of the ten spaces as he can to knock the pins down. One point is received for each pin knocked down with a health fact. A strike is scored whenever all ten spaces in a frame are completed. A two point bonus is awarded for a strike. A final score of 120 is excellent; 110–119 is very good; and 84—bowl again!!

Health concentration can replace matching type examinations, and provide fun while learning. Words or pictures are put on index cards. All cards are turned face down. The students take turns trying to uncover pairs. This activity could be played with health specialists. Pairs might be dentist-teeth; obstetrician-baby; opthalmologist-eyes; etc.

Games may be adapted from television game shows. For example, encourage students to develop research and speaking skills as they prepare *To Tell the Truth* about first aid. *What's My Line* can be used to review health occupations or changed to *What's My Organization,* when discussing voluntary health organizations.

Small groups of students can be asked to design "Bingo" games around specific health knowledge, e.g., Nutrition or Dental Health, or use regular scrabble games to spell out health related words.

Regular *scrabble games* can be used for spelling out health related words.

Puzzles

Crossword puzzles, unscrambling words and word search puzzles help familiarize students with health terms and their proper spelling.

Picture puzzles can be made by pasting a picture (such as various body organs) on cardboard and cutting around the picture. Use a black felt tip pen to mark puzzle pieces and cut them out. Let the students assemble the puzzle to review the structure of various organs. Students can also make puzzles and trade them with each other.

Creating Your Own Games

After you have used a variety of commercially prepared games in the class-room, try creating your own games. You will need to define your learning objectives, how long the game can last, the number of students involved and their goals, what materials will be needed, how the game will be played, and what determines when the game is over. After the game is played, discuss and evaluate the game to see what was learned and whether it can be improved.

Dramatization

Different types of *dramatization* can cause participants to identify with and become involved with the role they are playing. The value of such activities depends upon whether the students understand their roles, have background information, and enjoy this kind of communicating.

Story acting may be carried out in several ways:

1. Assign roles of individuals in familiar stories. Read the story aloud while students pantomime the story.

2. After reading the story and discussing the characters, put key words on the chalkboard and let the students present the play from memory. Choose stories that provide opportunities to sing, dance, and move around.

Through *role playing,* students can explore the different parts one could assume in a real life situation. The role play can be entirely spontaneous, or the teacher can assign specific roles.

Examples:

1. A quack selling health food at the fair.

2. A boyfriend and girlfriend discussing premarital sex.

3. A student and parent discussing dating.

The time limit may vary from a few minutes to an entire class period, but in any case it is essential that students identify with their roles. When the class discusses a character's feelings, the subject becomes more real and the students realize that they can use their own emotions as a guide to help them understand the feelings of others. You may want to let the class choose a problem it wishes to explore by role-playing. They can establish the situation and cast the characters in terms of their own concerns.

Simulation Games

Simulation games combine the decision-making and real life elements often found in role-playing, with the clearly specified rules for interaction and com-petition that are characteristics of games. A simulation game may or may not have a winner or winning teams.

Write to Pennant Educational Materials, 4680 Alvarado Canyon Road, San Diego, California, 92120, for their latest catalog. This company has developed some interesting simulation-type games dealing with values.

Real Things, Models, and Demonstrations

There is no shortage of real things to help you provide motivation when it comes to the teaching of health. They are often free for the asking or available at very little cost and effort. Books sometimes talk about modified real things, unmodified real things, and specimens. What is the difference?

Unmodified real things are just that . . . things that have not been altered except for having been removed from their original surroundings. They may work or be alive; they are of normal size. A live hamster or some medical and dental instruments are examples of unmodified real things.

Modified real things may include an "exploded skull." This is a real skull that has been separated and rearranged to clarify its structure. A human skeleton with painted portions to identify muscle attachments, or cross-sections of real objects, also fall into this classification.

Specimens, according to The American College Dictionary, are "a part of an individual taken as exemplifying a whole mass or number." Examples include biological specimens available in bottles, jars, or embedded in plastic, for safe and convenient study.

Animals

Small animals, birds, and reptiles are found living in many classrooms. Units on animal behavior, ecology, reproduction, and nutrition can all revolve around small living creatures.

Bones

Bones may sometimes be obtained from your meat man or poultry department. Skeletons of various animals may be purchased from biological supply houses as well.

Animal and human teeth are examples of real things that students find fascinating. Ask your dentist to save the teeth that he extracts. Display preserved animal organs for study and comparison. Set aside a corner of your room as a museum and display collected materials.

Food

Bring samples of food that students have probably never tasted into the classroom. Let students sniff the aroma of various herbs stored in glass jars. Show the students examples of how food is preserved (dried-raisins; smoked-sausage; salt curing-pork; dehydrated powdered milk; canned-vegetables; frozen-meat and vegetables).

Models

Models are modified real things. Some materials are too costly, large, dangerous or delicate to be used in the classroom—but they can be duplicated as models, reduced in size and cost, and simplified for classroom use.

Anatomical models, a human torso with removable organs, life-size mannequins, and a large model of teeth are commonly used models usually found without difficulty.

Demonstrations

Demonstrations, either by an expert, teacher or students, are effective in showing how something works and why it is important. When students give demonstrations, they have the opportunity to speak before a group, develop drawings and transparencies for clarification, and possibly prepare slides or tape recordings as well. The students may want to use real things, models, flip charts, or the chalkboard as a part of their demonstrations. It is essential that the room be so arranged that everyone can see, and that adequate time is available to cover important points as well as to allow questions at the end of the demonstration.

A good demonstrator remembers to speak clearly and loud enough to be heard; he concentrates on a few important ideas rather than telling all he knows; he is alert for signs of confusion and boredom; he varies his voice and the pace of his explanation; he conceals the visuals or devices he plans to use in an effort to build suspense; and he practices his demonstration so he will be able to proceed smoothly through a variety of steps.

Community Resources

The community has been called "a great human laboratory and an influential instructional medium." No matter where you live, there are valuable resource places and people who can enrich your school program; this is especially true when you are teaching about health.

Check with your central school district office and district media center to see whether an inventory of community resources exists. If it does not, you and your students can develop your own inventory. Collect material in loose-leaf form so that it may easily be updated. Your community resources inventory related to health instruction may include the local department of health, local voluntary health agencies, local industry and commercial associations such as life insurance companies (may have pamphlets about stress, safety), dairy council, and auto club.

Do not overlook fire stations, police stations, museums, bakeries, creameries, zoos, mental health agencies, and pharmacies. Find out which companies and organizations permit visits by school groups or offer speakers, pamphlets, films, etc., for students of middle and secondary school age.

Field Trips

Field trips can be very worthwhile if they fit naturally into curricular goals, are suitable for the student's grade level, and provide experiences which cannot be found in other media forms. You must consider whether student learning will exceed the time and trouble required to organize the trip. Before the trip, you must obtain permission from your school and from the students' parents as well as from the agency itself. Transportation, finances, and time schedules must be considered, as well as trip objectives, student responsibilities, safety standards, etc. The learning that takes place during field trip follow-up activities can be more beneficial than the trip itself, if students are permitted the opportunity to react to their experiences.

Guest Speakers

Well-informed people are often very interested in speaking before school classes; they may provide valuable first-hand information that is available nowhere else. Oral invitations should always be confirmed in writing and a definite time set for the visit. The speaker should clearly understand the purpose of his visit and be provided with written directions for reaching the school. The class should be prepared for the visit and encouraged to acknowledge specifically how information gained from the speaker has helped them. These essays or summaries of points learned may be included with their note of appreciation.

Health Fairs

Health fairs can be organized on either a small or large scale. They may have different objectives. Each student in a single class, grade or school may want to develop eye-catching booths that convey a special health message. Groups of students may work on puppet shows, skits, games, slide shows, experiments, and role playing activities which involve an aspect of health. The fair may be visited by other classes, schools, parents, and teachers.

In some areas, university health education majors team up with local middle and secondary school students and hold a health fair. They choose an overall theme for the fair, then section and group themes. The main theme is carried out in every aspect of the fair—decorations, booth handouts, lesson presentations, costumes, and name tags.

Health fairs may be used to acquaint students and their families with career opportunities in health; to increase knowledge about health agencies; to furnish information about health and health care; and to improve school-community relations.

Health Museums

There are institutions throughout the United States which are considered by the Association of Science-Technology Centers to be major health exhibitors. If one of these is in your area, a field trip to the museum would help in the construction of exhibits for a health fair.[11]

California:	California Museum of Science and Technology—Los Angeles; Lawrence Hall of Science—University of California, Berkeley
Connecticut:	Museum of Art, Science and Industry—Bridgeport
District of Columbia:	Museum of History and Technology (Smithsonian)
Florida:	Jacksonville Children's Museum
Georgia:	Fernback Science Center—Atlanta
Illinois:	Museum of Science and Industry—Chicago; Robert Crown Center for Health Education—Hinsdale
Iowa:	Des Moines Center of Science and Industry
Kansas:	Kansas Health Museum—Halstead
Massachusetts:	Museum of Science—Boston
Michigan:	Alfred P. Sloan, Jr. Museum—Flint
Minnesota:	Mayo Medical Museum—Rochester
North Carolina:	Charlotte Nature Museum—Charlotte
Ohio:	Cleveland Health Museum and Education Center; Center of Science and Industry—Columbus
Oregon:	Oregon Museum of Science and Industry—Portland
Pennsylvania:	Buhl Planetarium and Institute of Popular Science—Pittsburgh; Franklin Institute Science Museum—Philadelphia
Texas:	Dallas Health and Science Museum; Ft. Worth Museum of Science and History; Museum of Medical Science—Houston
Washington:	Pacific Science Center—Seattle

As with other instructional materials, the use of community resources involves planning if the experience is to be meaningful and pleasant.

Using Methods, Materials, and Media in the Classroom

A self-renewing teacher who is continually open, alive, and aware, recognizes and responds to the need to use many of the ideas that we have given you to have a creative classroom.

How can methods, materials, and media assist you in all phases of instruction and in developing a creative classroom?

Introduce new materials with newspaper articles, curious objects, colorful pictures, provocative films, field trip experiences, or speakers from your community. It is important that you choose resources that will stimulate enthusiasm and suggest directions for study.

During the *developmental* phase of study, students will locate, examine, assess and use or reject information in many different forms. Appropriate learning experiences may involve independent study, discussion, and decision-making activities, films and slides, recordings, pictures, biological specimens, torso with removable organs, and work with a microscope. Encourage students to write for free or inexpensive materials, and to explore in individual ways.

Questions are raised, and previous research and study activities are shared, during the *organizational* phase of instruction. Students can prepare written reports illustrated with tables or graphs; develop slide presentations; design bulletin boards and displays; create models and original transparencies; or construct mobiles.

Instruction may be *summarized* through class prepared displays, dramatizations, or group presentations. These projects may be shared with other classes or parents. Films are also used to summarize health topics.

The use of media is often overlooked when it is time for *evaluation*. Construct a buzz board so students can quiz themselves independently. Display various medical instruments, teeth, etc., for the students to identify. Ask your students to appraise the media they used and whether they think different methods would have been better.

Chapter Summary

To conclude our discussion of methods, materials, and media for use in the classroom, first let us say, do not be intimidated by the bewildering and vast array of things available for your use. Rather, as a self-renewing teacher, take time to explore those areas and create an exciting classroom where freedom to learn and to wonder is encouraged.

For quick review, we feel that this is best accomplished when the teacher understands and utilizes: (1) changeable display graphics; (2) graphic visual materials; (3) art projects; (4) common audio-visual aids that require special equipment; (5) activities that require writing, thinking, and discussion; (6) activities involving feelings and values; (7) games, dramatizations, and simulations; (8) real things, models, and demonstrations; and (9) community resources.

Further, the self-renewing teacher recognizes that methods, materials and media can be used in many facets of instruction: introduction, developmental, organizational, summary, and evaluation.

Notes

1. Gardner, John W. *Self Renewal . . . The Individual and The Innovative Society.* New York: Harper and Rowe, 1963, p. XIV.
2. Frymier, Jack R. *Motivation and Learning in School.* Bloomington, Indiana: The Phi Delta Kappa Educational Foundation, 1975, p. 6, 15.
3. Galloway, Charles M., Ed D. *Silent Language in the Classroom.* Bloomington, Indiana: The Phi Delta Kappa Educational Foundation, 1976, p. 22.
4. The American Heart Association. *Putting Your Heart Into the Curriculum—A Guide for Teachers and Youth Workers.* "Section C–4: How Do I Teach Effectively." The National Center, 7230 Greenville Avenue, Dallas, Texas 75231.
5. The American Heart Association. *Putting Your Heart Into the Curriculum—A Guide for Teachers and Youth Workers.* "Section C–3: Use of Audiovisuals." The National Center, 7230 Greenville Avenue, Dallas, Texas 75231.

6. The American Heart Association. *Putting Your Heart Into the Curriculum—A Guide for Teachers and Youth Workers*. "Section C–3: Use of Audiovisuals." The National Center, 7230 Greenville Avenue, Dallas, Texas 75231.

7. The American Heart Association. *Putting Your Heart Into the Curriculum—A Guide for Teachers and Youth Workers*. "Section C–13: Values Clarification." The National Center, 7230 Greenville Avenue, Dallas, Texas 75231.

8. Raths, Lewis, Merril Harmin, and Sidney Simon. *Values and Teaching*. Columbus, Ohio: Charles E. Merrill, 1966.

9. The American Heart Association. *Putting Your Heart Into the Curriculum—A Guide for Teachers and Youth Workers*. "Section C–13: Values Clarification." The National Center, 7230 Greenville Avenue, Dallas, Texas 75231.

10. The American Heart Association. *Putting Your Heart Into the Curriculum—A Guide for Teachers and Youth Workers*. "Section C–13: Values Clarification." The National Center, 7230 Greenville Avenue, Dallas, Texas 75231.

11. The American Heart Association. *Putting Your Heart Into the Curriculum—A Guide for Teachers and Youth Workers*. "Section C–29: Health Fairs/Exhibits." The National Center, 7230 Greenville Avenue, Dallas, Texas 75231.

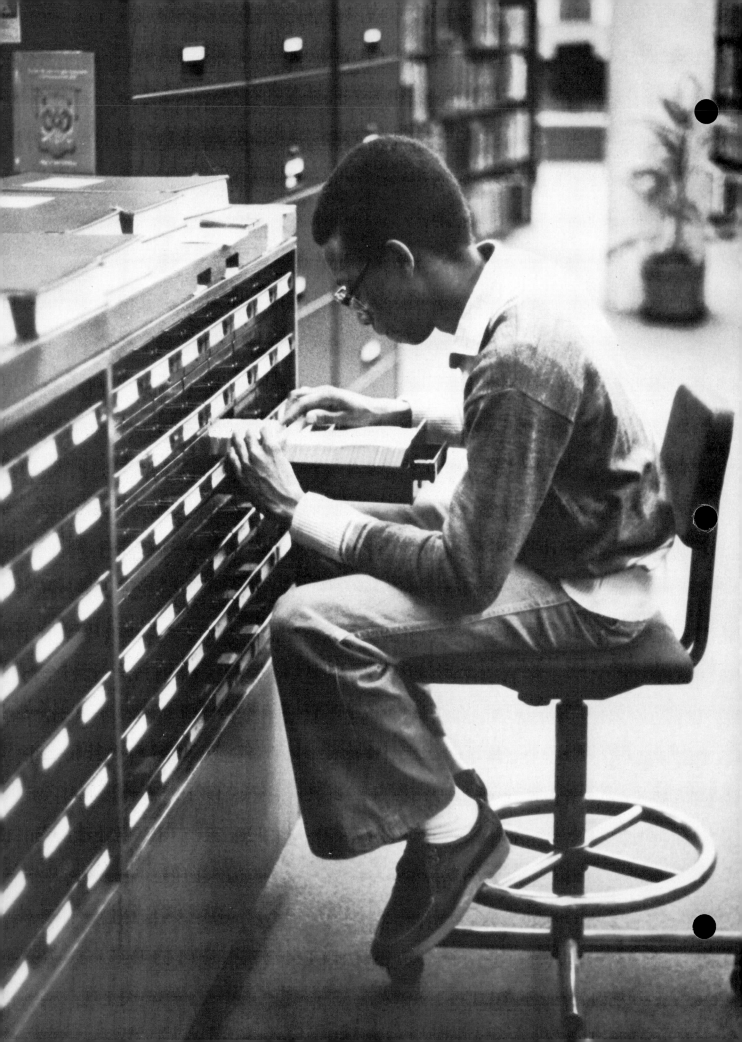

Resources

9

Numerous Resources Are Available

The field of health education is blessed with a wide variety of good, free, and inexpensive teaching aids. However, this requires considerable work on the part of the teacher to locate, select, and use the materials in an effective manner. The purpose of this chapter is to: (1) increase the reader's knowledge of the official, voluntary, and commercial agencies that are eager to provide the classroom teacher with health information; (2) provide a listing of valuable periodicals that will keep the secondary school teacher abreast of changes taking place in both the teaching and medical professions by providing abundant health content, methodology, and current research findings; (3) supply the teacher with more than 60 addresses of film sources; and (4) provide additional references under appropriate subject headings. In addition, many of the resources listed provide lesson plans, teaching guides, and curricula.

Requesting Materials

When contacting an agency or organization for materials, be certain to mention your particular area of interest, the type and quantity of materials desired, and the grade level of your classes. Try to request sample copies of their materials and/or an educational catalog of materials available, before requesting classroom quantities.

Reliability

Just as you would not think of showing a health film to your class without first previewing and evaluating its content, you must also evaluate the reliability of the various written materials that you wish to use. Numerous commercial organizations are as conscientious as such well-known organizations as the American Medical Association and the American Red Cross in promoting health before their own products; however, some materials are loaded with advertising and are probably unfit for use in the classroom. In appraising materials, first consider their source. Does the agency have a good reputation in the field of health? Why are they presenting the health information? Is the information based on scientific evidence, or meant simply to entertain? Is the material current and written at a level your students can comprehend? How do your colleagues and other medical experts regard the materials in question?

Official Health Agencies

Official health agencies include federal, state, county, and local branches of government which receive tax support and have been established by law to accomplish specific health maintenance and promotion activities. They may be able to provide pamphlets, speakers, films, posters, special exhibits, and health services.

Local Official Health Agencies

Write the name, address, and telephone number of the following agencies in the space provided:

1. Your local Board of Education: _____

   _____

   _____

2. Your city Health Department: _____

   _____

   _____

3. Your county Health Department: _____

   _____

   _____

State Official Health Agencies

Write the name, address, and telephone number of the following state agencies in the space provided:

1. Your state Department of Education: _____

   _____

   _____

2. Your state Department of Health: _____

   _____

   _____

3. Your state Department of Mental Health: _____

   _____

   _____

Federal Official Agencies

Federal agencies provide assistance in the form of information, field consultation, research data, and information on trends. They also have a great number of materials, publications, and instructional aids which are usually available at no charge when single copies are requested. The following agencies may prove helpful:

1. *National Center for Health Statistics.* U.S. Dept. of H.E.W., Washington, D.C. 20203.

2. *National Coordinating Council on Drug Abuse,* P.O. Box 19400, Washington, D.C. 20036.

3. *National Institute of Mental Health,* Barlow Building, Chevy Chase, Maryland 20015.

4. *National Interagency Council on Smoking and Health,* P.O. Box 3654, Central Station, Arlington, Virginia 22203.

5. *Superintendent of Documents*, U.S. Government Printing Office, Washington, D.C. 20025 (secure a catalog before ordering materials).

6. The United Nations World Health Organization, Geneva, Switzerland (New York, N.Y. 20006).

7. *U.S. Dept. of Transportation, National Highway Traffic Safety Administration.* Washington, D.C. 20590.

8. *U.S. Environmental Protection Agency,* Office of Public Affairs, Washington, D.C. 20460.

9. *U.S. Public Health Service,* HHS, Washington, D.C. 20201 (includes the National Institutes of Health).

Nonofficial Health Agencies

Nonofficial agencies generally include voluntary health agencies, professional associations, and commercial organizations, that have an express purpose of promoting health.

Voluntary Health Agencies

Voluntary Health Agencies exist to raise money for their particular cause. They are concerned with education, research, and defeating a specific disease entity. Depending on the agency, they may provide speakers, workshops, films and pamphlets. Before writing to the following voluntary agencies, check your telephone directory for a local, state, or district office to contact first.

Al-Anon Family Group Headquarters, Inc., P.O. Box 182, Madison Square Station, New York, N.Y. 10010

Alcoholics Anonymous, General Service Board, P.O. Box 459, Grand Central Station, New York, N.Y. 10017

Allergy Foundation of America, 801 Second Ave., New York, N.Y. 10017

Allied Youth, Rosslyn Building, 1901 Fort Myer Dr., Arlington, Va. 22209

American Association on Mental Deficiency, 5201 Connecticut Ave., N.W., Washington, D.C. 20015

American Cancer Society, Inc., 219 East 42nd St., New York, N.Y. 10017

American Diabetes Association, Inc., 600 Fifth Ave., New York, N.Y. 10020

American Foundation for the Blind, 15 West 16th Street, New York, N.Y. 10011

American Health Foundation, 320 East 43rd Street, New York, N.Y. 10017

American Hearing Society, 919 18th St., N.W., Washington, D.C. 20006

American Heart Association, The National Center, 7230 Greenville Ave., Dallas, Texas, 75231

American Institute of Family Relations, 5287 Sunset Blvd., Los Angeles, California 90027

American Lung Association, 1740 Broadway, New York, N.Y. 10019

American National Red Cross, 17th and D Streets, N.W., Washington, D.C. 20006

American Parkinson Disease Association, 147 East 50th St., New York, N.Y. 10022

Arthritis Foundation, 3400 Peach Tree Rd., N.E., Atlanta, Georgia 30326

Association for the Aid of Crippled Children, 345 East 46th St., New York, N.Y. 10017

Association for Education of the Visually Handicapped, 1604 Spruce St., Philadelphia, Pennsylvania 19103

Association for Family Living, 6 North Michigan Ave., Chicago, Illinois 60602

Better Vision Institute, 630 Fifth Ave., New York, N.Y. 10020

Child Welfare League of America, 67 Irving Place, New York, N.Y. 10003

Cleveland Health Museum, 8911 Euclid Avenue, Cleveland, Ohio 44106

Committee on Parenthood Education (COPE), P.O. Box 22025, San Diego, California 92122

Community Sex Information and Education Service, Inc., P.O. Box 2858, Grand Central Station, New York, N.Y. 10017

Epilepsy Foundation of America, Suite 1116, 733 15th St., N.W., Washington, D.C. 20005

Family Life Bureau, United States of Catholic Conferences, 1312 Massachusetts Ave., N.W., Washington, D.C. 20005

Family Service Association of America, 44 East 23rd St., New York, N.Y. 10010

Health Education Service, P.O. Box 7283, Albany, N.Y. 12224

Hogg Foundation for Mental Health, Will C. Hogg Building, The University of Texas, Austin, Texas 78712

Institute for Rational Living, Inc., 45 E. 65th St., New York, N.Y. 10021

Institute for Sex Research, Inc., University of Indiana, Bloomington, Indiana 47401

LaLeche League International, Inc., 9616 Minneapolis Ave., Franklin Park, Illinois 60131

Leonard Wood Memorial for the Eradication of Leprosy (American Leprosy Foundation), 1200 18th St., N.W., Washington, D.C. 20036

Leukemia Society of America, Inc., 211 East 43rd St., New York, N.Y. 10016

Margaret Sanger Research Bureau, 17 West 16th St., New York, N.Y. 10011

Maternity Center Association, 48 East 92nd St., New York, N.Y. 10028

Muscular Dystrophy Associations of America, Inc., 1790 Broadway, New York, N.Y. 10019

The Myasthenia Gravis Foundation, Inc., 2 East 103rd St., New York, N.Y. 10029

Narcotics Anonymous, Box 2000, Lexington, Ky. 40501

National Alliance Concerned with School-Age Parents, 7315 Wisconsin Ave., Suite 516E, Washington, D.C. 20014

National Association of Hearing and Speech Agencies, 919 18th St., N.W., Washington, D.C. 20006

National Association for Mental Health, Inc., 1800 N. Kent St., Arlington, Virginia 22209

National Association for Retarded Children, Inc., 2709 Avenue E, East, Arlington, Texas 76011

National Child Safety Council, 3146 Francis St., Jackson, Michigan 49203

National Committee Against Mental Illness, Inc., 1028 Connecticut Ave., N.W., Washington, D.C. 20036

National Congress of Parents and Teachers, 700 North Rush St., Chicago, Illinois 60611

National Coordinating Council on Drug Abuse, 1211 Connecticut Ave., N.W., Suite 212, Washington, D.C. 20036

National Council on Alcoholism, 2 Park Ave., New York, N.Y. 10016

National Council on Family Relations, 1219 University Ave., S.E., Minneapolis, Minnesota 55414

The National Foundation—March of Dimes, 1275 Marmaroneck Ave., White Plains, N.Y. 10605

National Cystic Fibrosis Research Foundation, 3379 Peachtree Rd., N.E., Atlanta, Georgia 30326

National Foundation for Neuromuscular Diseases, 250 West 57th St., New York, N.Y. 10019

National Hemophilia Foundation, 25 West 39th St., New York, N.Y. 10018

National Kidney Foundation, 116 East 27th St., New York, N.Y. 10016

National Multiple Sclerosis Society, 257 Park Ave., South, New York, N.Y. 10010

National Parkinson Foundation, Inc., 135 East 44th St., New York, N.Y. 10017

National Safety Council, 425 N. Michigan Avenue, Chicago, Illinois 60611

National Society for Crippled Children and Adults, 2023 West Ogden Ave., Chicago, Illinois 60603

National Society to Prevent Blindness, 79 Madison Ave., New York, N.Y. 10016

Nutrition Foundation, Inc., 99 Park Ave., New York, N.Y. 10016

Parents Without Partners, Inc. 7910 Woodmont Avenue, Washington, D.C. 20014

Planned Parenthood Federation of America, Inc. 810 Seventh Avenue, New York, N.Y. 10019

Population Crisis Committee, 1730 K St., N.W., Washington, D.C. 20006

Population Reference Bureau, Inc., 1735 Massachusetts Ave., N.W., Washington, D.C. 20036

Public Affairs Committee, Inc., 381 Park Ave., South, New York, N.Y. 10016

Sex Information Education Council of the U.S. (Siecus) 85 Fifth Avenue, New York, N.Y. 10001

United Cerebral Palsy Association, Inc., 321 West 44th St., New York, N.Y. 10036

Zero Population Growth, 367 State St., Los Altos, California 94022

Professional Health Associations

Professional Health Associations may exist at the local, state, national, or international level. They usually publish at least one journal and may help promote and interpret health research projects, establish guidelines for standards of excellence and competency for health professionals; and inform readers of progress in various health areas.

Action for Brain-Handicapped Children, Inc., 4020 Minnesota Blvd., Suite 305, Minneapolis, Minnesota 55416

Air Pollution Control Association, 4400 Fifth Ave., Pittsburgh, Pennsylvania 15213

American Academy of Pediatrics, Inc., 1801 Hinman Ave., Evanston, Illinois 60204

American Alliance for Health, Physical Education, Recreation, and Dance, Reston, Va. 22090

American Association for the Advancement of Science, 1515 Massachusetts Ave., N.W., Washington, D.C. 20036

American Association of Marriage, and Family Counselors, 102651 Croydon Circle, Dallas, Texas 75230

American College Health Association, 2807 Central St., Evanston, Illinois 60201

American Dental Association, Bureau of Dental Health Education, 211 East Chicago Ave., Chicago, Illinois 60611

American Dental Hygienists' Association, Suite 1616, 211 East Chicago Ave., Chicago, Illinois 60611

American Dietetic Association, 620 N. Michigan Ave., Chicago, Illinois 60611

American Genetic Association, 1028 Connecticut Ave., N.W., Washington, D.C. 20036

American Home Economics Association, 1600 20th St., N.W., Washington, D.C. 20009

American Hospital Association, 840 North Lake Shore Dr., Chicago, Illinois 60611

American Institute of Family Relations, 5287 Sunset Blvd., Los Angeles, California 90027

American Medical Association, Department of Health Education, 535 North Dearborn St., Chicago, Illinois 60610

American Nurses' Association, 2420 Pershing Rd., Kansas City, Missouri 64108

American Optometric Association, 7000 Chippewa, St. Louis, Missouri 63119

American Osteopathic Association, 212 East Ohio St., Chicago, Illinois 60611

American Pharmaceutical Association, 2215 Constitution Ave., N.W., Washington, D.C. 20037

American Physical Therapy Association, 1740 Broadway, New York, N.Y. 10019

American Podiatry Association, Council on Education, 3301 16th St., N.W., Washington, D.C. 20010

American Public Health Association, Inc., 1015 18th St., N.W., Washington, D.C. 20036

American Public Welfare Association, 1313 East 16th St., Chicago, Illinois 60637

American School Health Association, 1521 S. Water St., P.O. Box 708, Kent, Ohio 44240

American Social Health Association, 1740 Broadway, New York, N.Y. 10019

Association for Childhood Education International, 3615 Wisconsin Ave., N.W., Washington, D.C. 20016

Child Study Association of America, Inc., 9 East 89th St., New York, N.Y. 10028

Day Care and Child Development Council of America, Inc., 1401 K Street, Washington, D.C. 20005

National Alcoholic Beverage Control Association, 5454 Wisconsin Ave., Washington, D.C. 20015

National Association of Chiropodists, Council on Education, 3301 16th St., N.W., Washington, D.C. 20010

National Education Association, 1201 16th St., N.W., Washington, D.C. 20036

National Environmental Health Association, 1600 Pennsylvania, Denver, Colorado 80203

National Health Council, 1740 Broadway, New York, N.Y. 10019

National League for Nursing, 59th Street and Columbus Circle, New York, N.Y. 10019

National Recreation Association, 8 W. 8th St., New York, N.Y. 10011

National Safety Council, 425 North Michigan Ave., Chicago, Illinois 60611

National Sanitation Foundation, P.O. Box 1468, Ann Arbor, Michigan 48106

National Society for Medical Research, 1330 Massachusetts Ave., N.W., Washington, D.C. 20005

Rainbow Youth Spine Center 2065 Adelbert Road, Cleveland, Ohio 44106

Roswell Park Memorial Institute, Cigarette Cancer Committee, 666 Elm St., Buffalo, N.Y. 14203

Rutgers Center of Alcohol Studies, Rutgers-The State University, Box 560, New Brunswick, New Jersey 08903

Society for Nutrition Education (National Nutrition Education Clearing House), 2140 Shattuck Ave., Suite 1110, Berkeley, California 94704

Society for Public Health Education, 655 Sutter St., San Francisco, California 94102

Business and Commercial Organizations

There is a wealth of health education material offered by business enterprises for use in school health education. Interested in cleanliness and disease prevention? Contact soap companies and pharmaceutical corporations. Life insurance companies produce many teaching aids of great value. The National Dairy Council, the Cereal Institute, Inc., General Mills, Inc., the Florida Citrus Commission, and the Kellogg Company are known for their excellent nutrition materials.

Most firms are conservative with their advertising and may only include a credit line. Some firms, however, produce poorly written materials that contain excessive advertising and should not be used. The following represents only a partial listing of commercial organizations that have produced health materials for classroom use.

Abbott Laboratories, 14th and Eli LillySheridan Road, North Chicago, Illinois 60064

Aetna Life Affiliated Companies, Education Department, 151 Farmington Ave., Hartford, Connecticut 06115 (Safety)

American Automobile Association, Traffic Safety Department, Falls Church, Virginia 22042 (Safety)

American Institute of Baking, 400 East Ontario St., Chicago, Illinois 60611

American Meat Institute, 59 East Van Buren St., Chicago, Illinois 60605

Armour and Company, Public Relations Dept., 401 N. Wabash St., Chicago, Illinois 60690 (Nutrition)

Armour-Dial Company, Greyhound Tower, 111 W. Clarendon, . Phoenix, Arizona 85077 (Grooming)

Athletic Institute, 805 Merchandise Mart, Chicago, Illinois 60650

Automotive Safety Foundation, Ring Building, Washington, D.C. 20036

Avon Educational Services, Nine West Fifty Seventh St., New York, N.Y. 10019 (Grooming)

Ayerst Laboratories, New York, New York 10017

Baker Labs, Inc., East Troy, Wisconsin 53120 (Maternity Literature)

Beech Nut Baby Foods, 460 Park Avenue, New York, New York 10022

Better Vision Institute, 230 Park Ave., New York, New York 10017

Bicycle Institute of America, Inc., 122 East 42nd St., New York, N.Y. 10017

Blue Cross Association, 840 North Lake Shore Drive, Chicago, Illinois 60611

The Borden Company, Consumer's Service, 180 E. Broad Street, Columbus, Ohio 43215 (Dairy)

Calgon Company, Home Service Department, P.O. Box 1346, Pittsburgh, Pennsylvania 15230

Carnation Company, Medical Marketing, 5045 Wilshire Blvd., Los Angeles, California 90036

Cereal Institute, Inc., Educational Director, 135 South LaSalle Street, Chicago, Illinois 60603 (Food)

Channing L. Bete Co. Inc., 45 Federal Street, Greenfield, Massachusetts 01301 (Scriptograph pamphlets)

Church and Dwight Company, Inc., 70 Pine St., New York, N.Y. 10005

Colgate-Palmolive Company, 300 Park Avenue, New York, N.Y. 10022 (Dental Health)

Connecticut Mutual Life Insurance Co., 140 Garden St., Hartford, Connecticut 06105

Consumers Union of U.S., Inc., Mount Vernon, New York 10550

Cream of Wheat Corporation, Box M, Minneapolis, Minnesota 55413

Distilled Spirits Council of the U.S., Inc., 1300 Pennsylvania Building, Washington, D.C. 20004

Educational Activities, Inc., Box 392, Freeport, New York 11520 (Physical Fitness)

Eli Lilly Company, 740 South Alabama Street, Indianapolis, Indiana 46206 (Safety, Diabetes, Disease)

Equitable Life Assurance Society of the United States, Office of Community Services and Health Education, 1285 Avenue of the Americas, New York, N.Y. 10019

Evaporated Milk Association, 228 North LaSalle Street, Chicago, Illinois 60601 (Milk)

Florida Citrus Commission, P.O. Box 148, Lakeland, Florida 33802 (Citrus Fruits)

Ford Motor Company, Information Department, Dearborn, Michigan 48127 (Traffic Safety)

General Mills, Inc., Nutrition Service, P.O. Box 1113, Minneapolis, Minnesota 55401 (Nutrition)

Gerber Products Company, 445 State Street, Fremont, Michigan 49412

Gerico, Inc., 12520 Grant Drive, P.O. Box 33755, Denver, Colorado 80233

The Gillette Company, Personal Care Division, P.O. Box 61, Prudential Tower Building, Boston, Massachusetts, 02199 (Grooming)

Good Housekeeping Institute, 8th Avenue and 57th Street, New York, N.Y. 10019

Health Education Service, P.O. Box 7283, Albany, New York 12224

Health Information Foundation, Center for Health Administrative Studies, University of Chicago, 5555 South Ellis, Chicago, Illinois 60636

Health Insurance Institute, 277 Park Avenue, New York, N.Y. 10017

H. J. Heinz and Company, P.O. Box 57, Pittsburgh, Pennsylvania 15230 (Food Charts; Food Origins)

Johnson and Johnson Baby Products Company, Consumer and Professional Services, 220 Centennial Avenue, Piscataway, N.J. 08854

Johnson and Johnson, Educational Division, 501 George Street, New Brunswick, New Jersey 08903 (First Aid; Safety)

Kellogg Company, Department of Home Economics Services, 235 Porter St., Battle Creek, Michigan 49016 (Breakfast Pamphlets and Games)

Kimberly-Clark Corporation, The Life Cycle Center, Neenah, Wisconsin 54956

Kraft Cheese Company, 500 Peshtigo Court, Chicago, Illinois 60690 (Nutrition)

Lederle Laboratories, Division, American Cyanamid Company, Pearl River, New York 10965 (Child Health; Nutrition)

Lever Brothers Company, Educational Department, Public Relations Division, 390 Park Avenue, New York, N.Y. 10022

Licensed Beverage Industries, Inc., 155 E. 44th Street, New York, N.Y. 10017

Maltex Company, Burlington, Vermont 05401

Mead Johnson & Company, Public Relations Department, 2404 Pennsylvania Ave., Evansville, Indiana 47721

Mental Health Materials Center, 419 Park Avenue South, New York, New York 10016

Merck Sharpe & Dohme, Division of Merck & Co., Inc., West Point, Pennsylvania 19486

Metropolitan Life Insurance Company, Health and Welfare Division, 1 Madison Avenue, New York, N.Y. 10010 (Diseases; School Health Instruction)

Money Management Institute, Prudential Plaza, Chicago, Illinois 60601 (Consumer Health)

National Biscuit Company, 425 Park Avenue, New York, N.Y. 10022

National Board of Fire Underwriters, 85 John Street, New York, New York 10038 (Safety)

National Dairy Council, 6300 North River Road, Rosemont, Illinois 60018 (Nutrition, Dental Health, Consumer Health)

National Fire Protection Association, 60 Batterymarch Street, Boston, Massachusetts 02110 (Home Safety)

National Foot Health Council, 272 Union Street, Rockland, Massachusetts 02370

National Livestock and Meat Board, 36 South Wabash Avenue, Chicago, Illinois 60603 (Food Materials)

National Social Welfare Assembly, Inc., 345 E. 46th Street, New York, N.Y. 10017 (Health Comic Books)

Ocean Spray Cranberries, Inc., Executive Offices, Hanson, Massachusetts 02341 (Food Charts, Recipes)

Ortho Diagnostic, P.O. Box 178, Raritan, New Jersey 08869

Paper Cup and Container Institute, Public Health Committee, 250 Park Avenue, New York, N.Y. 10017

Personal Products Company, Assoc. Films, P.O. Box 117-R Ridgefield, New Jersey 07657 (Personal Hygiene)

Pet Milk Company, Inc., Office of Consumer Affairs, P.O. Box 392, St. Louis, Missouri 63166 (Nutrition)

Charles Pfizer and Company, Inc., The Education Services Department, 235 East 42nd Street, New York, N.Y. 10017

Pharmaceutical Manufacturers Association, 1155 15th Street, N.W., Washington, D.C. 20005 (General Health Topics)

Physicians Art Service, Inc. Patient Information Library, 343-B Serramonte Plaza Office Center, Daly California 94015

Procter and Gamble Company, P.O. Box 171, Cincinnati, Ohio 45201

Prudential Insurance Company of America, Public Relations and Advertising Department, Prudential Plaza, Newark, New Jersey 07010

Quaker Oats Co., Chicago, Illinois 60654

Ralston Purina Company Checkerboard Square, St. Louis, Missouri 63188

Reed and Carnick, Kenilworth, N.J. 07033

Roche Laboratories, Division of Hoffmann-LaRoche Inc., Nutley, New Jersey 07110

Ross Labs, 625 Cleveland Avenue, Columbus, Ohio 43215

Schering Laboratories, Kenilworth, New Jersey 07033

Scott Paper Company, Home Service Center, Philadelphia, Pennsylvania 19113 (Menstrual Hygiene)

Sealtest Foods, Consumer Service, 605 3rd Avenue, New York, N.Y. 10016 (Food Charts)

Searle Laboratories, P.O. Box 5110, Chicago, Illinois 60680

Smith, Kline and French Laboratories, 1500 Spring Garden Street, Philadelphia, Pennsylvania 19101

Soap and Detergent Association, 475 Park Ave., South, New York, N.Y. 10016

Sonotone Corporation, P.O. Box 200, Elmsforth, New York 10523

Spenco Medical Corporation, Box 8113, Waco, Texas 76710

E. R. Squibb & Sons, Division of Olin Mathieson Chemical Company, 909 Third Avenue, New York, N.Y. 10022

Sunkist Growers, P.O. Box 7888, Valley Annex, Van Nuys, California 91409 (Nutrition)

Swift and Company, Union Stockyards, Chicago, Illinois 60609

Tampax, Incorporated, Educational Director, 5 Dakota Drive, Lake Success, New York 11042 (Menstruation)

Toy Manufacturers Association of America, Inc., 200 Fifth Avenue, New York, N.Y. 10010

Travelers Insurance Company, Hartford, Connecticut 06115 (Growth/Posture)

Underwriters' Laboratories, Inc., 207 East Ohio Street, Chicago, Illinois 60611

United Fresh Fruit and Vegetable Association, 777 14th Street, N.W., Washington, D.C. 20005 (Nutrition)

United States Beet Sugar Association, Tower Building, Washington, D.C. 20005

Upjohn Company, 7000 Portage Road, Kalamazoo, Michigan 49002

Wheat Flour Institute, Supervisor of Distribution, 14 East Jackson Blvd., Chicago, Illinois 60604 (Breakfast Foods)

Wyeth Labs, P.O. Box 8299, Philadelphia, Pennsylvania 19101

Periodicals and Journals

The following journals may be obtained through membership in various professional organizations or borrowed from certain libraries. We have also listed several other periodicals that have proven useful from an informational viewpoint and are widely read by "non-professionals".

Professional Health Journals	**Professional Membership**
1. American Journal of Public Health	American Public Health Association
2. Health Education	American Alliance For Health, Physical Education and Recreation
3. Research Quarterly	American Alliance For Health, Physical Education, Recreation, and Dance
4. Journal of Health, Physical Education and Recreation	American Alliance For Health, Physical Education and Recreation
5. Health Education Quarterly	Society For Public Health Education
6. International Journal of Health Education	Society For Public Health Education
7. Journal of the American College Health Association	American College Health Association
8. Journal of School Health	American School Health Association

Other Journals of Interest

9. Adult Leadership	Adult Education Association of the United States of America (743 North Wabash Ave., Chicago, Illinois 60611)
10. American Journal of Nursing	American Nurses Association
11. Childhood Education	Association for Childhood Education International
12. Health Care Education	Health Education Media Association
13. Journal of the American Medical Association	American Medical Association
14. Journal of the National Education Association	National Education Association
15. Science	American Association for the Advancement of Science
16. Social Hygiene News	American Social Health Association
17. World Health	World Health Organization

Additional Health-Related Periodicals

18. Current Health—The Continuing Guide to Health Education	Curriculum Innovations, Inc., 501 Lake Forest Ave., Highwood, Illinois 60040
19. Family Health	Family Health, 1255 Portland Place, Boulder, Colorado 80302
20. Health Bulletin for Teachers	Metropolitan Life Insurance Co., 1 Madison Ave., New York, N.Y. 10010
21. Health Values: Achieving High Level Wellness	Charles B. Slack, Inc., 6900 Grove Rd., Thorofare, New Jersey 08086
22. Psychology Today	Psychology Today, P.O. Box 2990, Boulder, Colorado 80321

Film Sources

Agency for Instructional Television, Box A, Bloomington, Indiana 47401

Aims Instructional Media Services, P.O. Box 1010, Hollywood, California 90028

Alfred Higgins Productions, 9100 Sunset Blvd., Los Angeles, California 90069

American Education Films, 132 Laskey Drive, Beverly Hills, California 90210

Association Films, Inc., 25358 Cypress Avenue, Hayward, California 94544

Audio Arts, Portland, Oregon 97208

Avis Films, 2408 W. Olive Avenue, Burbank, California 91506

Bailey Films, Inc., 6509 De Longpre Avenue, Hollywood, California 90028

Barr Films, P.O. Box 5667, Pasadena, California 91107

BFA Educational Media, 2211 Michigan Avenue, Santa Monica, California 90404

Billy Budd Films, Inc., 234 E 57th Street, New York, N.Y. 10022

Brigham Young University, Provo, Utah 84601

Calvin Productions, 1105 Truman Road, Kansas City, Missouri 64106

Canadian National Film Board, 680 5th Avenue, New York, N.Y. 10019

Capitol Film Laboratories, Inc., 470 E Street, S.W., Washington, D.C. 20024

Carousel Films, 1501 Broadway, New York, N.Y. 10036

Cathedral Films, Inc., 2921 W. Alameda Avenue, Burbank, California 91505

Center for Mass Communication, Columbia University Press, 562 West 113th Street, New York, N.Y. 10025

Charles Cahill and Associates, P.O. Box 3220, Hollywood, California 90028

Churchill Films, 6671 Sunset Blvd., Los Angeles, California 90028

Classroom Film Distributors, Inc., 5120 Hollywood Blvd., Los Angeles, California 90027

CRM (McGraw-Hill) Educational Films, Del Mar, California 92014

Columbia University Press (Center for Mass Communication) 562 W. 113 Street, New York, N.Y. 10025

Consumer Report Films, Box XA 22, 256 Washington Street, Mt. Vernon, New York 10550

Coronet Instructional Films, 65 E. South Water St., Chicago, Illinois 60601

Ealing Corporation (BFA), 2211 Michigan Avenue, Santa Monica, California 90404

E. C. Brown Foundation, 1825 Willow Road, Northfield, Illinois 60093

Educational Activities, Inc., P.O. Box 392, Freeport, New York 11520

Educational Corporation, P.O. Box 517, Skokie, Illinois 60076

Encyclopedia Britannica Films, Inc., 1150 Wilmette Avenue, Wilmette, Illinois 60091

Environmental Control Administration, 12720 Twinbrook Parkway, Rockville, Maryland 20852

Eye Gate House, Inc., 146 Archer Avenue, Jamaica, New York 11435

Family Filmstrips, 5823 Santa Monica Blvd., Hollywood, California 90038

Film Distributing Company, Box 373, Mill Valley, California 94941

Filmfair Communications, 10946 Ventura Blvd., Studio City, California 91604

Films, Incorporated, 1144 Wilmette Avenue, Wilmette, Illinois 60091

Focus Education Inc., 3 E. 45th Street, New York, New York 10022

Guidance Associates, Pleasantville, New York 10570

Hank Newenhouse Films, 1825 Willow Road, Northfield, Illinois 60093

Human Relations Media Center, 22 Clemmons Square, Pound Ridge, New York 10576

Ideal Pictures Corporation, 321 W. 44th Street, New York, New York 10036

Image Publishing Corporation, P.O. Box 14 North Station, White Plains, New York 10603

International Film Bureau, Inc., 322 S. Michigan Avenue, Chicago, Illinois 60604

Jarvis Covillard Associates, P.O. Box 123, Culver City, California 91230

John Wiley and Sons, 605 Third Avenue, New York, New York 10016

Knowledge Builders, 625 Madison Avenue, New York, New York, 10000

Landford Publishing Company, P.O. Box 8711, San Jose, California 95125

Macmillan Films, Inc., 34 MacQuestan Parkway South, Mt. Vernon, New York 10550

McGraw-Hill Book Company, Inc., 330 West 42nd Street, New York, N.Y. 10036

Media Visuals, Inc., 342 Madison Avenue, New York, New York 10017

Modern Talking Picture Service, 45 Rockefeller Plaza, New York, New York 10020

Modern Learning Aids, Box 302, Rochester, New York 14603

Paulist Productions, 7575 Pacific Coast Highway, Pacific Palisades, California 90272

Perennial Education, 1825 Willow Road, Northfield, Illinois 60093

Picture Films Distributing Company, 43 West 16th Street, New York, New York 10011

Polymorph Films, 331 Newbury Street, Boston, Massachusetts 02115

Popular Science, 330 W. 42nd Street, New York, New York 10036

Pyramid Films, Box 1048, Santa Monica, California 90406

See-Saw Films, P.O. Box 262, Palo Alto, California 94302

Sid Davis Productions, 2429 Ocean Park Blvd., Santa Monica, California 90405

Society for Visual Education, Inc., 1345 Diversey Parkway, Chicago, Illinois 60614

Sterling Educational Films, 241 E. 34th Street, New York, New York 10016

Stuart Finley Productions, 3428 Mansfield Road, Fall Church, Virginia 22041

Sunburst Communications, Pound Ridge, New York 10576

Teaching Film Custodians, 25 W. 43rd Street, New York, New York 10036

Texture Films, Inc., 1600 Broadway, New York, New York 10019

Thorne Films, 1229 University Avenue, Boulder, Colorado 80302

Tribune Films, Inc., 38 West 32nd Street, New York, New York 10001

United World Films, 221 Park Avenue South, New York, New York 10003

Walt Disney Productions, 800 Senora Avenue, Gendale, California 91201

Warren Schloat Productions, Inc., 115 Tompkins Avenue, Pleasantville, New York 10570

Western Publishing Company, 830 Third Avenue, New York, New York 10022

Wexler Film Productions, 801 N. Seward Street, Los Angeles, California 90038

Young America Films, 330 W. 42nd Street, New York, New York 10036

The following publications are useful in determining what films exist for your particular subject and age level. Be sure to request a catalog of films that may be borrowed from your State Health Department as well.

Educational Film Guide. Edited by Josephine S. Antonini. H. W. Wilson Co., 950 University Avenue, New York, New York 10452. Annual supplements. Indexes and describes alphabetically by title and subject thousands of 16-mm motion pictures for all instructional areas.

Educators Guide to Free Films. Educators Progress Service, Randolph, Wisconsin 53956. Revised annually. Provides title, content description, length, running time, whether silent or sound, date of release, information on distributors, and limitations on distribution of currently available films that may be borrowed free of charge.

The Educational Media Index. McGraw-Hill Book Company, 330 West 42nd Street, New York, N.Y. 10036. Describes various instructional materials.

Instructional Television Motion Pictures: Descriptive Catalog Containing Series Data, Subject, and Use Level Index for 16-MM. Instructional Television Programs. NET Film Service, Audio-Visual Center, Indiana University, Bloomington, Indiana 47401. Lists and describes instructional television programs available to schools, organizations, and individuals for nontelevision and nontheatrical use.

Gives title, content description, length, film characteristics, grade classifications, and rental and purchase information.

Library of Congress Catalog: Motion Pictures and Filmstrips. Washington, D.C. 20540. Includes listings by title and a subject index of all the educational motion pictures and filmstrips released in the United States and Canada. Short annotations of each title are provided.

U.S. Government Films for Public Educational Use. Office of Education, U.S. Department of Health, Education, and Welfare, Washington, D.C. 20402. Available from the Superintendent of Documents, U.S. Government Printing Office, Washington, D.C. Price $2.75. Describes and indexes alphabetically by title and by subject motion pictures and filmstrips of U.S. government agencies and departments available for public use.

Filmstrips

Educators Guide to Free Filmstrips. Compiled and edited by Mary Foley Horkheimer and John W. Diffor. Educators Progress Service, Randolph, Wisconsin 53956. An annual listing of silent filmstrips, sound filmstrips, and slide sets that may be borrowed free of charge.

Additional References

The following references are provided for those persons interested in pursuing a topic in greater depth.

Defining Health Education

1. Dolfman, Michael L. "Toward Operational Definitions of Health," *Journal of School Health,* Volume 44, April, 1974, pp. 206-209.

2. Joint Committee on Health Education Terminology. "Definitions of Health Education," *School Health Review,* November-December, 1973.

3. Joint Committee on Health Education Terminology. "New Definitions", *Journal of School Health,* Volume 44, January, 1974, pp. 33-37.

Philosophy of Health Education

1. Association for the Advancement of Health Education plan of action, 1974-1975, "Blueprint For Progress," *Health Education,* Jan.-Feb., 1975, pp. 7-11.

2. Aubrey, Roger F., "Health Education: Neglected Child of the Schools," *Journal of School Health,* Volume 42, May, 1972, pp. 285-289.

3. Burt, John et al., "Philosophical Perspectives," *Health Education,* January-February, 1975, pp. 12-14.

4. Burt, John. "Rational Selection of Lifestyle Components," *School Health Review,* March-April, 1974, pp. 4-9.

5. Cooper, Theodore. "An Instrument of Prevention," *Public Health Reports,* Volume 91, May-June, 1976.

6. Douse, Mike. "Health Hints or Health Philosophy?" *Journal of School Health,* Volume 43, March, 1973, pp. 195-197.

7. Galli, Nicholas. "Foundations of Health Education," *Journal of School Health,* Volume 46, March, 1976, pp. 158-165.

8. Hoyman, Howard S. "New Frontiers in Health Education," *Journal of School Health,* Volume 43, Spetember, 1973, pp. 423-430.

9. Means, Richard K. "Can the Schools Teach Personal Responsibility For Health?" *Journal of School Health,* Volume 43, March, 1973, pp. 171-175.

10. Nolte, Ann. "The Relevance of Abraham Maslow's Work To Health Education," *Health Education,* May-June, 1976, pp. 25-27.

11. Pottebaum, Sharon. "A Philosophy of Health Education From Children's Literature," *Health Education,* May-June, 1977, pp. 6-7.

12. Salk, Jonas. "What Do We Mean By Health?" *Journal of School Health,* Volume 42, December, 1972, pp. 582-584.

100 Resources for Health and Education in the Classroom

1. Ahrens, Maurice R. "Methods Can Make a Difference," *Educational Leadership,* Vol. 3, No. 8 (May 1973), pp. 700-705.

2. Armsey, James W., and Norman C. Dahl. *An Inquiry into the Uses of Instructional Technology.* New York: The Ford Foundation, 1973.

3. Ashton-Warner, Sylvia. *Teacher.* New York: Bantam Books, Inc., 1964.

4. Barrett, Morris. *Health Education Guide: A Design for Teaching K-12,* 2nd edition, Philadelphia: Lea & Febiger, 1974.

5. Bender, Stephen J., Charles R. Schroeder, and Michael H. Hamrick, *Conceptual Approach to Health: A Guide to Intelligent Self-Direction* (Second Edition), Dubuque, Iowa, Kendall/Hunt, 1972.

6. Birney, Robert C., et al. *Fear of Failure.* New York: Van Nostrand-Reinhold Company, 1969.

7. Bloom, Benjamin S. et al., *Taxonomy of Educational Objectives—The Classification of Educational Goals, Handbook I: Cognitive Domain.* New York: David McKay Company, Inc., 1956.

8. Borton, Terry. *Reach, Touch and Teach.* New York: McGraw-Hill Book Company, 1970.

9. Brown, George Isaac. *Human Teaching for Human Learning: An Introduction to Confluent Education.* New York: The Viking Press, Inc., 1971.

10. Brown, James D., and Donald B. Stone. "Doomsday Prophets, Humanists, and Responsible Educators," *School Health Review,* Vol. 3, No. 4, July–August 1972, pp. 19–22.

11. Brown, M. B. "Knowing and Learning," *Harvard Educational Review 31,* Winter, 1961.

12. Brunner, Jerome S. "Learning and Thinking," *Harvard Education Review,* Vol. 29 (1959), pp. 184–192.

13. ———. *The Process of Education.* Cambridge, Mass.: Harvard University Press, 1960.

14. ———. *Towards a Theory of Instruction.* Cambridge, Mass.: Harvard University Press, 1966.

15. Collins, P. W.: Some philosophical reflections on teaching and learning, *The Record 71:* Feb., 1970.

16. Combs, Arthur W. (ed.) *Perceiving Behaving and Becoming.* Washington, D.C.: Association for Supervision and Curriculum Development, 1962.

17. Cook, Mrya B. *The Come-Alive Classroom.* West Nyack, N.Y.: Parker Publishing Co., 1967.

18. Coppen, Helen. *Aids to Teaching and Learning.* New York: Pergamon Press, 1969.

19. Dale, Edgar. *Audio-Visual Methods in Teaching.* New York: Dryden Press, 1954.

20. Davis, Harold S. (ed.) *Instructional Media Center.* Bloomington: Indiana University Press, 1971.

21. DeCecco, John P. *The Psychology of Learning and Instruction: Educational Psychology.* Englewood Cliffs, N.J.: Prentice-Hall, Inc., 1968.

22. DeKieffer, Robert E. *Media Milestones in Teacher Training.* Washington, D.C.: Educational Media Council, 1970.

23. Dennison, D.: Operant conditioning principles applied to health instruction, *The Journal of School Health 40:* Sept., 1970.

24. Derell, G. R. "Creativity in Education." *Clearing House,* Vol. 38 (October 1963), pp. 67–69.

25. Eiss, Albert F., and Mary Harbeck. *Behavioral Objectives in the Affective Domain.* Washington, D.C.: National Science Teachers Assoc., 1969.

26. Engs, Ruth C., H. Eugene Barnes, and Molly Wantz. *Health Games Students Play: Creative Strategies for Health Education.* Dubuque, Iowa: Kendall/Hunt Publishing Co., 1975.

27. Erickson, Carolton W., and David H. Curl *Fundamentals of Teaching with Audiovisual Technology.* New York: Macmillan Publishing Co., Inc., 1972.

28. Esbensen, Thorwald. *Working with Individualized Instruction.* Belmont, Calif.: Fearon Publishers, 1968.

29. Evaul, Thomas W. "The Automated Tutor," *Journal of Health, Physical Education and Recreation,* Vol. 35, No. 3 (March 1964).

30. Fairfield, Roy P. (ed.). *Humanistic Frontiers in American Education.* Englewood Cliffs, N.J.: Prentice-Hall, Inc., 1971.

31. Fantini, Mario, and Gerald Weinstein. *Making Urban Schools Work.* New York: Holt, Rinehart and Winston, Inc., 1968.

32. Faunce, R. C.: Teaching and learning in the junior high school, San Francisco, 1961, Wadsworth Publishing Co., Inc.

33. Flanagan, J. C.: How instructional systems manage learning, *Nation's Schools 86:* Oct., 1970.

34. Fodor, John T., And Gus T. Davis, *Health Instruction: Theory and Application,* Philadelphia, Lea & Febiger, 1966.

35. *Framework for Health Instruction in California Public Schools.* Sacramento: California State Department of Education, 1970.

36. Frels, L.: Behavioral changes in students, *The Journal of School Health 39:* June, 1969.

37. Gall, M. D.: The use of questions in teaching, *Review of Educational Research 40:* Dec., 1970.

38. Garner, C. W.: Nonverbal communication and the teacher, *School and Society 98:* Oct., 1970.

39. Garrison Cecil. *1001 Ideas for the Classroom Teacher*. Berkeley, Calif.: McCutchan Publishing Co., 1968.

40. Glasser, William, *Schools Without Failure,* New York, Harper & Row, 1969.

41. Gregory, Thomas B. *Encounters with Teaching*. Englewood, Cliffs, N.J.: Prentice-Hall, Inc., 1972.

42. Gronlund, Norman E. *Stating Behavioral Objectives for Classroom Instruction*. New York: Macmillan Publishing Co., Inc., 1970.

43. ————. *Preparing Criterion-Referenced Tests for Classroom Instruction*. New York: Macmillan Publishing Co., Inc., 1973.

44. Gunselman, Marshall (ed.). *What Are We Learning About Learning Centers?* Oklahoma City, Okla.: Eagle Media, 1971.

45. Havighurst, Robert J. *Developmental Tasks and Education,* 3rd ed. New York: David McKay Co., Inc., 1972.

46. Haviland, David S. *Multi-Media Classroom Revisited*. Troy, N.Y.: Center for Architectural Research, Rensselaer Polytechnic Institute, 1971.

47. Heit, Phil. "The Berkeley Model," *Health Education*. Vol. 8, No. 1, January–February, 1977, pg. 2.

48. Herrscher, Barton R. *Implementing Individualized Instruction*. Houston, Tex.: ArChem Company Pub., 1971.

49. Hoyman, Howard S., Ed.D. "New Frontiers in Health Education," *The Journal of School Health*. Volume XLIII, September, 1973, No. 7.

50. Hurt, Tom. "Conventional Versus Systems and Linear Versus Intrinsic Models for Developing Self-Instructional Materials for Health Education," *Journal of School Health,* Volume XLII, No. 9 (November 1972), pp. 542–547.

51. Juhasz, A. M.: Characteristics essential to teachers in health education, *The Journal of School Health 41:* Jan., 1971.

52. Kilander, H. Frederick, *School Health Education,* Toronto, Canada, The Macmillan Company, 1968.

53. Kohl, Herbert R. *The Open Classroom*. New York: Vintage Books, 1969.

54. Koran, John J., Earl J. Montague, and Gene E. Hall. "How to . . . Use Behavioral Objectives." *National Science Teachers Association,* 1969.

55. Krathwohl, David R., et al. *Taxonomy of Educational Objectives. Handbook II: Affective Domain.* New York: David McKay Company, Inc., 1964.

56. Lussier, Richard R. "Health Education and Student Needs," *The Journal of School Health* (December 1972).

57. Mager, Robert F. *Developing Attitude Toward Learning*. Palo Alto, Calif.: Fearon Publishers, 1968.

58. ————. *Preparing Instructional Objectives*. Palo Alto, Calif.: Fearon Publishing, 1962.

59. Mayshark, Cyrus, and Roy Foster, *Health Education in Secondary Schools,* St. Louis, C. V. Mosby, 1972.

60. Means, Richard K. *Methodology in Education*. Columbus, Ohio: Charles E. Merrill Publishing Co., 1968.

61. Metcalf, Lawrence (ed.). *Values Education: Rational Strategies and Procedures*. Washington, D.C.: NEA, 1971.

62. Meyers, R. E., and E. P. Torrance. "Can Teachers Encourage Creative Thinking?" *Education Leadership* (December 1961), pp. 156–159.

63. Miel, A. (ed.). *Creativity in Teaching: Invitations and Instances*. San Francisco: Wadsworth Publishing Company, 1961.

64. Miller, Richard. *Selecting New Aids to Teaching*. Washington, D.C.: Association for Supervision and Curriculum Development, 1971.

65. Montague, Earl J., and David P. Butts. "Behavioral Objectives." *The Science Teacher,* 35:33–35; March 1968.

66. Murphy, Judith, and Ronald Gross. *Learning by Television*. New York: Fund for the Advancement of Education, 1966.

67. Nelson, Leslie W. *Instructional Aids: How to Make Use of Them*. Dubuque, Iowa: Wm. C. Brown Company Publishers, 1970.

68. Nemir, Alma and Schaller, Warren E. *The School Health Program*. Philadelphia: W. B. Saunders Company, 1975.

69. New Mexico, Los Alamos. Los Alamos Schools. *Living Now, Transitional Health-Education, Curriculum Guide. Grades 7-12.*

70. New York, Albany: *Suggested Outlines for the Development of Courses of Study in Health Education for Junior and Senior High Schools.* New York State Department of Education, 1970.

71. Otto, Herbert. *Group Methods Designed to Actualize Human Potential.* Chicago: Stone-Brandel, 1967.

72. Parker, J. Cecil, and Louis J. Rubin. *Process as Content: Curriculum Design and the Application of Knowledge.* Skokie, Ill.: Rand McNally & Co., 1966.

73. Pennsylvania, Philadelphia. The School District of Philadelphia. *Health Education, Grades 10-11-12. (Senior High School).* 1968, 218 pp.

74. Popham, W. James, and Eva Baker. *Establishing Instructional Goals.* Englewood Cliffs, N.J.: Prentice-Hall, Inc., 1970.

75. ———. *Systematic Instruction.* Englewood Cliffs, N.J.: Prentice-Hall, Inc., 1970.

76. Postman, Neil, and Charles Weingartner, *Teaching as a Subversive Activity,* New York, Delacorte Press, 1969.

77. Prentice, Marjorie. "Systematic Instruction," *Educational Leadership,* Vol. 30, No. 8 (May 1973), pp. 706-709.

78. Rash, J. Keogh. *The Health Education Curriculum,* Bloomington, Ind., Indiana University Press, 1965.

79. Raths, Louis E., Merrill Harmin, and Sidney B. Simon. *Values and Teaching: Working with Values in the Classroom.* Columbus, Ohio: Charles E. Merrill Publishing Co., 1966.

80. Read, Donald A., and Walter H. Greene, *Creative Teaching in Health,* New York, Macmillan, 1971.

81. Rogers, Carl. *Freedom to Learn.* Columbus, Ohio: Charles E. Merrill Publishing Co., 1969.

82. Saxe, Richard W. *Schools Don't Change.* New York: Philosophical Library, 1967.

83. School Health Education Study, *Health Education: A Conceptual Approach to Curriculum Design,* St. Paul, Minn., 3M Education Press, 1967.

84. Schramm, Wilbur. *Programmed Instruction Today and Tomorrow.* New York: Fund for the Advancement of Education, 1962.

85. Schrank, Jeffrey. *Teaching Human Beings: 101 Subversive Activities for the Classroom.* Boston: Beacon Press, 1972.

86. Schultz, Morton J. *The Teacher and Overhead Projection.* Englewood Cliffs, N.J.: Prentice-Hall, Inc., 1965.

87. Simon, Sidney B., Leland W. Howe, and Howard Kirschenbaum. *Value Clarification: A Handbook of Practical Strategies for Teachers and Students.* New York: Hart Publishing Co., Inc., 1972.

88. Sleet, David A., "The Use of Games and Simulations in Health Instruction," *California School Health,* Vol. 9, January 1975, pp. 11-14.

89. Sleet, David A., and R. Stadsklev, "Annotated Bibliography of Simulation/Games in Health Education," *Health Education Monographs,* Vol. 5(1), Spring 1977.

90. Sorochan, Walter. *Personal Health Appraisal,* New York, John Wiley & Sons, 1976.

91. Stevens, John O. *Awareness: Exploring, Experimenting, Experiencing.* Lafayette, Calif.: Real People Press, 1971.

92. Tanzman, Jack. *Using Instructional Media Effectively.* West Nyack, N.Y.: Parker Publishing Co., 1971.

93. Taylor, Calvin W., and Frank E. Williams (ed.). *Instructional Media and Creativity.* New York: John Wiley & Sons, Inc., 1966.

94. Tennessee, Chattanooga. Hamilton County Department of Education. *Nutrition Education Guide Grades 7-12.*

95. Thelen, Herbert A. *Education and the Human Quest.* Chicago: The University of Chicago Press, 1972.

96. Tickton, Sidney. *To Improve Learning.* New York: R. R. Bowker Co., 1970.

97. Virginia, Norfolk. Norfolk City Schools. *Building Healthier Youth.* Free.

98. West Virginia, Charleston. Kanawha County Schools. *Health Education Units for Grade 7.* 1971.

99. Willgoose, Carl, *Health Teaching in Secondary Schools,* Philadelphia, W. B. Saunders, 1977.

100. *WOW Health Education Curriculum Guide* (Washington State Department of Public Instruction, Olympia; Wisconsin State Department of Public Instruction, Madison; Oregon State Department of Education, Salem) 1975.

Testing and Evaluation

1. Ahmann, J. S., and Marvin D. Glock. *Evaluating Pupil Growth,* 2nd ed. Boston: Allyn & Bacon, Inc., 1963.

2. Burton, William, et al. *Education for Effective Thinking.* New York: Appleton-Century-Crofts, 1960.

3. Cheffers, John T. F., Edmund J. Amidon, and Ken D. Rodgers. *Interaction Analysis: An Application to Nonverbal Activity,* Minneapolis: Association for Productive Teaching, 1974.

4. Colebank, Albert D. *Health Behavior Inventory: Junior High,* Monterey, California: California Test Bureau, Revised. (There are 24 health attitude items, 25 health behavior items, and 50 health knowledge items, for a total of 100 multiple choice questions.)

5. *Cooperative Health Education Test* (AAHPER), 1972. Educational Testing Service, Box 999, Princeton, New Jersey 08540. (Junior High)

6. Curtis, Paul Ramsey. "Testing in Tomorrow's Schools," *Educational Leadership,* Vol. 17 (May 1960).

7. Daly, William C. "Test Scores: Fragment of a Picture," *Elementary School Journal,* Vol. 60 (October 1959).

8. Educational Testing Service. *Making the Classroom Test: A Guide for Teachers.* Princeton, N.J.: Educational Testing Service, 1961.

9. Fast-Tyson *Health Knowledge Test,* Kirksville, Missouri, 1975. Available from Charles G. Fast, c/o Northeast Missouri State University 63501. (Senior High)

10. Green, Lawrence. Heit, Phil. Iverson, Donald. Kolbe, Lloyd. and Kreuter, Marshall. "The School Health Curriculum Project: Its Theory Measurement and Implementation Experience," *Health Education Quarterly,* Spring, 1980.

11. Holt, John. *How Children Fail.* New York: Dell Publishing Co., Inc., 1964.

12. Johns, Edward B., Juhnke, Warren L. and Pollock, Marion B. *Health Behavior Inventory,* Los Angeles, California: Tinnon-Brown Publishing Company, 1974. (Senior High)

13. Karmel, Louis. *Measurement and Evaluation in the Schools.* New York: Macmillan Publishing Co., Inc., 1970.

14. Kilander, H. Frederick. *Information Test on the Biological Aspects of Human Reproduction,* 3rd edition, Staten Island, New York, 1968. (A 33-item multiple choice test—junior high).

15. Kilander, H. Frederick. *Information on Drugs and Drug Abuse,* 3rd edition, Staten Island, New York. Revised. (25-question multiple choice—junior high).

16. Kilander, H. Frederick. *Information Test on Smoking and Health,* Staten Island, New York. Revised. (A 25-item test for junior high school through college levels. Single copies available from Dr. Glenn Leach at Wagner College).

17. Kilander, H. Frederick. *Kilander Health Knowledge Test,* 7th edition, Staten Island, New York: Dr. Glenn Leach, Wagner College. Revised. (A high school instrument of 100 multiple choice questions).

18. Kilander, H. Frederick. *Nutrition Information Test,* 5th edition, Staten Island, New York, 1968. (A 33-item multiple choice test with norms set up from junior high school to college. Also available from Dr. Leach).

19. Kirschenbaum, Howard, et al. *Wad-Ja-Get?* New York: Hart Publishing Co., Inc., 1971.

20. LeMaistre, E. Harold, and Pollock, Marion B. *Health Behavior Inventory: Senior High,* Monterey, California: California Test Bureau, Revised. (75 multiple choice items).

21. McHugh, Gelolo. *Sex Knowledge Inventory,* rev., Durham, N.C.: Family Life Publications, Inc., 1970. (High School)

22. Morgan, H. Gerthon. "What Is Effective Evaluation," *NEA Journal*, Vol. 48 (November 1959).

23. Nelson, Clarence. *Measurement and Evaluation in the Classroom.* New York: Macmillan Publishing Co., Inc., 1970.

24. Pollock, Marion B. *Mood Altering Substances: A Behavior Inventory,* Los Angeles, California: Tinnon-Brown Publishing Company, 1968. (75 miltiple choice items).

25. Schwartz, William F. *Achievement Test on Syphillis and Gonorrhea,* Durham, N.C.: Family Life Publications, Inc., Revised. (This is the original 25-item venereal disease test set up for programmed instruction, published by the American Alliance for Health, Physical Education and Recreation.)

26. Sanders, Norris M. *Classroom Questions.* New York: Harper & Row, Publishers, Inc., 1966.

27. Secarea-Olsen. *Evaluation Instrument for Appraising Health Knowledge of Seventh Grade Students,* Champaign, Illinois, 1974. Available from Larry K. Olsen, Department of Health and Safety, University of Illinois 61820.

28. Solleder, Marion K. "Evaluation in the Cognitive Domain," *Journal of School Health,* 42:16-20, January, 1972.

29. Solleder, Marion K. *Evaluation Instruments in Health Education,* Revised. Washington, D.C.: American Alliance for Health, Physical Education and Recreation.

30. Thompson, Clem W. *Thompson Smoking and Tobacco Knowledge Test,* rev., Mankato State College, Mankato, Minn. (Junior High)

31. Torrance, E. Paul. *Education and the Creative Potential.* Minneapolis: University of Minnesota Press, 1963.

32. Tuthill, Robert W., et al., "Evaluating a School Health Program Focused on High Absence Pupils: A Research Design," *American Journal of Public Health,* January 1972, pp. 40-42.

33. Veenker, Harold C. *Health Knowledge Test for the Seventh Grade,* Lafayette, Indiana: Purdue University. Revised.

34. Vincent, Raymond J. "New Scale for Measuring Attitudes,"*School Health Review,* 6:19-21, March/April, 1974.

35. Vincent, Raymond J. "Selected Instructional and Behavioral Objectives for a Tenth Grade Drug Education Program," *The Journal of School Health* (June 1971), pp. 310-313.

36. Yarber, William A. "A Comparison of the Relationship of the Grade Contract and Traditional Grading Methods to Changes in Knowledge and Attitude," *Journal of School Health,* 44:395-399, September, 1974.

Mental Health and Self-Concept

1. Adams, James F., "Adolescents' Identification of Personal and National Problems," *Adolescence,* Fall 1966, pp. 240-250.

2. Allensmith, Wesley, and George W. Goethals. *The Role of the Schools in Mental Health.* New York: Basic Books, Inc., Publishers, 1961.

3. Alschuler, Alfred (ed.). "New Directions in Psychological Education," *Educational Opportunities Forum.* New York State Department of Education, Albany, N.Y., June 1969.

4. Baker, Frank. "From Community Mental Health to Human Service Ideology," *American Journal of Public Health,* June 1974, pp. 576-581.

5. Beck, Aaron T., et al., "Classificiation of Suicidal Behaviors," *Archives of General Psychiatry,* July 1976, pp. 835-837.

6. Berkman, Paul L. "Life Stress and Psychological Well-being; A Replication of Langner's Analysis in the Midtown Manhattan Study," *Journal of Health and Social Behavior,* March 1971, pp. 35-45.

7. Bernard, Harold W., *Mental Health in the Classroom,* New York, McGraw-Hill, 1970.

8. Blackham, Garth J., *The Deviant Child in the Classroom,* Belmont, California: Wadsworth, 1967.

9. Blum, Lucille Hollander, "The Discotheque and the Phenomenon of Alone-Togetherness," *Adolescence,* Winter 1966-67, pp. 351-366.

10. Brill, Norman Q., "Social Problems and Psychiatric Illness," *Military Medicine,* February 1975, pp. 98-107.

11. Brenner, Meyer Harvey, *Mental Illness and the Economy,* Cambridge, Mass., Harvard University Press, 1973.

12. Brocher, Tobias, "Work, Stress and Human Values," paper presented at the American Public Health Association, November 1975.

13. Cahn, Lorynne, and Robert Petersen. "Education and Mental Health: A Need for Interdisciplinary Involvement," *Journal of School Health,* Vol. XLIII, No. 4 (April 1973), pp. 218-220.

14. Cameron, Norman A. *Personality Development and Psychopathology.* Boston: Houghton Mifflin Company, 1963.

15. Carroll, Jerome F. X., "Understanding Adolescent Needs," *Adolescence,* 3:12, Winter 1968/69, pp. 380-394.

16. Clarke, Kenneth. "The Relevance Perspective in Drug Education," *School Health Review,* Vol. 3, No. 2 (March-April 1972), pp. 5-7.

17. Coelho, George, David A. Hamburg, and John E. Adams, *Coping and Adaptation,* New York, Basic Books, 1974.

18. Cole, Luella, *Psychology of Adolescence,* New York, Holt, Rinehart and Winston, 1959.

19. Coleman, James C., *Personality Dynamics and Effective Behavior,* Chicago, Scott, Foresman, 1960.

20. Covi, Lindo, et al., "Drug and Psychotherapy Interactions in Depression," *American Journal of Psychiatry,* May, 1976, pp. 502-508.

21. Donnelly, John, "The Generation Gap," *Mental Health Talks-1969.* Hartford, Conn.: Connecticut Mutual Life, 1969, pp. 3-10.

22. Draper, Edgar, "A Developmental Theory of Suicide," *Comprehensive Psychiatry,* January-February 1976, 63-80.

23. Dressler, David, James M. Donovan, and Ruth A. Geller, "Life Stress and Emotional Crisis—The Idiosyncratic Interpretation of Life Events," *Comprehensive Psychiatry,* July-August 1976, pp. 549-558.

24. Dubos, Rene, *Mirage of Health,* Garden City, Doubleday (Anchor Books), 1961.

25. Dubos, Rene, *So Human an Animal,* New York, Scribner, 1968.

26. Dunham, H. Warren, "Society, Culture and Mental Disorder," *Archives of General Psychiatry,* February 1976, pp. 147-156.

27. Dunn, H. L., *High Level Wellness,* Washington, D.C., Mt. Vernon, 1961.

28. Ellis, Albert. "Teaching Emotional Education in the Classroom," *School Health Review* (November 1969).

29. Erikson, Erik. *Identity, Youth and Crisis,* New York, W. W. Norton, 1968.

30. Foulds, G. A., and A. Bedford, "The Relationship Between Anxiety-Depression and the Neuroses," *British Journal of Psychiatry,* 128, 1976, pp. 166-168.

31. Frisk, M., et al., "Psychological Problems in Adolescents Showing Advanced or Delayed Physical Maturation," *Adolescence,* 1:2, Summer, 1966, pp. 126-140.

32. Ginott, Haim, *Between Parent and Teenager.* New York, MacMillan, 1969.

33. Ginzberg, Eli, *Technology and Social Change,* New York, Columbia University Press, 1964.

34. Glasser, William, *Schools Without Failure,* New York, Harper & Row, 1969.

35. Hauser, Stuart T., "The Content and Structure of Adolescent Self-Images," *Archives of General Psychiatry,* January 1976, pp. 27-32.

36. *Health Curriculum Guide in Mental and Social Health.* Fall River, Mass.: Fall River School Department, 1971.

37. Heath, Douglas H. *Humanizing Schools.* New York: Hayden Book Company, Inc., 1971.

38. Hodge, James R., "How Patients Get Better Through Psychiatry," *Medical Times,* January 1976, pp. 83-86.

39. Hountras, Peter T., *Mental Hygiene,* Columbus, Charles E. Merrill, 1961.

40. James, Muriel, and Dorothy Jongeward. *Born to Win.* Reading, Mass.: Addison-Wesley Publishing Co., Inc., 1971.

41. Johnson, David W., *Reaching Out,* Englewood Cliffs, N.J., Prentice-Hall, 1972.

42. Joint Commission on Mental Illness and Health. *Action for Mental Health.* New York: Basic Books, Inc., Publishers, 1961.

43. Jones, Richard M. *Fantasy and Feeling in Education.* New York: New York University Press, 1968.

44. Jourard, Sidney M. *Healthy Personality.* New York: Macmillan Publishing Co., Inc., 1974.

45. Kaplan, Louis. *Education and Mental Health.* New York: Harper & Row Publishers, Inc., 1971.

46. Kaplan, Louis, *Mental Health and Human Relations in Education,* New York, Harper & Row, 1959.

47. Kiev, Ari, "Cluster Analysis Profiles of Suicide Attempters," *American Journal of Psychiatry,* February 1976, pp. 150-153.

48. Konopka, Gisela, "Mental Depression a Serious Disease," *San Diego Union,* October 6, 1975.

49. Kovacs, Maria, Aaron T. Beck, and Arlene Weissman, "The Communication of Suicidal Intent," *Archives of General Psychiatry,* February 1976.

50. Lawrence, T.: An evaluation of the emotional health of secondary school pupils, *The Journal of School Health 35:* Sept., 1965.

51. Leonard, George. *Education and Ecstasy.* New York: Delta Books, 1968.

52. Lowenfield, Viktor. *Creative and Mental Growth,* 6th ed. New York: Macmillan Publishing Co., Inc., 1975.

53. Lowental, Uri, "Suicide—The Other Side," *Archives of General Psychiatry,* July 1976, pp. 838-842.

54. Luft, Joseph. *Group Processes: An Introduction to Group Dynamics.* Palo Alto, Calif.: National Press Books, 1970.

55. Lyon, Harold C., Jr., *Learning to Feel—Feeling to Learn.* Columbus, Ohio: Charles E. Merrill Publishing Co., 1971.

56. MacMillan, Donald L. *Behavior Modification in Education.* New York: Macmillan Publishing Co., Inc., 1973.

57. Mantz, Genelle K. "Can Mental Health Be Taught," *Journal of School Health,* Vol. XLII, No. 7 (September 1972), pp 398-399.

58. Maslow, Abraham H. *Motivation and Personality.* New York: Harper & Row, Publishers, Inc., 1970.

59. Maslow, Abraham H., *Toward a Psychology of Being,* New York, Van Nostrand Reinhold, 1968.

60. May, Rollo, *Man's Search for Himself,* New York, W. W. Norton, 1953.

61. Mead, Margaret, "Mental Health in our Changing Culture," *Mental Hygiene,* Summer, 1972, pp. 6-81.

62. "Mental Health in the Classroom," *The Journal of School Health,* Vol, XXVIII, No. 5a (May 1968, special issue).

63. Mishara, Brian L., Harvey A. Baker, and Janju T. Mishara, "The Frequency of Suicide Attempts: A Retrospective Approach Applied to College Students," *American Journal of Psychiatry,* July 1976, pp. 841-843.

64. Morgan, Jack C., "Adolescent Problems and the Mooney Problem Check List," *Adolescence,* Spring 1969, pp. 111-125.

65. Musa, Kathleen E., and Mary E. Roach, "Adolescent Appearance and Self-Concept," Adolescence, 8:31, Fall 1973, pp. 385-394.

66. Muuss, Rolf E., "Jean Piaget's Cognitive Theory of Adolescent Development," *Adolescence,* 2:6, Summer 1967, pp. 285-310.

67. Myers, Jerome K., et al., "Life Events and Mental Status: A Longitudinal Study," *Journal of Health and Social Behavior,* December 1972, pp. 398-405.

68. Palmore, Erdman, and Clark Luikart, "Health and Social Factors Related to Life Satisfaction," *Journal of Health and Social Behavior,* March 1972, pp. 68-80.

69. Rahe, Richard, H., et al., "Psychosocial Predictors of Illness Behavior and Failure in Stressful Training," *Journal of Health and Social Behavior,* December 1972, pp. 393-397.

70. Ramsdell, Les C., "An analysis of the health interests and needs of West Virginia high school students— a report," *The Journal of School Health,* October 1972, pp. 477-480.

71. Renshaw, Domeena C., "Depression in the 1970's," *Diseases of the Nervous System,* June, July 1973, pp. 241-245.

72. Ridenour, Nina, *Mental Health Education,* New York, Mental Health Materials Center, 1969.

73. Ringness, Thomas A., *Mental Health in the Schools,* New York, Random House, 1968.

74. Rogers, Carl R., *On Becoming a Person,* Boston, Houghton Mifflin, 1961.

75. Romey, William D. *Risk-Trust-Love: Learning in a Humane Environment.* Columbus, Ohio: Charles E. Merrill Publishing Co., 1972.

76. Rubin, Eliz., "A Psycho-educational Model for School Mental Health Planning," *The Journal of School Health,* November 1970, pp. 489-493.

77. Rucker, W. Ray, V. Clyde Arnspiger, and Arthur J. Brodbeck, *Human Values in Education,* Dubuque, Iowa, Wm. C. Brown Company, 1969.

78. Rutter, Michael, et al., "Adolescent Turmoil: Fact or Fiction?" *Journal of Child Psychology and Psychiatry,* 17, 1976, pp. 35-56.

79. Salzman, Leon, "Adolescence: Epoch or Disease?" *Adolescence,* 8:30, Summer 1973, pp. 247-256.

80. Selye, Hans, *The Stress of Life,* New York, McGraw-Hill, 1959.

81. Sieg, Ann, "Why Adolescence Occurs," *Adolescence,* 6:23, Fall 1971, pp. 337-348.

82. Teper, Lynn. "Emotional Education," *School Health Review,* Vol. 3, No. 2 (March-April 1972), p. 24.

83. ———. "Role Playing as a Tool in Mental Health Education," *School Health Review* (February 1971), p. 31.

84. Thomas, Alexander, and Stella Chess, "Evolution of Behavior Disorders into Adolescence," *American Journal of Psychiatry,* May 1976, pp. 539-542.

85. Thorpe, Louis. *The Psychology of Mental Health.* New York: The Ronald Press Company, 1960.

86. Toffler, Alvin, *Future Shock,* New York, Random House, 1970.

87. Toolan, James M. "Depression in Children and Adolescents," in Gerald Caplan and Serge Lebovinf, *Adolescence: Psychosocial Perspectives,* New York: Basic Books, 1969, pp. 264-269.

88. Vaillant, George E. "Natural History of Male Psychological Health," *Archives of General Psychiatry,* May, 1976, pp. 535-545.

89. Weiner, Irving B. *Psychological Disturbance in Adolescence.* New York, Wiley Interscience, 1970.

90. Weiner, Irving B., and Andrew C. Del Gaudio, "Psychopathology in Adolescence," *Archives in General Psychiatry,* February 1976, pp. 187-193.

Adolescent Behavior

1. Adams. Understanding Adolescence. Current Developments in Adolescent Psychology. 3rd ed. Boston, Allyn & Bacon, 1976.

2. Caplan, Gerald and Serge Levocivi, editors, *Adolescence: Psychosocial Perspectives,* New York, Basic Books, 1969.

3. Cole, Luella, Psychology of Adolescence, New York, Holt, Rinehart and Winston, 1959.

4. Conger. Adolescence and Youth. Psychological Development in a Changing World. 2nd ed. New York, Harper and Row, 1977.

5. Fine, Louis L., M.D. *What's A Normal Adolescent? A Guide for the Assessment of Adolescent Behavior.* Clinical Pediatrics, Vol. 12:1, January 1973.

6. Gallager, J. Rosswell. *The Adolescent's Personality: Implications for Treatment.* Rhode Island Medical Journal 38:491, September 1955.

7. Gallager, J. Rosswell & Harris, Herbert J. *Emotional Problems of Adolescents.* New York, Oxford University Press, 1976.

8. Griffra, Mary, "Demystifying Adolescent Behavior," *American Journal of Nursing,* Volume 75, No. 10, October 1975, pp. 1724-1727.

9. Grinder. Adolescence. 2nd ed. New York, John Wiley, 1978.

10. Josselyn, Irene. *The Adolescent and His World.* New York, Family Service Assoc., 1972.

11. Miller, Derek. *Adolescence: Psychology, Psychopathology and Psychotherapy.* New York, Jason Aronson, 1974.

12. Rodgers, Dorothy, *The Psychology of Adolescence,* Englewood Cliffs, N.J., Prentice-Hall, 1972.

13. Seligman, Roslyn, M.D. and Others. "The Effect of Earlier Parental Loss in Adolescence," *Archives of General Psychiatry,* Volume 31, October, 1974, pp. 475-479.

14. Semmens & Krantz. The Adolescent Experience. A Counseling Guide to Social and Sexual Behavior. London, Macmillan-Collier, 1970. (PL)

Adolescence: Physical Growth and Development

1. Anderson, Frances, R.N., "The developmental experience of adolescence," *Issues in Comprehensive Pediatric Nursing,* May/June, 1976, pp. 1-16, McGraw-Hill, New York.

2. Dwyer, Johanna, and Jean Mayer, "Psychological Effects of Variations in Physical Appearance During Adolescence," *Adolescence,* 3:12, Winter 1968/69, pp. 353-380.

3. Frisch, Rose, and McArthur, Janet, "Menstrual Cycles: Fatness as a Determinant of Minimum Weight for Height Necessary for Their Maintenance or Onset," *Science,* Volume 185, September 1974, pp. 949-951.

4. Hettinger, Theodore, *Physiology of Strength,* Springfield, Mass., Charles C. Thomas, 1961.

5. Hurlock, Elizabeth B., *Adolescent Development,* New York, McGraw-Hill, 1955.

6. Katchadourian, Herant. *The Biology of Adolescence.* W. H. Freeman and Company, San Francisco, 1977.

7. Kilpatrick, W. Kirk, "McLuhan: Implications for Adolescence," *Adolescence,* 6:22, Summer 1971, pp. 235-258.

8. Klein, Karl K., *The Knees: Growth-Development and Activity Influences,* Greeley, Colo., All-American Productions and Publications, 1967.

9. Konopka, Gisela, "Requirements for Healthy Development of Adolescent Youth," *Adolescence,* 8:31, Fall, 1973, pp. 291-316.

10. Reiter, Edward, M.D. and Root, Allen, M.D., "Hormonal Changes of Adolescence," *Medical Clinics of North America,* Volume 59, No. 6, November 1975, pp. 1289-1303.

11. Reiter, Edward, M.D., and Root, Allen, M.D., "Physical Growth and Development During Puberty," *Medical Clinics of North America,* Volume 59, No. 6, November 1975, pp. 1305-1317.

12. Root, Allen, MD. "Endocrinology of Puberty: Normal Sexual Maturation," *The Journal of Pediatrics,* Volume 83, No. 1, July 1973, pp. 1-19.

13. Tanner, J. M., *Growth at Adolescence,* Oxford, England, Blackwell Scientific Publications, 1962.

14. Tichy, Anna, and Malasanos, Lois, "The Physiological Role of Hormones in Puberty," *The American Journal of Maternal and Child Nursing,* November/December 1976, pp. 384-388.

Toward High Level Wellness

1. Ardell, Donald B. *High Level Wellness—An Alternative to Doctors, Drugs and Disease.* Rodale Press, 1977.

2. Benson, Herbert, *The Mind/Body Effect.* New York: Simon and Schuster, 1979.

3. Benson, Herbert. *The Relaxation Response.* New York: Avon, 1975.

4. Bloomfield, Harold H., M.D. and Robert B. Kory. *The Holistic Way to Health and Happiness.* New York: Simon and Schuster, 1978.

5. Cooper, Cary L., and Roy Payne, eds. *Stress at Work.* New York: John Wiley and Sons. 1978.

6. Cooper, Kenneth. *The New Aerobics.* New York: Bantam, 1977.

7. Fixx, James E. *The Complete Book of Running.* New York: Random House, 1977.

8. Friedman, Meyer and Roger H. Rosenman. *Type A Behavior and Your Heart.* New York: Alfred A. Knopf, 1974.

9. Green, Alyce and Elmer. *Beyond Biofeedback.* Meninger Foundation.

10. Getchell, Bud, *Physical Fitness: A Way of Life,* New York, John Wiley and Sons, 1976, p. 224.

11. Keck, Bob. *The Spirit of Synergy.* Abingdon, 1978.

12. Leonard, George, "The Holistic Health Revolution," *New West.* May 10, 1976, pp. 40-49.

13. Lynch, James J. *The Broken Heart: The Medical Consequences of Loneliness.* New York: Basic Books, 1977.

14. Maness, William. "What Do You Really Know About Exercise?" *Today's Health,* 53:14-17, November, 1975.

15. McCamy, John, M.D. and James Presley. *Human Life Styling— Keeping Whole in the Twentieth Century.* New York: Harper and Row, 1975.

16. Morehouse, Laurence E., and Augustus T. Miller, *Physiology of Exercise,* Saint Louis, C. V. Mosby, 1963.

17. Newman, Mildred and Bernard Berkowitz. *How to Be Your Own Best Friend.* New York: Ballantine, 1971.

18. Pelletier, Kenneth R. *Mind as Healer, Mind as Slayer: A Holistic Approach to Preventing Stress Disorders.* New York: Delta, 1977.

19. Rarick, Lawrence G., *Physical Activity.* New York, Academic Press, 1973.

20. Sorochan, Walter D., *Personal Health Appraisal.* New York, John Wiley and Sons, Inc., 1976.

21. Vickery, Donald M. *Life Plan for Your Health.* Reading, Massachusetts: Addison Wesley, 1978.

22. Williams, Robert L. and James D. Long. *Toward a Self-Managed Life Style,* 2nd ed. Boston: Houghton Mifflin Co., 1979.

Nutrition

1. Bagert, L. Jean, George M. Briggs, and Doris Howes Galloway, *Nutrition and Physical Fitness,* Philadelphia, W. B. Sanders, 1966.

2. Berland, Theodore, "Rating the Diets," Skokie, Ill., *Consumer Guide,* 1974.

3. Cooper, Lenna, and Helen S. Mitchell, *Nutrition in Health and Disease,* Philadelphia, J. B. Lippincott, 1963.

4. Fiedler, Dolores E., Dorothea M. Lang, and Judy M. Carlson, "Pathology in the Healthy Female Teenager," *American Journal of Public Health,* 63:962-965, November 1973.

5. Frankle, Reva and F. K. Heussentamin. "Food Zealotry and Youth," *American Journal of Public Health,* 64:11-16, January, 1974.

6. Jones, Kenneth L., Louis W. Shainberg, and Curtis O. Byer, *Foods, Diet, and Nutrition,* San Francisco, Canfield Press, 1975.

7. LaSalle, Dorothy, and Gladys Geer, *Health Instruction for Today's Schools,* Englewood Cliffs, N.J., Prentice-Hall, 1963.

8. Lewin, Robert. "Starved Brains: New Research on Hunger's Damage," *Psychology Today,* 9:29-34, September, 1975.

9. Mayer, Jean. *A Diet for Living,* New York: McKay, 1975.

10. Mayer, Jean. "Fat Babies Grow into Fat People," *Family Health,* 60:24-27, March 1973.

11. Mayer, Jean, "Introduction: Obesity," *Journal of Postgraduate Medicine,* 51:66, May 1972.

12. Mayer, Jean, *Overweight: Causes, Cost and Control,* Englewood Cliffs, N.J., Prentice-Hall, 1968.

13. Peckos, Penelope, R. D., "The Treatment of Adolescent Obesity," *Issues in Comprehensive Pediatric Nursing,* May/June, 1976, pp. 17-30, McGraw-Hill, Inc., New York.

14. Schwartz, Nancy E., "Nutritional Knowledge, Attitudes, and Practices of High School Graduates," *Research,* 66:29-31, January 1975.

15. "The State of Nutrition Today," *FDA Consumer,* 7:13-17, November, 1973.

16. Stare, Frederick J. and Johanna Dwyer, "An Eye to the Future: Health Eating for Teenagers," *Journal of School Health,* 39:595-599, November 1969.

17. U.S. Senate (Select Committee on Nutrition and Human Needs). *Nutrition and Health: an Evaluation of Nutritional Surveillance in the United States.* Washington, D.C. Government Printing Office.

Drugs, Alcohol and Tobacco

1. Berland, Theodore. "Should Children Be Taught to Drink," *Today's Health,* Vol. 47, No. 2 (February 1969), pp. 46-49.

2. Bland, Hester Beth, and Rugh R. Shibuga. "Drug Education and the Curriculum," *Journal of School Health,* Vol. XLII, No. 6 (June 1972).

3. Bland, H. B.: "Problems related to teaching about drugs, *The Journal of School Health 39:* Feb. 1969.

4. Bowen, O. R.: The Medicolegal conflict in drug usage, *The Journal of School Health 39:* March, 1969.

5. Brecher, Edward M. *Licit and Illicit Drugs,* Boston: Little, Brown and Company, 1972.

6. Burgess, Louise, *Alcohol and Your Health,* Los Angeles, Charles Publishing, 1973.

7. Cahalan, Don, and Ira H. Cisin. "American Drinking Practices: Summary of Findings from a National Probability Sample," *Quarterly Journal of Studies on Alcohol,* Vol. 29 (March 1968), pp. 130-151.

8. ———, and Robin Room. "Problem Drinking Among American Men Aged 21-59," *American Journal of Public Health,* Vol. 62, No. 11 (November 1972), pp. 1472-1482.

9. Carrol, Charles, *Alcohol: Use, Nonuse and Abuse,* Dubuque, Iowa, Wm. C. Brown, 1975.

10. Cherry, Nicola, and Kathy Kiernan, "Personality scores and smoking behavior," *British Journal of Preventive Social Medicine,* 30, 1976, pp. 123-131.

11. Clarke, Kenneth. "The Relevance Perspective in Drug Education," *School Health Review,* Vol. 3, No. 2 (March-April 1972), pp. 5-7.

12. Cornacchia, Harold, David Bentel, and David Smith, *Drugs in the Classroom: A Conceptual Model for School Programs,* St. Louis, C. V. Mosby, 1973.

13. Daniel, Ralph. "Alcohol Education vs. Alcoholism Education," *Journal of Alcohol Education,* Vol. 13, No. 1 (Spring 1967), pp. 44-45.

14. deLone, Richard H. "The Ups and Downs of Drug-Abuse Education," *Saturday Review of Education* (November 11, 1972).

15. Demone, Harold W. "Implications from Research on Adolescent Drinking," *Alcohol Education: Conference Proceedings.* Washington, D.C.: U.S. Department of Health, Education, and Welfare (March 1966), pp. 16-19.

16. Diehl, Harold S. *Tobacco and Your Health.* New York: McGraw-Hill Book Company, 1969.

17. Farnsworth, Dana L. "Drug Use for Pleasure: A Complex Social Problem," *Journal of School Health,* Vol. XLIII, No. 3 (March 1973), pp. 153-158.

18. Fisher, Gray, and Irma Strantz. "An Ecosystems Approach to the Study of Dangerous Drug Use and Abuse with Special Reference to the Marijuana Issue," *American Journal of Public Health,* Vol. 62, No. 10 (October 1972), pp. 1407-1414.

19. Fort, Joel, *Alcohol: Our Biggest Drug Problem,* New York, McGraw-Hill 1973.

20. Fox, Vernelie. "Alcoholism In Adolescents," *Journal of School Health,* Vol. XLII, No. 1 (January 1973), pp. 32-35.

21. Fulton, Gere B. "Drug Abuse Education—Tell It Like It Is," *School Health Review,* Vol. 3, No. 4 (July-August 1972), pp. 33-37.

22. Girdano, Dorothy and Daniel Girdano, *Drugs—A Factual Account,* Reading, Mass., Addision-Wesley, 1976.

23. Globetti, Gerald, "Social Adjustment of High School Students and Problem Drinking," *Journal of Alcohol Education,* Vol. 13, No. 2 (Fall 1967), pp. 21-39.

24. Hanson, David J. "Social Norms and Drinking Behavior: Implication for Alcohol and Drug Education," *Journal of Alcohol and Drug Education,* Vol. 18, No. 2 (Winter 1973), pp. 18-24.

25. Hauck, John H., "Addiction: Food, Alcohol and Drugs," *Mental Health Talks— 1969,* Hartford, Conn.: Connecticut Mutual Life, 1969, pp. 12-19.

26. Henke, Lorraine J. "Student-to-Student Teaching About Tobacco Smoking," *School Health Review,* Vol. 4, No. 1 (January-February 1973), pp. 17-18.

27. Johnson, Kit G. "Survey of Adolescent Drug Use I—Sex and Grade Distribution," *American Journal of Public Health,* Vol. 61, No. 12 (December 1971), pp. 2418-2431.

28. ———, et al. "Survey of Adolescent Drug Use II Social and Environmental Factors," *American Journal of Public Health,* Vol. 62, No. 2 (February 1972), pp. 164-166.

29. Jones, Kenneth L., Louis W. Shainberg, and Curtis O. Byer, *Drugs: Substance Abuse,* San Francisco, Canfield Press, 1975.

30. Kaplan, John. *Marijuana—The New Prohibition.* New York: Pocket Books, 1971.

31. Keller, Mark. "Alcohol in Health and Disease: Some Historical Perspectives," *Annals of the New York Academy of Science,* Vol. 133 (1966), pp. 820-827.

32. Kelson, Saul R., et al. "The Growing Epidemic: A Survey of Smoking Habits and Attitudes Among Students in Grades 7 through 12." *American Journal of Public Health,* 15:923:938, September 1975.

33. Lucia, Salvatore P. (ed.). *Alcohol and Civilization.* New York: McGraw-Hill Book Company, 1963.

34. Maddox, George L., and B. C. McCall. *Drinking Among Teenagers: A Social Interpretation of Alcohol Use by High School Students.* New Brunswick, N.J.: Rutgers Center of Alcohol Studies, 1964.

35. Matchett, William Foster. "Who Uses Drugs? A Study in a Suburban Public High School," *The Journal of School Health,* Vol. XLI, No. 2 (February 1971).

36. Mayright, Gerald F. "Considerations in the Development of the School Drug Policy," *Journal of School Health,* Vol. XLII, No. 8 (October 1972), pp. 435-440.

37. McCarthy, Raymond G., *Alcohol Education for Classroom and Community.* New York, McGraw-Hill, 1964.

38. Merki, D. J.: What we need before drug abuse education, *The Journal of School Health 39:* Nov., 1969.

39. Miles, Samuel A. (ed.). *Learning About Alcohol.* Washington, D.C.: American Association for Health, Physical Education and Recreation, 1974.

40. Nickerson, Carl J. "An Examination of Five Difficult Issues Related to School Drug Problems," *Journal of School Health,* Vol. XLII, No. 8 (October 1972), pp. 441-445.

41. Notaro, Carol, R. N., "Adolescents and Alcohol," *Issues in Comprehensive Pediatric Nursing.* May/June, 1976, pp. 52-58, McGraw-Hill, Inc., New York.

42. Pittman, David J., and Charles R. Snyder (eds.). *Society, Culture and Drinking Patterns.* New York: John Wiley & Sons, Inc. 1962.

43. Ray, Oakley S. ed., *Drugs, Society, and Human Behavior,* St. Louis, C. V. Mosby, 1972.

44. Schonfield, Jacob, "Differences in Smoking, Drinking and Social Behavior by Race and Delinquency Status in Adolescent Males," *Adolescence,* Winter, 1966-67.

45. St. Pierre, Richard, and Carrie Lee Warren. "Smoking and Obesity: The Behavior Ramifications," *Journal of School Health,* 45:406-409, September, 1975.

46. Stacey, Barrie, and John Davies. "Drinking Behavior in Childhood and Adolescence: An Evaluative Review," *Journal of Alcohol and Drug Education,* Vol. 17, No. 3 (Spring 1972), pp. 1-11.

47. Todd, Frances, *Teaching about Alcohol,* New York, McGraw-Hill, 1964.

48. Weinswig, N. H. Doerr, D. N., and Weinswig, S. E.: Drug abuse education, Phi Delta Kappan 50: Dec., 1968.

49. Weitman, Morris, et al. "Survey of Adolescent Drug III. Correlations Among Use of Drugs," *American Journal of Public Health,* Vol. 62, No. 2 (February 1972), pp. 166-170.

50. Windham, Gerald O., James D. Preston, and Harold B. Armstrong. "The High School Student in Mississippi and Beverage Alcohol," *Journal of Alcohol Education,* Vol. B, No. 1 (Spring 1967), pp. 1-12.

Disease

1. American Cancer Society, 1979, *Cancer Facts and Figures,* New York.

2. Bahnson, Calus Behne, "Epistemiological Perspectives of Physical Disease from the Psychodynamic Point of View," *AJPH,* November 1974, pp. 1034-1040.

3. *Before Illness Strikes* (pamphlet), Interhealth Life Extension Institute, 2970 Fifth Avenue, San Diego, Calif.

4. Behan, R. W., "Quality of Life Can Be Determined," *Journal of Environmental Health,* March/April 1971, pp. 501-507.

5. Belson, Abby A., "Predictive Medicine," *Family Health,* January 1975.

6. "Biochemical Profiles," *Statistical Bulletin,* New York, Metropolitan Life, December 1969.

7. Boyer, John L., "Heart Attack-Prevention Starts with Children," *Journal of Physical Education,* March-April, 1972, pp. 103-05.

8. Brown, William. "Acquired Syphillis." *American Journal of Nursing* (April 1971), 713-715.

9. Bylinsky, Gene, "Science Is on the Trail of the Fountain of Youth," *Fortune,* July 1976, pp. 134-40.

10. Caldwalader, Mary H., "Early Warnings of Future Disease," *Smithsonian Magazine,* May 1974.

11. Caldwalader, Mary H., "Changes as Stress," (reprint) *Time,* March, 1971.

12. Cassel, John, "An Epidemiological Perspective of Psychosocial Factors in Disease Etiology," *AJPH,* November 1974, pp. 1040-1043.

13. Clarke, Blake, "A Checkup May Save Your Life," *Readers Digest,* March 1972.

14. Commoner, Barry, "Cancer as an Environmental Diaease," *Hospital Practice,* February 1975, pp. 82-84.

15. *Control of Communicable Diseases in Man,* 11th ed. New York: American Public Health Association, 1970.

16. deCastro, Fernando J., et al., "Hypertension in Adolescents," *Clinical Pediatrics,* January 1976, pp. 24-26.

17. Deschin, C. S.: Teenagers and venereal disease, *Children 9:* March, 1962.

18. "Diet Linked to Fight Breast Cancer," *The San Diego Union,* May 30, 1976.

19. "Disease," *All About Science* 3:6, September 12, 1974.

20. Dubos, Rene, *So Human an Animal,* New York, Scribner, 1968.

21. Edelson, Edward, *Early Disease Detection—A New Way to Health* (Pamphlet No. 467), New York Public Affairs Committee, 1971.

22. "Emotions and Cancer: The Link Is Becoming More Apparent," *The San Diego Union,* July 11, 1976.

23. Evans, Jane, R.N., and Singleton, Elaine, R.N. "Acne: the scourge of adolescence," *Issues in Comprehensive Pediatric Nursing,* July/August, McGraw-Hill, Inc., New York, 1976, pp. 60-68.

24. Fiedler, Dolores E., Dorothea M. Long, and Judy M. Carlson, "Pathology in the 'Healthy' Female Teenager," *AJPH,* November 1973, pp. 962-965.

25. Gardner, Pierce, "Reasons for Antibiotic Failures," *Hospital Practices,* February 1976, pp. 41-45.

26. Greenberg, Bernard G., "The Changing Scene in Public Health," *APHA,* June 1974, pp. 534-37.

27. Hawryluk, Orest, "Chronic Disease Patterns in United States Army Officers," *Military Medicine,* February 1975, pp. 89-93.

28. *Health and Disease,* New York: Time, Incorporated, 1965.

29. *How Often Do You Need a Health Examination—Planning for Health* (pamphlet), Los Angeles: Kaiser Foundation Health Plan, Fall 1973.

30. Interhealth, *Prospective Medicine,* (pamphlet), San Diego, Interhealth.

31. Jones, Herbert, Dorothy Nowack, and Jean Heindel. "Which Methodology for Venereal Disease Education?", *School Health Review,* Vol. 3, No. 2 (March-April 1972), pp. 8-9.

32. Ladou, Joseph, John N. Sherwood, and Lewis Hughes, "Health Hazard Appraisal in Patient Counseling," *Preventive Medicine,* February 1975, pp. 177-80.

33. Lenz, Philomene. "Women—The Unwitting Carriers of Gonorrhea." *American Journal of Nursing* (April 1971), 716-719.

34. Lewis, Howard R. and Martha E., Lewis, "Does Your Personality Invite Disease," *Science Digest,* December 1972.

35. *Life and Death and Medicine,* San Francisco, W. H. Freeman, 1973.

36. "Life-Style Linked to Divorce Rate," *The San Diego Union,* February 25, 1973.

37. Loggie, Jennifer M. H., "Hypertension in Children and Adolescents," *Hospital Practice,* June 1975, pp. 81-92.

38. McInnis, Mary E. *Essentials of Communicable Disease.* St. Louis: C. V. Mosby Co., 1975.

39. Pless, Ivan B., and Klaus J., Roghmann, "Chronic Illness and Its Consequences: Observations Based on Three-Spidemologic Surveys," *The Journal of Pediatrics*, September 1971, pp. 351-59.

40. Schwartz, William F., *Teachers Handbook on Venereal Disease Education*, Washington, D.C. Government Printing Office, 1965.

41. Sharpe-Subak, Genell, "The Venereal Disease of the New Morality," *Today's Health*, March 1975.

42. Simmons, James S., *Public Health in the World Today*, Cambridge, Mass., Harvard University Press, 1949.

43. Syme, S. Leonard, "Behavioral Factors Associated with the Etiology of Physical Disease: A Social Epidemiological Approach," *AJPH*, November 1974, pp. 1043-1045.

44. Tavormina, J. B., et al., "Chronically Ill Children: A Psychologically and Emotionally Deviant Population," *Journal of Abnormal Child Psychology*, 4:2, 1976, pp. 99-110.

45. Tizes, Reuben, "Tuberculosis in Suburbia—New Indices for an Old Disease," *AJPH*, December 1972, pp. 1586-1589.

46. "Your Childhood Family Life Helps Determine Disease You May Develop as Adult," *Enquirer*, April 13, 1976.

First Aid and Safety

1. Contact your local AAA Club or write to: AAA Foundation for Traffic Safety, 8111 Gatehouse Road, Room 328, Falls Church, Virginia 22042, and request their *Catalog of Traffic Safety Materials.*

2. Arnold, Peter. *Checklist for Emergencies.* Garden City, New York: Doubleday & Company, Inc., 1976.

3. Bishop, W. R.: How did they happen? *Safety Education 42:* April 1963.

4. Brennan, William T. and Ludwig, Donald J., *Guide to Problems and Practices in First Aid and Emergency Care.* Dubuque: Wm. C. Brown Publishing Co., 1976.

5. Clarke, Kenneth S. "Values and Risk-Taking Behavior: The Concept of Calculated Risk," *Health Education,* 6:26-29, November/December 1975.

6. Dzenowagis, J. G.: Health and safety problems of the school noon hour, *The Journal of School Health 31:* Sept. 1961.

7. Dzenowagis, J. G.: College sports—accidents, injuries, *Safety Education 41:* March 1962.

8. Engs, Ruth C., S. Eugene Barnes, and Molly Wantz. *Health Games Students Play: Creative Strategies for Health Education,* Dubuque, Iowa: Kendall-Hunt Publishing Co., 1975, Chapter 12.

9. Florio, A. E., and Stafford, G. T.: *Safety education,* ed. 3, New York, 1969, McGraw-Hill Book Co.

10. Fox, B. H., and Fox, J H., editors: Alcohol and traffic safety, Bethesda, Md., 1963, U.S. Department of Health, Education, and Welfare.

11. Haddon, W., et al.: *Accident research—methods and approaches,* New York, 1964, Harper & Row Publishers.

12. Huelke, D. F.: Automobile accidents, *Bulletin of National Association of Secondary School Principals 52:* May 1968.

13. Kraus, Jess F., et al. "The Effectiveness of a New Touch Football Helmet to Reduce Head Injuries," *Journal of School Health,* 40:496-500, November 1970.

14. Licht, Kenneth F. "Safety and Accidents—A Brief Conceptual Analysis, and a Point of View," *Journal of School Health,* 45:530-534, November 1975.

15. Mayshark, Cyrus, "Curriculum Development and Research for Safety Education," *Health Education,* 7:28-32, May-June 1976.

16. Nader, R.: *Unsafe at any speed,* New York, 1965, Grossman Publishers Inc.

17. Parrish, H. M., et al.: Epidemiological approach to preventing school accidents *The Journal of School Health 37:* May 1967.

18. Rinear, Charles E. "Emergency Care in the Inner City," *Health Education,* 6:6-10, May/June 1975.

19. Rosenfied, H.: Guilty, *Safety Education 42:* April, 1963.

20. Seaton, D.C., et al.: *Administration and supervision of safety education,* New York, 1968, Macmillan Co.

21. Smith, V.: A study of injuries, *The Journal of School Health 41:* Feb. 1971.

22. Spadofora, J.: Accidents: the number one killer, *Safety Education 42:* May 1963.

23. Stack, H. J., and Elkow, J. D.: *Education for safe living,* ed. 4, New York, 1966, Prentice-Hall, Inc.

24. Strasser, J. E., et al.: *Fundamentals of safety education,* New York, 1964, The Macmillan Co.

25. Suggested school safety policies, Washington, D.C., 1964, American Association for Health, Physical Education, and Recreation.

26. Thygerson, Alton L. "Safety In Health Education: Some Precautions," *Journal of School Health,* 44:508-511, November 1974.

27. Willgoose, Carl E. "Educating for Safety," *Instructor,* 81:62-63, February 1971.

Human Sexuality

1. Abidin, Richard R., *Parenting Skills: Trainer's Manual and Workbook,* New York, Human Science Press, 1976.

2. Ager, Joel W., et al. "Vasectomy: Who Gets One and Why?" *American Journal of Public Health,* 64:680-684, July 1974.

3. Anderson, Claudia, R.N., "Adolescent Pregnancy," *Issues in Comprehensive Pediatric Nursing.* May/June 1976, pp. 44-49, McGraw-Hill, Inc., New York.

4. Blaufarb, Marjorie. "Rap Sessions, Sexuality Resource People, & Teacher Team Training," *School Health Review,* Vol. 3, No. 2 (March-April 1972), pp. 20-23.

5. Brown, Jacquelyn, R.N., and Clancy, Barbara, R.N., "Meeting the needs of teens regarding their sexuality," *Issues in Comprehensive Pediatric Nursing.* November/December, 1976, pp. 29-43, McGraw-Hill, Inc., New York.

6. Bruers, Clint E., and J. Thomas Fisher, *Growth Patterns and Sex Education,* Kent, Ohio, The American School Health Association, 1967.

7. Burt, John J. and Linda Meeks. *Education for Sexuality: Concepts and Programs for Teaching,* 2nd edition, W. B. Saunders Co., Philadelphia, Pa., 1975.

8. Bracher, Marjory. "The Martinson Report: Implications for Sex Education," *Journal of School Health,* Vol. XXXVII, No. 10 (December 1967) pp. 491-496.

9. Calderone, Mary S. "The Development of Health Sexuality," *Journal of Health, Physical Education and Recreation,* Vol. 37, No. 7 (September 1966), pp. 23-27.

10. Calderone, M. S.: Sex—health or disease, *The Journal of School Health 35:* June 1965.

11. Calderone, Mary S., *Sexuality and Human Values,* New York, Human Science Press, 1967.

12. Casler, Lawrence, *Is Marriage Necessary?,* New York, Human Science Press, 1974.

13. Cohn, Frederick. *Understanding Human Sexuality,* Englewood Cliffs, N.J.: Prentice-Hall, Inc., 1974.

14. Couch, G. B.: Youth Looks at sex, *The Journal of School Health 37:* Sept. 1967.

15. Dalrymple, Willard. *Sex Is for Real.* New York: McGraw-Hill Book Company, 1969.

16. Daly, Michael. "The Unwanted Pregnancy." *Clinical Obstetrics and Gynecology* (September 1970), 713-726.

17. Daniels, Ada M. "Reaching Unwed Adolescent Mothers." *American Journal of Nursing* (February 1969), 332-335.

18. Davis, Lucille and Grace, Helen. "Anticipatory Counseling of Unwed Pregnant Adolescents." *Nursing Clinics of North America,* (December 1971), 581-590.

19. Fulton, Gere B. "Sex Education: Some Issues and Answers," *Journal of School Health,* Vol. 40 (May 1970), pp. 263-286.

20. Furstenberg, Frank F. *Unplanned Parenthood: The Social Consequences of Teenage Childbearing.* The Free Press, New York, 1976.

21. Gendel. E. S., and Green, P. B.: Sex education controversy; a boost to new and better programs. *The Journal of School Health 41:* Jan. 1971.

22. Gordon, Sol. "What Adolescents Want to Know." *American Journal of Nursing,* (March 1971), 534-535.

23. Graf, Christina, R.N., "Sex and the Adolescent," *Issues in Comprehensive Pediatric Nursing.* May/June, 1976, pp. 31-41, McGraw-Hill, Inc., New York.

24. Hinton, Gertrude, D. M., *Teaching Sex Education: A Guide for Teachers,* Palo Alto, Calif., Fearon Publishers 1969.

25. Hoyman, H. S.: Our most explosive sex education issue: birth control, *The Journal of School Health 39:* Sept. 1969.

26. Jensen, Gordon, and Rauh, Joseph, "Counseling Adolescents on Sex Problems," *Interact,* Volume 1, No. 4, Searle.

27. Jensen, Gordon, D. and Robbins, Mina. *Ten Reasons Why "Sex Talks" With Adolescents Go Wrong.* Medical Aspects of Human Sexuality, July 1975.

28. Johnson, Eric W. *Love and Sex in Plain Language.* Philadelphia: J. B. Lippincott Co., 1965.

29. Johnson, Lois, "Problems with Contraception in Adolescents: The Successful Use of an Intrauterine Device," *Clinical Pediatrics,* Volume 10, No. 6, June 1971, pp. 315-319.

30. Johnson, Warren R. *Human Sexual Behavior and Sex Education,* 2nd ed. Philadelphia: Lea & Febiger, 1968.

31. Johnson, R. Winifred. "Sex Education and the Nurse." *Nursing Outlook* (November 1972), 32-35.

32. Juhasz, Anne McCreary. "Understanding Adolescent Sexual Behavior in a Changing Society." *Journal of School Health* (March 1972), 149-154.

32 a. Kaplan, Robert. Meeks, Linda and Segel, Jay. *Group Strategies in Understanding Human Sexuality,* Dubuque: Wm. C. Brown Company Publishers, 1978.

33. Katchadourian, Herant, and Donald T. Lunde. *Fundamentals of Human Sexuality.* New York: Holt, Rinehart and Winston, Inc., 1972.

34. Kirkendall, Lester, and Wesley Adams. *The Students' Guide to Marriage and Family Life Literature* Dubuque, Iowa: Wm. C. Brown Company Publishers, 1971.

35. Kinch, Robert A. H. *The Physician's Role in Counseling the Sexually Active Teenager,* Consultant, July 1975.

36. Klemers, Richard, and Rebecca Smith. *Teaching About Family Relationships,* Minneapolis: Burgess Publishing Co., 1975.

37. Lieberman, E. James, M.D. and Peck, Ellen. *Sex and Birth Control: A Guide for the Young.* Thomas Y. Crowell Company, New York, 1973.

38. Lin, Barbara B., et al. "A Peek at Sex Education in a Midwestern Community," *Journal of School Health,* Vol. XLII, No. 8 (October 1972), pp. 462-465.

39. Louko, Kenneth R., and Paul E. Wagner, "Signs of Sexual Difficulties in Adolescents," *Medical Aspects of Human Sexuality,* July 1976, pp. 104-118.

40. Maddock, James W., "Sex in Adolescence: Its Meaning and its Future," *Adolescence,* Fall 1973, pp. 325-342.

41. Malo-Juvera, Dolores. "What Pregnant Teenagers Know About Sex." *Nursing Outlook* (November 1970), 32-35.

42. McCary, James Leslie. *Human Sexuality,* 2nd edition, New York: Van Nostrand, 1973.

43. Menken, Jane. "The Health and Social Consequences of Teenage Childbearing." *Family Planning Perspectives,* Vol. 4, No. 3 (July 1972), 45-53. (35 cents from: The Center for Family Planning Program Development, 515 Madison Avenue, N.Y., N.Y. 10022).

44. Osofsky, Howard J. and Osofsky, Joy D. "Let's Be Sensible About Sex Education." *American Journal of Nursing* (March 1971), 532-535.

45. Pannor, Reuben. "The Forgotten Man." *Nursing Outlook* (November 1970), 36-37.

46. Pannor, Reuben. "The Teen Age Unwed Father." *Clinical Obstetrics and Gynecology* (June 1971), 466-472.

47. Perren, Mark and Thomas E. Smith, *Ideas and Learning Activities for Family Life and Sex Education,* Dubuque, Iowa, Wm. C. Brown Company Publishers, 1972.

48. Rauh, Joseph, M.D., et al., "Contraception for the Teenager," *Medical Clinics of North America,* Volume 59, No. 6, November 1975, pp. 1407-1418.

49. Rauh, Joseph, M.D., "The Management of Adolescent Pregnancy and Prevention of Repeat Pregnancies," *HSMHA Health Reports,* Volume 86, No. 1, January 1971, pp. 66-73.

50. Reiss, Ira L. "The Dilemma of Sex Education in the Public Schools," in Donald Read (ed.), *New Directions in Health Education.* New York: Macmillan Publishing Co., Inc., 1971.

51. ———, (ed) "The Sexual Renaissance in America," special issue, *The Journal of Social Issues,* Vol. XXII, No. 2 (April 1966).

52. *Sex Education:* SIECUS Discussion Guide No. 1, Revised 1975. Publications Office, 122 East 42nd St., New York, N.Y. 10017.

53. *Sex Education—A Working Design for Curriculum Development and Implementation, Grades K-12,* The Education Council, 131 Mineola Blvd., Mineola, N.Y. 11501.

54. Simon, S.B.: Nourishing sexuality in the schools, *The National Elementary Principal 50:* Feb. 1971.

55. Sorensen, Robert C. *Adolescent Sexuality in Contemporary America.* New York: The World Publishing Company, 1972.

56. Stephenson, John, M.D., "Approaching Adolescents about Sexual Matters," *Clinical Pediatrics,* Volume 9, No. 4, April 1970, pp. 232-236.

57. Taylor, Diana, "A New Way to Teach Teens About Contraceptives," *The American Journal of Maternal and Child Nursing,* November, December 1976, pp. 378-383.

58. Webb, Gilbert, M.D., "Care of the Pregnant Adolescent," *Pediatric Annals,* January 1975, pp. 99-107.

59. Willke, Dr. J C., and Mrs. J. C. Willke, *Sex Education, The How-To for Teachers,* Cincinnati, Ohio: Hiltz Publishing Co., 1970.

Consumer Health and Medical Care

1. Baugh, Robert J., and Carolyn B. Noe, "National Health Care: Consumer's Delight or Dilemma?" *Health Education,* 6:11-13, November/December 1975.

2. Editors of Consumer Reports, "National Health Insurance: Which Way to Go?" *Consumer Reports,* 40:118-124, February 1975.

3. Editors of Consumer Reports, "The Safe Approach to Laxatives," *Consumer Reports,* August 1975, p. 508.

4. Editors of Consumer Reports, "Chiropractors: Healers or Quacks," *Consumer Reports,* Sept. 1975, p. 542.

5. Consumer Union Editors. The Medicine Show. Orangeburg, N.Y.: *Consumer Reports* 1974.

6. Cornacchia, Harold. *Consumer Health,* St. Louis: C. V. Mosby Co., 1976.

7. Dubos, Rene, *Mirage of Health,* Garden City, N.Y.: Doubleday, (Anchor Books), 1961.

8. Editorial, "The Escellence Deception in Medicine," *Hospital Practice,* April 1976, pp. 11-11.

9. Gallager, Heald & Garell, *Medical Care of the Adolescent.* 3rd Edition. New York, Appleton-Century Crofts, 1976, Chap. 1, 4, 5, 22.

10. Goleman, Daniel, "The Tranquility Box: A Consumer's Guide to Biofeedback Machines," *Psychology Today,* 9:132-135, November 1975.

11. Hammar, S. L., M.D., "The Approach to the Adolescent Patient," *Pediatric Clinics of North America,* Volume 20, No. 4, November 1973, pp. 779-788.

12. Hammar, S. L. and Holterman, V. *Interviewing and Counseling Adolescent Patients.* Clinical Pediatrics, 9:1, January 1970.

13. Howell, Keith A. "Death and the Consumer," *Health Education,* 6:15-18, November/December 1975.

14. Moody, Howard. "Demythologizing Medicine: Redefining Health Care," *Christianity and Crisis,* 35:219-224, September 1975.

15. Punke, Harold H. "Caffeine in America's Food and Drug Habits," *Journal of School Health,* 44:550-558, December 1974.

16. Quinn, Nancy and Anne R. Somers, "The Patient's Bill of Rights," *Nursing Outlook*, 22:240-245, April 1974.

17. Rosen, S. "Beware of the 'Quackupuncturist' Who Operates for Profit," *Today's Health*, 52:6-7, 66-67, August 1974.

18. Schaller, Warren E. and Charles R. Carroll. *Health, Quackery, and the Consumer*. Philadelphia: W. B. Saunders Co., 1976.

19. Smith, Ralph L. *At Your Own Risk: The Case Against Chiropractic*, New York: Pocket Books. 1969.

20. Stephenson, John, M.D., "Communication in Adolescent Medicine: Some Facilitating and Time-Saving Aids and Approaches," *Clinical Pediatrics*, Volume 9, No. 9, September 1970, pp. 558-564.

21. Weaver, Peter. "Are You Using Credit Wisely?" *Today's Health*, 53:42-44, November 1975.

Environmental Health

1. *A Guide for Teaching: Humans and Their Environment (Ecology) 1 (grade 12)*, San Diego City Schools, 1973.

2. Bresler, Jack B., *Environments of Man*, Reading, Mass. Addison-Wesley, 1968.

3. Bundy, McGeorge. *Managing Knowledge to Save the Environment*, New York: The Ford Foundation, 1970.

4. Cole. H. S. D., et al., *Models of Doom: A Critique of the Limits of Growth*, New York, Universe Books, 1973.

5. Commoner, Barry, *The Closing Circle*, New York, Bantom Books, 1974.

6. Ehrlich, Paul R., *The Population Bomb*, New York, Sierra Club/Ballantine, 1971.

7. Ehrlich, Paul. "Eco-catastrophe," *Ramparts*, September 1969.

8. Goldsmith, John R., "Air Pollution and Disease," *Hospital Practice*, May 1970, pp. 61-71.

9. Gurley, John, "The Crisis of Capitalism," *Los Angeles Times*, March 28, 1976.

10. Hawkins, Donald E., and Dennis A. Vinton. *The Environmental Classroom*, Englewood Cliffs, N.J.: Prentice-Hall, Inc., 1973.

11. Holdren, John and Philip Herrera. *Energy*. New York, Sierra Club, 1971.

12. Kormondy, Edward J. *Concepts of Ecology*, Englewood Cliffs, N.J., Prentice-Hall, 1976.

13. Marters, Gilbert M., *Introduction to Environmental Science and Technology*, New York, John Wiley & Sons, 1974.

14. Marx, Leo. "American Institutions and Ecological Ideals," *Science*, November 27, 1970.

15. Meadows, Dennis L., *The Limits to Growth*, New York, Universe Books, 1972.

16. Moncrief, Lewis W., "The Cultural Basis for Our Environmental Crisis," *Science*, October 1970, pp. 508-512.

17. Pohlman, Edward, *Population*, New York, Mentor Books, 1973.

18. Pryor, Larry, "Solutions to Energy Crisis Could Threaten Life-Styles," *Los Angeles Times*, June 3, 1973.

19. Sargent, Frederick, "The Human Habitat," *Archives of Environmental Health*, October 1972, pp. 229-223.

20. Schiff, Maurice, "Nonauditory Effects of Noise," *Transactions*, September-October 1973.

21. Sesser, Stanford N. "The National Debates an Issue: The Economy vs. The Environment," *The Wall Street Journal*, November 3, 1971.

22. Stapp, William B. *Environmental Education: Strategies Toward A More Liveable Future*, New York: Halsted Press, 1975.

23. Turner, Alvis S. "The Environment of One World," *American Journal of Public Health*, 65:523-524, May 1975.

24. Vivian, Eugene and E. L. Henderson. "Environmental Education," *Instructor*, 50:52-61, January 1971.

25. Waldbott, George L. *Health Effects on Environmental Pollutants*, St. Louis, C. V. Mosby, 1973.

26. Watts, Kenneth E. F., "A Tragedy of Errors," *Science Review*, November 25, 1972, pp. 56-60.

27. Willgoose, Carl E. "Health Aspects of the Conservation-Recreation Effort," *Journal of School Health*, 38:359-365, June 1968.

28. Yannacone, Victor John Jr., *Energy Crisis: Danger and Opportunity*, New York, West Publishing Co., 1974.

Education for Aging and Dying

Aging

1. Beverley, Virginia E. "Lifelong Learning—A Concept Whose Time Has Come," *Geriatrics*, August, 1976.

2. Beverley, Virginia E. "Reading, Writing, and 'rithmetic—Adapted to retirees' needs," *Geriatrics*, September 1976.

3. Beverley, Virginia E. "Organizations for Seniors—What They Stand For, What They Offer," *Geriatrics*, November 1976.

4. Bernard, Allen. "The Geriatric Boondoggle." *Medical Opinion*, May, 1971.

5. Burdman, Robert. "The Media and Health Needs of the Elderly," *Health Education*, July/August 1975.

6. Gilmore, Anne. "Attitudes of the Elderly to Marriage," *Gerontologia Clinica*, Vol. 15, #2, 1973.

7. Graber, Richard F. "Aging in 2025: Telling It Like It's Going To Be," *Geriatrics*, February 1976.

8. Ivester, Connie and Karl King. "Attitudes of Adolescents Toward the Aged," *The Gerontologist*, February 1977.

9. Kawabori, Chisato. "The Aged: An Opportunity for the Educator," *Health Education*, July/August 1975.

10. Krueger, Esther S. "Freedom To Age Graciously," *Health Education*, July/August 1975.

11. Prehoda, Robert W., "Our Children May Live to be 200 Years Old," *The Futurist*, February 1969.

12. Ramoth, Janis. "A Plea for Aging Education," *Health Education*, July/August 1975.

13. Rao, Dodda B., M.D. "The Team Approach to Integrated Care of the Elderly," *Geriatrics*, February 1977.

14. Reichel, William, "Multiple Problems in the Elderly," *Hospital Practice*, March 1976, pp. 103-08.

15. Reif, Susan Dempsey. *Into Aging—A Simulation Game*. Charles B. Slack, Inc., 6900 Grove Rd., Thorofare, N.J. 08086 (1978).

16. Saul, Shura. *Aging: An Album of People Growing Old*. John Wiley and Sons, Inc., New York, 1974.

17. Spinazzola, Angelo. "Sexual Patterns in the Process of Aging." *Health Education*, July/Aug. 1975.

18. Twaddle, Andrew C., "Aging, Population Growth and Chronic Illness," *Journal of Chronic Diseases*, 1968, pp. 417-21.

19. Wallace, Bill C. "Aging: Health Education's Responsibility," *Health Education*, July/Aug. 1975.

20. Woodruff, Diana S. and James E. Birren. *Aging—Scientific Perspectives and Social Issues*. New York: D. Van Nostrand Company, 1975.

21. U.S. Dept. of Labor, Bureau of Labor Statistics, Washington, D.C. 20212—Occupational Outlook Quarterly Special Issue: "Working with Older People." Fall 1976.

Death and Dying

22. Beletz, Elaine E. and Mary Meng. "The Grievance Process," *American Journal of Nursing*. February 1977.

23. Becker, Ernest. *The Denial of Death*. New York, The Free Press, 1973.

24. Caine, Lynn. *Widow—The Personal Crisis of a Widow in America*. William & Morrow Co., 1974.

25. Egleson, Jim and Janet. *Parents Without Partners*. New York: Ace Star Books, 1961.

26. Everett, Marianne. "Helping Parents Teach About Death," *Health Education*, July/Aug. 1976.

27. Freireich, Emil J., M.D. "Death With Dignity?" *The Cancer Bulletin*, Nov./Dec. 1974.

28. Grollman, Earl A. (Editor) *Explaining Death to Children*. Boston: Beacon Press, 1967.

29. Hendin, David. *Death as a Fact of Life*, New York, Warner 1974.

30. Kobrzycki, Paula. "Dying With Dignity at Home," *American Journal of Nursing*, Aug. 1975.

31. Koop, E. Everett, M.D. *The Right to Live: The Right to Die*. Wheaton, Illinois: Tyndale House Publishers, Inc., 1976.

32. Kubler-Ross, Elizabeth. *Death—The Final Stage of Growth*, New Jersey, Prentice-Hall, 1975.

33. Kubler-Ross, Elizabeth. *On Death and Dying.* New York, Macmillan, 1969.

34. Kubler-Ross, Elizabeth. *Questions and Answers on Death and Dying.* New York, Collier, 1974.

35. Leviton, Dan. "Death, Bereavement and Suicide Education," in Donald A. Read (ed.), *New Directions in Health Education,* New York: Macmillan Publishing Co., Inc., 1971, p. 179.

36. Lifton, Robert J. and Eric Olson, *Living and Dying,* New York, Bantam, 1975.

37. McMahon, Joan D. "A Unit for Independent Study in Death Education," *School Health Review,* Vol. 4, No. 4 (July-August 1973), pp. 27-34.

38. Mitford, Jessica, *The American Way of Death,* Conn., Fawcett Publications, 1963.

39. Moody, Raymond A., M.D. *Life After Life* and *Reflections on Life After Life,* New York: Bantam Books, Inc., 1977.

40. Shneidman, Edwin S. *Death: Current Perspectives.* Palo Alto, Calif.: Mayfield Publishing Co., 1976.

41. Tuccille, Jerome, *Here Comes Immortality.* New York, Stein and Day, 1973.

Chapter Summary

All health educators need to be aware of the multitude and variety of materials that can be incorporated in the school health program. The types of materials available as well as the procedures used to obtain these materials can help improve the quality of school health education.

Among the resources one can contact to obtain materials are: official health agencies, nonofficial health agencies, periodicals which are located in libraries, professional organizations, as well as colleges and universities.

The health educator can organize, search for materials by categorizing health topics, then contact a resource for a specific topic. For example, if one is searching for information concerning a teaching unit on breast cancer, the American Cancer Society can be contacted to provide pamphlets, brochures or speakers regarding this topic. Often health educators do not make use of the numerous free and available resources in their local communities.

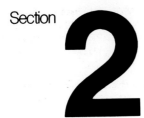

Creative Lessons for Teaching in the Middle and Secondary Schools

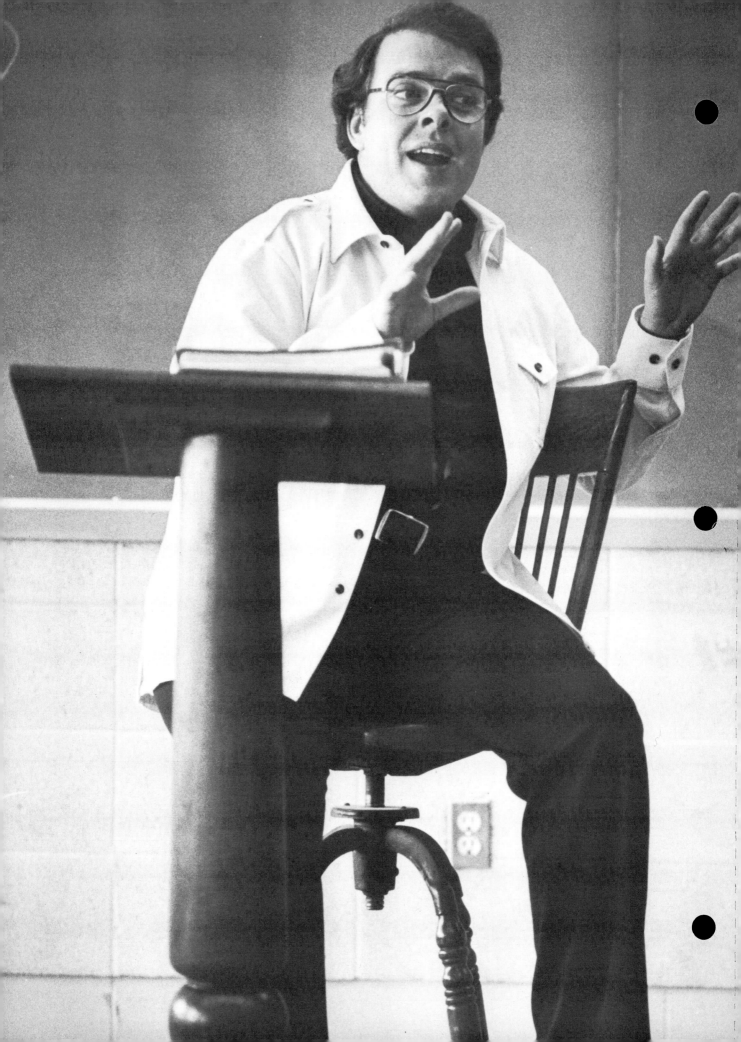

10

Teaching Health Science to Middle and Secondary School Students

Adolescence

Adolescence is the traditional period between childhood and adulthood. "Estimates by the United States Bureau of the Census for 1972 show that 45 percent of the 209 million population in the United States were less than 25 years of age. Within this category there were 42 million between the ages of 10 and 19 who could unequivocally be labelled adolescents. Projections of present trends indicate that the number of adolescents in the United States may reach 54 million by the year 2000."[1]

Developmental Tasks

It is important to have an understanding of adolescence when teaching health to the middle or secondary school student. Their development physically, socially, intellectually, and emotionally will influence their health behavior and their decisions as well as their ability to learn.

Robert Havighurst, author of *Developmental Tasks and Education,* emphasizes the impact of different developmental tasks on the life of the adolescent. He defines a developmental task as "a task which arises at or about a certain period in the life of the individual, successful achievement of which leads to his happiness and to success with later tasks, while failure leads to unhappiness in the individual, disapproval by the society, and difficulty with later tasks."[2]

Havighurst's developmental tasks for the 12–18 year old are identified in the following chart.

Developmental Tasks of Adolescence[3]
About 12 to about 18 years

1. Achieving new and more mature relations with age mates of both sexes.

2. Achieving a masculine or feminine social role.

3. Accepting one's physique and using the body effectively.

4. Achieving emotional independence of parents and other adults.

5. Achieving assurance of economic independence.

6. Selecting and preparing for an occupation.

7. Preparing for marriage and family life.

8. Developing intellectual skills and concepts necessary for civic competence.

9. Desiring and achieving socially responsible behavior.

10. Acquiring a set of values and an ethical system as a guide to behavior.

Growth and Development

At the same time that the adolescent is attempting to meet these developmental tasks, (s)he is experiencing an increased rate of growth, a rapidly expanding physique, a changing metabolism, as well as other biological changes. This means that the health status of adolescents will probably be accompanied by some psychological and social changes related to normal adolescent processes.

The Role of the Teacher

The middle and secondary school teacher needs to appreciate the physical, mental, and social changes occurring in the students. The instructor also needs to be aware of the potential health problems in this group. And finally, the teacher needs to relate the characteristics of the students and their potential health problems as well as their interests to the classroom. Let us examine each of these.

Characteristics of Students

Physical

Depending on the grade level structure of the school system, a middle or a secondary school student might be in a health education class between the ages of 12 and 18. The physical differences in these students because of the variability of sex and age is quite noticeable. Thus, the middle or secondary school student can be described only within a continuum with respect to physical likeness and physical difference.

Generally changes begin in females first at about the age of eight. At this time the pituitary gland begins to secrete the hormone FSH which influences the body in growth and sexual characteristics. Hormonal secretions in males generally lag two years behind that of females.

Puberty

Puberty is the period of adolescence when these glandular secretions begin to influence the body, and noticeable changes occur. The onset of puberty varies. Generally, the beginning of puberty is estimated to be around the age of eleven in females and around the age of thirteen in male.

Puberty is accompanied by the following physiological changes in the female: breasts begin to develop, the buttocks become fuller with fat deposits, hair develops under the arms and on the legs and pubic region, the skin becomes softer, and menstruation begins.

Puberty is accompanied by the following physiological changes in the male: the voice deepens, hair grows in the pubic region, under the arms and on the face, and the body becomes more muscular and triangular in shape, with the genitals enlarging.

The diverse responses of hormone levels result in varied periods of growth among adolescents. It is possible for an adolescent to have a growth spurt of four inches in one year. Because of this rapid increase in height, many adolescents slouch and have very poor posture. In addition, the adolescent who is developing rapidly needs extra sleep. A tired student might be less effective in the classroom only because (s)he is developing rapidly.

By the twelfth grade, most adolescents have reached adult height with the long bones completing their growth. The heart has generally reached its adult size.

Mental and Emotional

Adolescence has often been referred to as a turbulent, stormy period. The rapid physical growth and the varied nature of hormonal secretions often leave the adolescent feeling somewhat anxious. The adolescent may be puzzled by these varied changes. The reassurance of the teacher is helpful.

A healthy self-concept is a major focal point of concern during this period. Due to physical changes, the adolescent may find it difficult to deal with body image and self acceptance. The teacher who explains these changes in appearance and in mood as natural, helps the adolescent feel more comfortable and self-accepting.

The adolescent is also examining life and its meaning. It is not uncommon to hear youngsters discuss philosophy and to hear them question the older generation. These questions are normal and not a sign of a rebellious or belligerent youngster. The adolescent is also able to think more analytically and to intellectualize about a variety of concerns.

Social

In addition to the physical, mental, and emotional changes accompanying adolescence, we also notice a new approach toward the social life. The adolescent wants to be thought of as an adult. (S)he emulates and imitates adults who are liked and admired. At the same time, the peer group takes on greater importance and there is a tendency to want to be accepted by the group. The so-called "clique" may dictate socially acceptable rules and regulations.

The pressure to be socially acceptable is perhaps one of the most difficult factors of adolescent life. The adolescent is sensitive to ridicule and to the comments of others. Unfortunately, popularity is valued, sometimes at any cost. This need for acceptance among peers may influence health behaviors among adolescents. The middle and secondary school teacher needs to help the adolescent examine how (s)he makes decisions.

Dating is an integral part of the social life of the adolescent. Females begin to show an interest in males before the males reciprocate this interest. In high school, the interest is nearly equal. This preoccupation with dating is accompanied by an increased interest in physical appearance and dress. A discussion of grooming and ways to enhance personal appearance will most likely be of interest to the middle and secondary school student.

Rapid growth, developing mental faculties, turbulent emotional periods, and increased social awareness are common for the adolescent. There are certain health concerns related to growth that are common in this age group.

Problems related to Growth

Because of the impact of growth and bodily changes on the adolescent, problems related to growth are perhaps the most worrisome to the student and subsequently to the parents. However, in most cases the adolescent who lags behind or zooms ahead of peers is perfectly normal.

Delayed Onset of Puberty

One of the most common reasons for a visit to the physician by the adolescent female is the lagging onset of puberty. In particular the female and her parents may be concerned about delayed menstruation. In most cases, reassurance is the only treatment. In few, but occasional cases, the female has a poorly functioning thyroid gland, and some form of hormone therapy is needed. Most physicians avoid treatment with hormones if possible.

Some females complain about menstrual cramps. These cramps may be accompanied by headaches, nausea and vomiting. Sometimes cramping is attributed to disease, other times to physical abnormality, and most likely to emotional attitudes and fears. The teacher can do a great deal to dispel myths about menstruation and to help the student accept herself.

The adolescent male is also concerned about his growth; this is also the most frequent reason for a visit to the physician. Penis size is one of the main concerns of males. Also, with increased glandular secretions, wet dreams are common, and masturbation becomes a common sexual outlet. In some cases, the male develops benign breast tissue. This is bothersome as well as anxiety producing. The tissue will disappear when the male glands become more mature.

The concerns of the adolescent male may also be alleviated by a reassuring teacher and by adequate information about sexuality and growth and development.

Bones and Joints

There are few muscular or skeletal problems found in adolescents. Complaints about aches in the back or in the joints can usually be alleviated by improving posture. Regular daily exercise is also helpful.

There are two maladies which sometimes result from rapid growth. Sometimes the head of the femur or the thigh bone will slip in the hip joint, and the adolescent will limp. This will require the assistance of a physician.

Sometimes the adolescent will tear the cartilage fibers around the knee joint. The resulting knee pain is quite common and also requires the assistance of a physician.

Acne

Acne is another growth related problem of adolescence. The typical troublesome pimples and blackheads are caused by fluctuating hormones, emotional turmoil, infections somewhere else in the body, fatigue, and a poorly balanced diet. The habits of teens may irritate the acne further. Females may use cosmetics that irritate the skin and males may irritate the skin shaving. The teacher can encourage the student to cleanse the skin properly, get a good night's sleep, and select a balanced diet.

Diet

Malnutrition is not uncommon among adolescents. While developing physically, there is a need for protein, calcium, and particularly for the female, iron. The iron is needed to produce red blood cells. The stores of iron in the body can be easily depleted by rapid growth and by the onset of menstruation.

Lack of adequate nutrients may contribute to problems of growth, menstrual difficulties, and feelings of tiredness.

Infections

The adolescent is usually healthy when it comes to threats of infection. Generally they have been immunized during elementary school years or have developed natural immunity by having had some of the childhood diseases.

Infectious mononucleosis is a viral infection that may afflict the teenager. The virus affects the lymph glands and may have an accompanying sore throat, fever, and general feeling of tiredness. It may take several weeks to recover from mono. With complete recovery there is immunity.

Tuberculosis is a bacterial infection that may afflict teens more seriously than other age groups because it is thought to be related to glandular changes and to rapid growth. Tuberculin testing is recommended yearly for ages 10–19. Tuberculosis spreads rapidly in the body and it is highly contagious.

Mumps may be severe if acquired during the teenage years. If mumps occur after puberty, the virus may spread to the reproductive organs. Orchiditis, the inflammation of the testes, may occur and result in permanent sterility. Fortunately, there is a vaccine for those who did not have mumps during childhood.

The sexually transmissible diseases are rapidly increasing in incidence in adolescents. It is estimated that about two million adolescents acquire one of these diseases each year. This estimate is most likely low, the actual incidence being much higher.

Chronic Disease

In addition to infectious diseases, many adolescents have chronic diseases such as diabetes, epilepsy, or asthma. The teacher needs to have adequate information on the special needs of students who have chronic diseases. This information should be a part of the school health record. The teacher may also need to consult with the school nurse or with the student's parents.

Stress

The rapidly changing status of the adolescent physically, socially, intellectually, and emotionally creates a variety of pressures causing stress. Perhaps one of the main characteristics which differentiates one adolescent from another is the means chosen to deal with these stressors.

Some adolescents will learn to feel comfortable with themselves and to accept their feelings as normal. This self acceptance and resulting self-esteem may contribute to sound health practices.

Other adolescents faced with a variety of stressors to cope with may turn to other alternatives. Drugs, cigarettes, marijuana, obesity, delinquency, to mention a few, might be used as alternative means to cope.

The Challenge

The middle and secondary school teacher can assist the adolescent in dealing with physical, social, intellectual, and emotional changes. In addition, the teacher can help the student develop healthy attitudes toward living and healthy behaviors to practice. Through the identification of alternatives to healthy lifestyle and the careful examination of each alternative, the adolescent learns to control and direct the future, to take personal responsibility for health.

The remaining chapters in this text deal with the alternatives to health behavior that are of concern to adolescent students.

Chapter Summary

Adolescence is the traditional period between childhood and adulthood. During this time period the adolescent has different developmental tasks to achieve and (s)he experiences rapid growth and development.

Middle and secondary school teachers need to appreciate the physical, mental and emotional and social changes in the students to facilitate the learning process.

The physical characteristics of adolescents are triggered by puberty when glandular secretions begin to influence the female and the male. Delayed puberty is the primary reason for a visit to the physician. Some of the concerns adolescents have about physical changes include menstruation, masturbation, penis size, and wet dreams.

The mental and emotional status of adolescence is greatly influenced by fluctuating hormonal levels. This often results in feelings of anxiety. Social forces also have an influence on adolescent feelings. Adolescents tend to emulate admired adults and feel the pressure of the peer group.

Some of the health problems of adolescence are aches in the back and joints, acne, malnutrition, mononucleosis, tuberculosis, mumps, sexually transmissible diseases, and chronic diseases.

Middle and secondary school teachers can help the adolescent develop self-acceptance and can provide the information needed to make healthy decisions.

Notes

1. Hiliary E. C. Millar, M.D., *Approaches to Adolescent Health Care in the 1970s.* United States Department of Health, Education, and Welfare; Public Health Service, Health Services Administration; Bureau of Community Health Services; Rockville, Maryland, 20852, page 1.
2. Robert J. Havighurst, *Developmental Tasks and Education.* New York: David McKay Company, 1972, page 2.
3. Robert J. Havighurst, *Developmental Tasks and Education.* New York: David McKay Company, 1972, pages 45–82.

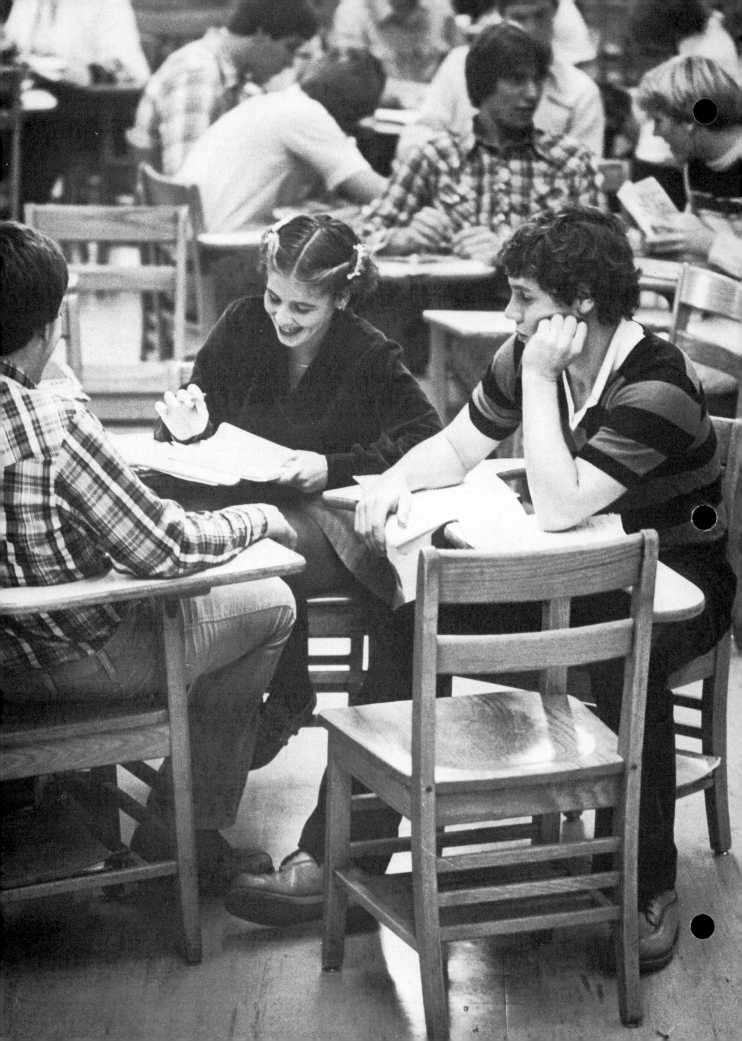

11

Teaching about Mental Health and Self Concept

Prior to the study of the alternatives to a healthy life style, it is our belief that middle and secondary school students need some personal skills. These personal skills will enable the students to learn more about themselves and will give them the tools needed in the process of making healthy life style decisions. This chapter includes an outline of Suggested Topics for Teaching About Mental Health and Self Concept, Three Detailed Sample Lessons that have been used with middle and secondary school students, and additional Selected Learning Activities.

The first lesson, **Communication Skills,** helps the students develop skills in relating clearly. The students are exposed to five levels of communication and learn that the level of communication which is chosen affects the type of relationship that develops—open or closed. The students learn the three components of an "I message"—a message that entails personal responsibility. We feel that students need to be able to express *I* or responsibility taking messages if they are communicating feelings to others. In addition to these tools, the students develop the skill of active listening.

The second lesson, **Developing Assertive Behavior,** also focuses on communication. The students learn what it means to be assertive, nonassertive, and aggressive and see how these types of behaviors facilitate or impede meeting their needs. Middle and secondary students who develop assertive behavior will be more likely to make their own decisions, rather than being pressured by peers. We also believe that assertive behavior will provide some defense to prevent the later development of psychosomatic illnesses.

The third lesson, **Coping Kit,** is a practical but complete lesson for middle and secondary school students. It discusses the many facets of mental health. Good mental health is defined and a mental health quiz is included. This is followed by a careful examination of the stress and stressors most common among middle and secondary school students together with a discussion of alternative means of coping. The students also learn about the mental health services available.

Mental Health and Self Concept
 I. Factors Related to Developing Positive Mental Health and Self Concept
    A. Hereditary
    B. Environment
 II. Growth and Evolution of Personality
    A. Freud's views on behavior
    B. Maslow and self-actualization
 III. The Secondary School Youth-Developing Self-Identity
    A. Erikson's stages of human development
    B. Sexual self-identification in the teenage male
    C. Sexual self-identification in the teenage female
    D. Adult values vs. peer group values
    E. Same sex and opposite sex relationships
 IV. Achieving Positive Mental Health
    A. Dealing with stress
    B. Adapting to change
    C. Accepting one's feelings
 V. Learning to Adapt
    A. Developing communication skills
    B. Developing and achieving goals and objectives
    C. Defense mechanisms
 VI. Barriers To Achieving Positive Mental Health
    A. Neuroses
    B. Depression
    C. Schizophrenia
    D. Paranoia
    E. Psychosomatic disorders
    F. Suicide - causes and prevention
 VII. Treatment of Mental Disorders
    A. The role of psychoanalysts
    B. The practice of psychotherapy
    C. Behavior modification
    D. Drug treatment
    E. Self-help groups
    F. Fad therapies

Mental Health and Self Concept
Communication Skills

Objectives

1. The student will be able to define communication.

2. The student will be able to role play each of the five levels of communication identified by John Powell: cliché conversation, reporting the facts about others, my ideas and judgments, my feelings (emotions) "gut level," and peak communication.

3. The student will be able to list and explain the five rules for gut level communication.

4. The student will be able to list the three parts of an *I* message and will be able to give examples of *I* messages in writing and while role playing.

5. The student will be able to demonstrate active listening when presented with role simulations from the teacher.

Sources

1. Dr. Thomas Gordon. *Teacher Effectiveness Training.* New York: David McKay Company, Inc., 1974.

2. Robert Kaplan, Linda Meeks, and Jay Segal. *Group Strategies in Human Sexuality: Getting in Touch.* Dubuque, Iowa: William C. Brown Company Publishers, 1978.

3. John Powell, S. J., *Why Am I Afraid to Tell You Who I Am?* Illinois: Argus Communications, 1969.

4. Hugh Prather. *Notes to Myself (My struggle to become a person.)* Utah: Real People Press, 1970.

Content and Procedures

Communication

Communication is a process by which someone or something is made common, when it is shared.[3] Communication is how we relate to the world around us and how that world relates to us. Communication is very important to our mental health and to building and maintaining a healthy self concept.

When we communicate effectively with another person, several things happen:[4]

1. I become aware of You- I discover you.
2. I make you aware of me- I uncover myself.
3. I am ready to change during our conversation and I am willing to reveal my changes to you.

This kind of process is not easy for everyone and it may be more or less difficult, depending upon the situation. It involves a great deal of caring, trust, and personal risk-taking. If I am going to do these things I am going to need to care enough about you to listen so I can "discover you." I am also going to need to trust you as I "uncover myself." And I am going to need to trust you as I reveal how I am "changing during our conversation."

But can I trust you? I am going to need to risk myself, and this frightens me. John Powell, author of *Why Am I Afraid to Tell You Who I Am?*, discusses this fear in his book. He says "I am afraid to tell you who I am because if I tell you who I am, you may not like who I am, and it's all I have.[3]

What does this statement mean to you? Have you ever felt this way? (Stop and have student discussion.)

The fears that we experience and the risks that honest self-communication would involve may seem so intense that we can choose not to communicate openly, honestly, and effectively. You will remember that in our previous lessons we discussed the fact that there are many alternatives from which to choose our behavior. We can choose to communicate on several different levels.

Levels of Communication

Overlay of five levels of communication:

---

5. Cliché Conversation

4. Reporting the facts about others

3. My ideas and judgments

2. My feelings (emotions) "gut level"

1. Peak communication

John Powell identified five levels of communication in his book. We will look at the fifth level first. The fifth level represents the least willingness to communicate ourselves to others. The successive, descending levels indicate greater and greater success in the adventure.[3]

Levels of Communication*

5. Cliché Conversation

When we use cliché conversation, there is no sharing of persons at all.

Examples: "How are you?" "How is your family?" "Going to the football game?" (Have the students give examples)

A. _____

B. _____

C. _____

4. Reporting the Facts about Others

When we report the facts about others, we are content to tell others what so and so has said or done. We do not express any personal comments about these facts.

Examples: "Mary's mother won't let her date until she is 16." "I heard that John smokes pot."
(Have the students give examples)

A. _____

B. _____

C. _____

3. My Ideas and Judgments

On this level, I will risk telling you some of my ideas and judgments and decisions. If I feel that you do not accept my ideas, judgments, and decisions, I will stop talking.

Examples: "I am not going to vote for Mary for homecoming queen." "I don't want John for a friend anymore."
(Have the students give examples)

A. _____

B. _____

C. _____

2. My Feelings (Emotions) "Gut Level"

When I use gut level communication, I express the feelings that underlie my ideas, judgments, and convictions.

Examples: "I think you are intelligent and I feel jealous." "I am embarrassed when I can't answer a question in my math class."
(Have the students give examples)

A. _____

B. _____

C. _____

*Reprinted from *Why Am I Afraid To Tell You Who I am?* by John Powell © 1969 Argus Communications. Used with permission from Argus Communications, Niles, Illinois.

1. **Peak Communication**

   Peak communication is difficult to describe. Among friends or between partners in marriage there will come from time to time a complete emotional and personal communion.

   Examples: Many married persons report that at the birth of one of their children, they (the couple) were so "high" that they felt in complete emotional and personal communion.

   (Ask the students if any of them has ever had an experience where they felt that there was peak communication.)

   A. _____

   B. _____

   C. _____

We have just examined five different levels of communication. We mentioned that peak communication or a complete emotional and personal communion is not an everyday occurrence. But "feelings" or "gut level" communication can be.

By using "feelings" communication we can promote our health in several ways. One of these has to do with illness. When we keep things bottled inside us we develop headaches, ulcers, stomach aches, etc. When we use "feelings" communication we let these feelings come out and we deal with them.

Also, when we use "feelings" communication, we can come closer to others because we are sharing on a more intimate level.

We have given some examples of gut level or "feelings" communication. Let's look at this type of communication more closely so that we can develop some skills to make it easier to relate in this manner.

I Messages

Feelings communication can be established by using "*I* messages." *I* messages are statements about the self, revelations of inner feelings and needs, information not processed by others.[1]

To have the greatest impact, an *I* message must have three components.[1] (Show the students the following overlay about *I* messages. This overlay is summarized from Gordon's book.)

I Messages

1. The first component involves the identification of a specific behavior.

2. The second component describes the effect that the behavior causes.

3. The third part of the I message states the feelings generated by the effect.

   I messages contain a behavior, an effect, and a feeling.

Here are some examples of *I* messages:

1. When you picked me up late for the football game, I knew that I would miss the band coming in and I was angry.

2. When you broke the date with me, it was too late to get another date and I was furious staying home.

When we use *I* messages we are trying to communicate carefully where we are at with others. *I* messages take responsibility and are stated in the first person.

Hugh Prather says "If you tell me the way you see it, rather than the way it is, that helps me to more fully discover the way I see it." Thus, *I* messages open the way to effective communication on the feelings level.

When communicating on the "feelings" level there are some helpful guidelines. These guidelines are also found in John Powell's book.

Guidelines for Feelings Communication*

1. Feelings level communication must never imply a judgment of the other.

    Let's look back at our first example. When we use *I* messages we describe how we feel. "When you picked me up late for the football game, I knew that I would miss the band coming in and I was angry." This is more effective than if we placed a judgment on the other person. "When you picked me up late for the football game, I knew that I would miss the band coming in and I knew how selfish you really are." The second statement will most likely put the person on the defensive.

2. Emotions are not moral (good or bad). It is o. k. to feel angry, hurt, loving, sad, or whatever. We are expressing how we feel.

    Listen carefully to what Hugh Prather, psychologist, says about this. "I am beginning to think that there are no destructive feelings, only destructive acts, and that my actions become destructive only when I condemn and reject my feelings. If I say I don't want to feel a certain way I disregard the fact that I do feel that way and that the feelings are in me. Feeling a certain way is one feeling; not wanting to feel that way is another feeling and it does not cause the first feeling to stop. I can change my response to a feeling, but I can no more get rid of it than I can get rid of myself. When I disown a feeling, I do not destroy it I only forfeit my capacity to act it out as I wish.[4]

3. Feelings (emotions) must be integrated with the intellect and will.

    In the mentally healthy person, emotions are not kept inside nor do they assume control. They are recognized -what is it that I am feeling? Do I want to act on this feeling or not?

4. In gut level or feelings communication, emotions must be reported.

    To communicate effectively, we are going to need to take some risks. We are going to need to share exactly how we are feeling.

5. With rare exceptions, emotions must be reported at the same time that they are being experienced.

    It is difficult to recapture a feeling once it has passed into my personal history.

So far we have been concerned with communicating on a feelings level and with developing our ability to express our feelings. To enhance communication we also need to be a good listener when someone else is expressing feelings to us.

*Reprinted from *Why Am I Afraid To Tell You Who I Am?* by John Powell © 1969 Argus Communications. Used with permission from Argus Communications, Niles, Illinois.

Feedback

Feedback is the process by which we give information back to another person by any reaction, observation, opinion, clarification, supportive comment, or nonverbal behavior.[2]

One way that we can be a good listener on the feelings level is to practice the art of active listening. Active listening is a skill by means of which we try to make certain that we understand the feelings conveyed in a conversation.

Often when two people talk, the person talking will not express the feeling. The person listening might respond to the talk but not to the feeling. In active listening, the listener tries to make certain that he has heard the feeling part of the message clearly.

"Mary picked me up late for the football game again. It really bugs me when she is always late."

(Response) You really feel annoyed when Mary is late for the game?

Being a careful listener is important because it conveys the fact that you care, as well as helping to clarify what has really been said.

Evaluation

Refer to the behavioral objectives for the suggested ways to evaluate student performance on this lesson.

Mental Health and Self Concept
Developing Assertive Behavior

Objectives

1. When presented with different problem situations, the student will be able to role play responses that demonstrate assertive, nonassertive, and aggressive behavior.

2. The student will be able to write an essay about developing assertive behavior, mentioning at least 10 points made during the lesson.

Sources

1. Neal Ashby "Stop Putting Up With Put Downs," *Today's Health.* July/August, 1975, page 15.

2. "What Is Your Aggravation Quotient?" *Go To Health.* New York: Dell Publishing Company, Inc., copyright 1972 by Communications Research Machines, Inc., page 19.

Content and Procedures

Examining Behavior

Today we are going to examine our behavior, to look at how we react to aggravating situations. I am giving each one of you a questionnaire titled "What Is Your Aggravation Quotient?" I would like you to take about 15 minutes to complete this questionnaire. Give your first and your gut level response. No one but you will see your answers.

What Is Your Aggravation Quotient?*

Read through the following situations, then circle the response that most closely approximates what you think you would do.

1. You have scrimped and saved to spend your weekly allowances to go to the State Fair with a friend. There is one exhibit that is so popular that the lines of people waiting to enter have been endless. You are really interested in this particular exhibit. You stand in line over two hours. You are within several feet of the entrance with only minutes to spare before closing time when a troop of Boy Scouts is escorted by their leader to the front of the line. Your response would be to:
   a. say loudly that the Scout leader is setting a bad example for his troop;
   b. give up and leave the line;
   c. rush to the front of the line and demand entrance;
   d. politely inform the leader of his inconsiderate action;
   e. signal to an attendant and ask that he direct the leader and the Boy Scout troop to the end of the line;
   f. remain in line, seething inwardly.

2. You are sitting in a packed movie theater. The movie has just reached the most exciting part. Two girls behind you begin to discuss how they think the movie will end. It is hard for you to watch and enjoy the movie with their loud discussion. You would:
   a. tell them to shut up or get out;
   b. try to ignore their loud talk;
   c. show them that you are annoyed by turning around and giving them dirty looks;
   d. call an usher to put an end to it;
   e. turn around and ask them to please be quiet;
   f. move to another seat.

3. Your family has just moved to a new neighborhood. You are all quite pleased with the location and with your new house. After living there for several days, a teenager who lives next door invites himself over. It becomes very obvious to you that he is very lonely and really doesn't have any friends. The visits are o.k. at first, but soon you find yourself listening for long periods of time to all of his problems. You would:
   a. very firmly tell him that you need some privacy and time for yourself and ask him to leave immediately;
   b. try to conceal your boredom by a show of concern;
   c. tell him to see the school guidance counselor;
   d. interrupt him and say that you are expecting some friends, that you have to go somewhere, or some similar excuse;
   e. tell him that you are busy now and that when you have time you will go over to his house;
   f. not know what to do.

4. You are out to lunch with a person of the opposite sex whom you like quite a lot. You would like to get to know this person better, but he/she is blowing cigarette smoke in your face. You would:
   a. rise from the table and say, "You're making me sick.";
   b. grin and bear it so that you don't risk not getting to know this person better;
   c. begin a discussion about cigarette smoking, explaining smoking etiquette and all of the statistics that you have read about smoking and lung cancer;
   d. explain that you do not like cigarette smoke and ask him/her to blow the smoke in the other direction;
   e. ask the person to stop smoking during your lunch;
   f. jokingly fan the smoke away from your face with a menu, cough, or make other gestures to express your annoyance.

Adapted from "What Is Your Aggravation Quotient?" *Go to Health*. New York: Dell Publishing Company, 1972.

5. A good friend of yours is staying at your house while his/her parents are on vacation. Unfortunately, your friend has a habit of using swear words. Your parents do not use swear words, and they are very much offended by teenagers who do. During dinner on the first night of your friend's visit, he/she tells a story and uses a four letter word. Both your father and your mother look upset. You would:
   a. cut him/her off abruptly and tell him to either stop swearing or leave the table;
   b. excuse yourself and leave the table:
   c. at the first pause, suggest that he/she see the school guidance counselor about the need to swear;
   d. apologize to your parents for his/her language and explain the behavior as being due to the generation gap;
   e. make an excuse for both of you to leave the table and tactfully tell your friend that his/her language is upsetting your parents;
   f. try to cover for your friend by monopolizing the conversation.

6. It's your birthday and some of your friends have decided to treat you to dinner at the best restaurant in town. You are delighted and, not having had a steak in weeks, you order your favorite filet mignon, medium. The others are served before you and all seem quite satisfied with their dinner. When the waiter brings your steak you are disappointed to find that it has been overcooked. You react by:
   a. calling the manager and complaining about the poor service;
   b. remaining silent to avoid spoiling your birthday celebration;
   c. loudly criticizing the waiter and asking your friends not to leave a tip;
   d. pointing out that the steak is well done and asking the waiter to bring a medium broiled steak;
   e. waiting for the waiter to notice that you are not eating.

7. The student who sits next to you during home room has very bad breath. You have noticed it for several weeks and thought that she would do something about it. You would:
   a. tell her the trouble she's having making friends is because of her terrible breath;
   b. leave mints and gum on your desk hoping she will take some;
   c. really become disgusted and ask your teacher to move her to another desk;
   d. tell her that she has bad breath and that she should visit a dentist or doctor to get rid of it;
   e. offer her gum and mints, telling her that you've found them helpful when you have had bad breath;
   f. be somewhat uncomfortable sitting by her but try hard to ignore it.

8. You are on a camping trip with several friends. Each of you has to share sleeping quarters with someone. The friend that you share a bed with snores loudly. You are a light sleeper. You would:
   a. wake him/her up each time the snoring begins and discuss how awful it is;
   b. try to get used to it;
   c. inform him/her that if the snoring does not stop you are going home;
   d. nudge him/her gently until he/she changes positions;
   e. tell him/her that you cannot sleep because of the snoring and discuss together what can be done about the problem;
   f. use ear plugs.

9. The teacher you have for history class has assigned several projects to be done in groups. Each time there is an assignment and groups are selected, the teacher appoints a group leader. You are working on a project that is very important to you and to your grade. Your group leader blocks rather than helps the group. You have been trying to work around all of the mistakes that the group leader has been making, but you are losing patience. You would:
   a. go to your teacher, tell the teacher about the problem, and say that if something is not done you will quit working on the assignment;
   b. work harder to make up for the lack of work and the mistakes of the group leader;
   c. show the stupidity of your group leader by making fun of his ideas during group meetings;
   d. discuss the problem with other students in your group to try to find ways to make the situation better;
   e. tell the group leader that you are not happy with the way he/she runs the group;
   f. try to get into another group.

10. You are taking the final for your most difficult class. The teacher has put you on the honor system. You are in the middle of the exam when you notice that your closest friend is cheating. With grading done on a curve, a superior paper could really affect your chance of getting a good grade, which you need to go on to college. You would:
   a. tell the teacher that your friend was cheating;
   b. resent your friend's cheating but remain quiet;
   c. copy your friend's answers so that his/her cheating won't hurt you;
   d. tell your friend that if he/she does not stop cheating you will tell the teacher;
   e. remain silent during the exam, but after the exam tell your friend how disappointed and upset you are;
   f. not tell your friend how upset you were about his/her cheating, but drop the friendship.

11. You have finally gotten your driver's license. Your parents have said that you need to help make payments when the car is broken down. To do this, you use the money you have saved. You have just spent $200 to have your car thoroughly checked and repaired. As you are driving home, you notice steam pouring out from under the hood. Suddenly, the car stops running. It costs $25 to have the car towed to the gas station where an attendant tells you that the cooling system is not working. You had been told earlier that the car was "as good as new." Now you are told that you need to spend another $75. You would:
   a. tell the man who looked at your car earlier that he is a crook and demand that he fix the car for free;
   b. tell the second repair man to go ahead with the work and hope that it is the end of your problems;
   c. make a sign that says "lousy service" and that night stick it in the ground in front of the service station;
   d. tell the first repair man that you feel he is responsible for the breakdown and that you do not think that you should pay for the repair;
   e. tell the first repair man that the next time your car needs service you will take it somewhere else;
   f. take the car to another garage hoping that they will do the job right.

12. It is very late on Friday afternoon and you are going to celebrate your father's birthday at dinner. You go into the only good store near your home to quickly find a gift. You have picked out a gift and are standing by the cash register. Not more than five feet away are three sales girls chatting to one another and doing their best to ignore you. You would:
   a. walk out of the store with the gift without paying for it;
   b. wait for one of them to see you;
   c. very loudly proclaim your disgust and demand to be waited on;
   d. approach one of the salesgirls and ask her to wait on you;
   e. go to the manager and inform him that if the service doesn't improve you will have to stop shopping at this store;
   f. give up and leave the store.

13. Today you have the car and get to drive to school. At your school there is very limited space for student parking. You drive around the lot for twenty minutes looking for a space. You finally find a space where someone is pulling out. You wait patiently for them to back out. Just as you begin to back into the space, another student with a small car starts to pull into the spot from behind. You:
   a. wait until he leaves his car and then let the air out of his tires;
   b. get so discouraged that you get sick and go home;
   c. back up and honk your horn until he moves on;
   d. back up so he is unable to park and wait for him to pull out;
   e. back up so he can't enter and explain that you've been waiting a long time for the space and that he should find his own;
   f. give up and look for another parking place.

14. You are invited to a party at a friend's house and you are told that there will be a special surprise when you get there. You really like the friend although you don't know all of the guests who will be there. When you arrive you find out that the surprise is an assortment of drugs to help you all "get high." You are very uncomfortable. You would:
   a. tell the guests at the party that they are immoral and that you are leaving;
   b. take some of the drugs so that you did not look foolish;
   c. call the police;
   d. explain to your friend that you are uncomfortable with drugs and that you are going to leave the party;
   e. leave the party and call your friend later and explain that you were disappointed that there were drugs at the party;
   f. pretend that you were sick and leave the party.

15. The guy (girl) you are dating invites you over to his/her house after school. His (her) parents are not at home leaving you with privacy. You are enjoying kissing and hugging. He/she suggests that you have sex with each other for the first time. You would:
    a. jump up and say "I didn't know that you were like that";
    b. not want to have sex but go ahead and participate so you wouldn't disappoint him/her;
    c. discuss the immorality of premarital sexual behavior;
    d. explain that you are not comfortable with the idea and discuss some limits;
    e. suggest that you discuss your sexual relationship under less threatening circumstances;
    f. say that you need to go home.

(Pause for 15 minutes.)

Now I would like you to add up the number of responses that you have for each letter and jot them down on a piece of paper. Example:

_____ A
_____ B
_____ C
_____ D
_____ E
_____ F

In each of the problem situations presented, two reactions were given that could be characterized as aggressive, two that are nonassertive, and two that are assertive. It will be interesting for you to examine your responses to these situations and to learn how you respond. We will discuss all three behaviors.

Aggressive Personality[2]

If a majority of your responses are A or C you are selecting aggressive responses to aggravating situations. What does this mean? It generally means that you feel the need to assert yourself but that you confuse the natural expression of your rights with encroaching upon the rights of others.

If you have 5–7 A or C responses you are probably aggressive only in certain situations such as when you feel someone is taking advantage of you or you are frustrated, due to interference with your attaining your goal.

Would anyone like to share with us an aggressive response that he or she selected? (Follow with questions about why this response was chosen, did this response help the situation, etc.)

Nonassertive Personality[2]

If a majority of your responses are B or F you are selecting nonassertive responses to aggravating situations. What do you think we mean by a nonassertive response? Look at your B or F responses and see what you think.

When we demonstrate nonassertive behavior we repress our feelings for fear of hurting others or being hurt by them.

The smoking example can be used. If you are bothered by cigarette smoke and you "grin and bear it," you are not expressing how you feel. You are choosing to hold your feelings inside.

Nonassertive behavior is very closely linked to many psychosomatic illnesses such as ulcers, headaches, back ailments. What happens is that the feelings which are bottled up inside rather than expressed directly, are indirectly expressed as an ache or a pain.

If you have selected 5 to 7 B or F answers you may demonstrate nonassertive behavior in certain situations. Sometimes we select nonassertive responses when we are unable to think of a way to deal with behavior.

Assertive Personality[2]

If the majority of your responses are either D or E, you are selecting assertive behavior and most likely you feel very confident in your ability to direct your own life.

You know that by communicating your own feelings in a friendly and honest manner your interpersonal relationships will be enhanced and your desired goals achieved.

You feel happy with yourself for being able to confront your anxiety about a situation and deal with it in a manner that is consistent with your true feelings.

Developing Assertive Behavior[1]

Because of the mental health and self concept benefits of assertive behavior, not to mention the improved interpersonal relationships, assertiveness training workshops are being held in various places.

Assertiveness training is based on the premise that nonassertive and aggressive responses are learned and so they can be unlearned. Assertiveness training programs teach participants to use new techniques when dealing with aggravating situations.

Learning assertive behavior or unlearning nonassertive and aggressive behavior can be accomplished in three steps.

The first step involves examining your current behavior. How do you usually react to aggravating or intimidating situations?

The second step is to look at the behavior that you are not comfortable with. In aggravating situations we often react out of fear. Ask yourself about this fear. What is it that I am afraid of? What is the likelihood of it happening? If it does happen how awful would it really be?

The third step involves putting skills to use. It is very helpful to:

1. State directly what you want or don't want;

2. Speak firmly and confidently—the nonverbal is also very important, voice, body posture, facial expression;
   We often say "no" verbally, but nonverbally give our permission or approval. Can you think of situations where you may have done this?

3. If you aren't successful, be persistent:
   a. repeat your statement,
   b. "you don't seem to be listening";

4. Spell out some consequences if necessary "I feel that what I am asking is reasonable, I will lose respect for you if you don't pay attention to me";

5. In some cases of leadership, you need to demand what you want:
   a. "I'm not going to argue, I insist."

Perhaps the most important lesson to be taught is to avoid the use of "should." Don't rage inwardly because someone is not behaving the way he "should." Instead state the kind of behavior you expect.
a. I was here first, it's my turn.
b. I can't concentrate on my work with that music playing.

Materials

Make a copy of "What Is Your Aggravation Quotient?" for each student.

Evaluation

The evaluation is clearly stated in the behavioral objectives. For the first objective, ask each student to write down a personally aggravating situation on an index card. The students do not need to put their names on the cards. The cards can be shuffled and given to small groups for the role play evaluation.

The following questions might be used for a unit test on mental health and self concept.

1. A person who releases hostilities on innocent victims is demonstrating:
   a. assertive behavior
   b. aggressive behavior
   c. repressive behavior
   d. nonassertive behavior
   e. all of the above

2. You may appear self-confident and in command, but you are actually alienated and react strongly to the slightest threat to your rights:
   a. assertive behavior
   b. aggressive behavior
   c. repressive behavior
   d. nonassertive behavior
   e. all of the above

3. Respect for authority to the point where your rights become subordinate to the desires of others:
   a. assertive behavior
   b. aggressive behavior
   c. hostile behavior
   d. nonassertive behavior
   e. all of the above

4. You know that by communicating your own feelings in a friendly and honest manner your interpersonal relationships will be enhanced:
   a. assertive behavior
   b. aggressive behavior
   c. hostile behavior
   d. nonassertive behavior
   e. all of the above

5. In most cases you feel timid, anxious, and unable to act on your own convictions or you feel guilty about doing so:
   a. assertive behavior
   b. aggressive behavior
   c. hostile behavior
   d. nonassertive behavior
   e. all of the above

6. Assertiveness training is based on the idea that inappropriate responses to aggravating situations is:
   a. learned behavior
   b. undesirable behavior
   c. can be unlearned
   d. responsible for psychosomatic illnesses
   e. all of the above

7. The first step in training for assertive behavior:
   a. stating directly what you want or don't want
   b. rethinking your responses to aggravating or intimidating situations
   c. becoming dominant the first time someone steps on you
   d. expressing a need to a loved one
   e. all of the above

Objectives

1. The student will be able to identify three broad descriptions of the mentally healthy person and three statements which further clarify each broad description.

2. When given a problem situation to evaluate, the student will be able to apply the problem-solving approach (clearly define problem, identify solutions, evaluate solutions, select the best solution, try it, evaluate).

3. The student will be able to describe how a friend might assist in the problem solving-approach.

4. The student will be able to identify at least five things that one can do to help oneself when one has the "blues."

5. The student will be able to identify the ten danger signals of mental health.

6. The student will be able to describe four characteristics of a person considering suicide.

7. The student will be able to identify eight behaviors that indicate suicide symptoms.

8. The student will be able to identify at least five things to do when someone close openly expresses an interest in suicide.

9. The student will be able to give the phone number of the National Youth Emergency Hotline.

Sources

1. National Association of Mental Health. *Mental Health is 1, 2, 3*. Washington, D.C.: National Association for Mental Health, 1968.

2. National Association for Mental Health, "Ten Danger Signals," 1800 North Kent Street, Arlington, Virginia 22209.

3. "Point of No Return: Teenagers and Suicide," *Current Lifestudies*. Volume 2, No. 7, March 1979, pages 4-13.

Content and Procedures

What Is Mental Health

Have you ever asked yourself what it means to be mentally healthy? or, how do you know if you have good mental health? After all, each of us has to cope with a variety of situations. The presence of a difficult situation in our life does not mean that we are not mentally healthy.

Stop for a minute and write down what it means to you to be mentally healthy. . . . . who would like to share with the class their answer to this question?

Now I am going to give you a handout that describes "what is good mental health." It is taken from the National Association for Mental Health from a publication titled *Mental Health Is 1, 2, 3*. Let's look carefully at the description of the person who has good mental health. We can see that there are three broad descriptions of the mentally healthy person and then several statements which further clarify each broad description. The three broad areas are:

1. The mentally healthy person feels comfortable about himself.
2. The mentally healthy person feels right about other people.
3. The mentally healthy person is able to meet the demands of life.

Take a minute to read through each description and put a check in front of each statement that describes you. You will keep this for yourself, unless you would like to share something you have checked or left blank with me or with your classmates.

Would anyone like to share something that he learned by looking at this list closely and thinking about himself?

I would like to share something that I feel about mental health. I would like to say that I think that we need to look at our mental health frequently to assure that we are in top running order.

I find that I am faced with new situations, new people, new challenges, and that I need to adapt and to meet many different demands of daily living.

Some mental health experts have defined the mentally healthy person as "the person who effectively uses the problem-solving approach to living and who learns to successfully cope as problems arise."

Problem Solving

What does this mean? It simply means that each of us has problems or difficulties and that we need to develop; the art of problem-solving and to apply problem-solving to difficulties as they arise in our daily living.

This is how problem-solving works:

1. First of all you notice that things are not going as smoothly as you would like them to. As we mentioned before, you might notice that you do not feel comfortable with yourself, that you do not feel right about other people, or that you are not able to meet the demands of life, i.e., school, the team, the group.

2. The first thing that you do when you use the problem-solving approach in your daily living, is to define what you see as the problem or difficulty. It is a good idea to clearly state the problem in writing. Writing the problem will help you to clarify it and to focus more clearly on what is bothering you.

3. After you have defined your problem, let your imagination go to work without making any decisions. Write down every possible solution you can think of. Remember, do not make any judgments. Get every possible idea in front of you.

4. After you have listed all the solutions that you can possibly think of, go through your list. What do you think of each idea? Which solution is the easiest? Which solution will work the best? Are there any drawbacks to the solution?

5. Select the solution that you are most satisfied with—the one which answers the most of the questions that we just discussed.

6. Try this solution to see how it works.

7. After you have tried the solution, ask yourself: Am I satisfied with this solution? Do I feel more comfortable with myself? Do I feel right about the people who may be involved? Do I feel that I am now able to meet the demands of daily living? If the solution that you selected worked well for you then you can retain it. If it did not, begin again. Define the problem, then reflect and try a new solution.

To the teacher: Ask the students for different examples of problems and have the class apply the problem solving approach.

Friends May Help

We have just learned the problem-solving approach. I wanted to repeat something that I said. The mentally healthy person learns to employ problem solving to difficult situations as they arise in daily living. Thus, the more you practice this approach, the more natural it will become. You will feel and be more effective in your life style.

Sometimes, however, you have difficulty with one of the steps in the problem solving approach. Here are some of the difficulties that each of us might experience, add any that you can think of:

1. It is difficult to see the problem clearly. You are having a hard time defining the problem, it is unclear and confusing.

2. You feel that there are some alternatives, some ways to deal with the problem that you cannot think of.

3. You are having difficulty evaluating each alternative carefully and objectively.

Can you think of any other difficulties?

Sometimes it is helpful to talk to a friend, someone whom you trust, about a difficult situation. Your friend might be able to help you in a variety of ways:

1. Sometimes by just listening, a friend helps us to discover more about the problem, alternatives, and solutions.

2. A caring friend will be helpful when you are feeling "down in the dumps."

3. Your friend might share some ideas, helping you to define the problem more clearly and to identify more alternatives.

Friends are important. There is one thing to remember, however. You should always make the decision. It may be helpful to talk things over with a friend, but it is always your responsibility to make the decision on how to solve a problem.

The same guidelines apply when you are helping one of your friends. You may be helpful by listening, caring, defining the problem, sharing ideas or solutions, and helping to evaluate, but you should let your friend choose his or her solution to the problem.

So far, we have talked about dealing with a problem directly by oneself and discussing a problem with a friend or someone else you trust, perhaps your teacher, your parents, your coach.

What Is Good Mental Health?

Directions: Put a check in front of each statement that describes you. This handout is reprinted from the National Association for Mental Health, *Mental Health is 1, 2, 3*. Washington, D.C.: National Association for Mental Health, 1968.

_____ 1. *I feel comfortable about myself.*

_____ 2. I am not bowled over by my own emotions—by my fears, anger, love, jealousy, guilt, or worries.

_____ 3. I can take life's disappointments in their stride.

_____ 4. I have a tolerant, easygoing attitude toward myself as well as others; I can laugh at myself.

_____ 5. I neither underestimate nor overestimate my abilities.

_____ 6. I can accept my own shortcomings.

_____ 7. I have self-respect.

_____ 8. I feel able to deal with most situations that come my way.

_____ 9. I get satisfaction from the simple, everyday pleasures.

_____ 10. _I feel right about other people._

_____ 11. I am able to give love and to consider the interests of others.

_____ 12. I have personal relationships that are satisfying and lasting.

_____ 13. I expect to like and trust others, and take it for granted that others will like and trust me.

_____ 14. I respect the many differences I find in people.

_____ 15. I do not push people around, nor do I allow myself to be pushed around.

_____ 16. I can feel I am part of a group.

_____ 17. I feel a sense of responsibility to my neighbors and fellow men.

_____ 18. _I am able to meet the demands of life._

_____ 19. I do something about my problems as they arise.

_____ 20. I accept my responsibilities.

_____ 21. I shape my environment whenever possible; I adjust to it whenever necessary.

_____ 22. I plan ahead but do not fear the future.

_____ 23. I welcome new experiences and new ideas.

_____ 24. I make use of my natural capacities.

_____ 25. I set realistic goals for myself.

_____ 26. I am able to think for myself and make my own decisions.

_____ 27. I put my best effort into what I do, and get satisfaction out of doing it.

Tips While Working on Problems

While you are working on a problem that is posing you some difficulty you may feel down in the dumps. This feeling is one of depression, the most common emotional problem. When you experience depression and it is not severe, you can do many different things to make yourself feel better. While you are involved in the problem-solving approach also try the following:

1. Change your routine. Avoid monotony by going to school a different way, calling a friend you have not talked to for a while, eating something different for lunch, rearranging your room.

2. Discuss your temporary depression with your best friend, your parents, your teacher, or your school counselor.

3. Do something nice for someone else. Visit someone who is sick or help a youngster with a problem.

4. List all of the things that you do well and all of the things that you like about yourself.

5. Pay close attention to your grooming habits. Get out of bed as soon as you wake up, and get dressed.

6. Try to get exercise and fresh air each day.

Community or Other Mental Health Service

Sometimes the problems of living become so difficult that normal responses to life situations are interrupted and a person is left with behaviors that are not conducive to positive mental health. Since we all experience problems of living, you might ask "What behaviors indicate that I may need some extra kind of help?"

The National Association for Mental Health identifies ten danger signals:[2]

1. A general and lasting feeling of hopelessness and despair.

2. Inability to concentrate, making reading, writing, and conversation difficult.

3. Changes in physical activity like eating, sleeping, sex.

4. A loss of self-esteem which brings on continual questioning of personal worth.

5. Withdrawal from others, not by choice but from an immense fear of rejection by others.

6. Threats or attempts to commit suicide.

7. Extreme sensitivity to words and actions of others, and general irritability.

8. Misdirected anger and difficulty in handling most feelings.

9. Feelings of guilt and self blame.

10. Extreme dependency.

If feelings and behaviors such as these persist, then counseling may be helpful. There are several places where you can receive good counseling:

1. your school counselor;
2. a community mental health center;
3. your church;
4. a qualified counselor in private practice.

What can you expect to happen when seeking outside help? What are some of the questions that people have about such counseling? While specific practices may differ, the following information is typical of many counseling situations:

1. You will call for an appointment, giving your name, address, and nature of the difficulty.

2. All information which you give will be kept confidential unless you agree in writing that the information can be shared. Everything that you say to a counselor is confidential, (including your parents).

3. When you meet with your counselor you will discuss your problem in more detail. A counselor is a trained professional who will once again help you to see the problem more clearly, develop many solutions, evaluate the alternatives, and select one to try.

4. You cannot expect a counselor to give you the solution to a problem or to select the alternative for you to try. The counselor assists you in finding what will work best for you.

5. Sometimes the counselor will refer you to another person or agency that might better assist you with your difficulty.

Teenagers have many different problems or life situations facing them. It is not uncommon for a teenager to be confused and to need to use the problem-solving approach frequently. It is also very common for teenagers to have a friend with whom to share some of these situations. And it is very acceptable for a teenager to see a counselor when difficulties persist.

As mentioned previously, effective coping or problem solving means examining many alternatives or solutions to a problem and selecting one that will work the best.

Teenage Suicide

There is one alternative to problems of living that is selected by approximately 5000 teenagers between the ages of 15 and 24 each year. This alternative to difficulties is tragic—it is suicide, an irreversible alternative or solution.

The suicide rate for teenagers and young adults has tripled in the last twenty years. Charlotte Ross, director of the San Mateo Suicide Prevention Center said that "the yearly suicide rate for persons between the ages of 15 and 24 years old is now almost 5000. We have validated attempts by kids as young as six or seven years old," she said. "The reasons for suicide among young people could be loss of a parent, a divorce, breaking up with a girlfriend or boyfriend or loss of self esteem, health or faith," she said.[3]

Suicide is one solution to a problem. At one point or another everyone thinks about committing suicide. However, in each of the cases we have just mentioned (loss of parent, etc.) can you think of other solutions to the problem that are not as tragic or irreversible as suicide?

Characteristics of Someone Thinking about Suicide

Dr. Calvin Frederick of the National Institute of Mental Health offers a good deal of important information about suicide. He says that a person considering suicide may:[3]

1. talk a lot about suicide in general or someone else's suicide;

2. ask a lot of questions about life after death;

3. give away a prized possession, hinting that (s)he won't be needing it anymore;

4. talk a lot about revenge or getting even with his or her parents.

Dr. Frederick thinks that it is important that each of us notices behaviors which may indicate suicide symptoms. Notice when a person close to you:[3]

1. acts depressed;

2. keeps away from friends;

3. stops communicating with parents, or indicates there is trouble at home;

4. begins smoking heavily;

5. acts irritable or anxious;

6. changes behavior drastically—a person who usually is busy becomes apathetic and isolated, a quiet person suddenly becomes loud;

7. loses interest in school work;

8. changes sleeping and eating habits drastically.

What to Do

Further, when someone close to you openly expresses suicide, here are some guidelines:[3]

1. Really listen to the person. Don't pass it off with "Oh, you can't mean that." Quietly hear the person out.

2. Don't be judgmental. Avoid statements like "you must be crazy to think that."

3. Give reassurance that feelings of depression are temporary and will pass.

4. Mention that if a person chooses to die, the situation cannot be reversed.

5. Don't challenge the person in an attempt to shock him or her out of suicidal ideas.

6. Point out that while life exists, there is always a chance for solving problems, but that death is final.

These points tie in closely with the problem-solving approach. Suicide is just one of the many alternatives to select when facing a difficult situation or problem. When evaluating the pros and cons of this choice, it is not a good one. There is a National Youth Emergency Hotline for youth who are thinking about this as a choice, or for youth who just want to discuss any problem of living. The number is toll free:

800–621–4000
800–972–6004 (if you live in Illinois)

To the Teacher: Arrange for someone from your community hotline to come and talk to your class. After the visit, your students can role play using telephones and simulating calls for help to the hotline. Students should be able to propose at least five things to do when someone calling the hotline mentions suicide.

Coping Kit Activity

Have each student make a coping kit. Have the students use as much originality as possible in designing a kit and deciding what it should include. Example: The Franklin County Mental Health and Retardation Board developed a MENTAL HEALTH: 1977 OWNER'S MANUAL. It was designed like a car owner's manual with "important operating, maintenance, and service information." Your students will think of many clever ideas for summarizing the material from this lesson.

Evaluation

Each of the objectives identified can be tested easily with a short completion test. You might like the students to select a personal problem to work with for the completion of the second objective. This will help the student apply what (s)he has learned in the test situation.

Mental Health and Self Concept

_____ Make a list of what you consider to be the ten most distressing events in the life of a teenager.

_____ Make a list of at least ten things you love to do.

1. Place the letter "A" after those activities you enjoy when you're alone.
2. Place the letter "P" after those activities you enjoy with other people.
3. Place the symbol $ after each activity that costs more than ten dollars.
4. Place the letter "R" after those activities that involve personal risk.
5. Place the letter "M" after each activity that your mother also enjoys.
6. Place the letter "F" after each activity that your father also enjoys.
7. Make a checkmark after each activity you think you will still enjoy doing five years from now.

_____ Discuss pictures of people showing various emotions. Do you think it's all right to cry? Play the song or read the poem, "It's All Right to Cry," from _Free To Be . . . You and Me._

_____ Discuss cheating—What does it gain? Whom does it hurt?

_____ Describe a tension you have experienced lately. What did you do to relieve it?

_____ Investigate a specific phobia. Aerophobia—fear of fresh air; agoraphobia—fear of open places; androphobia—fear of men; algophobia—fear of pain.

_____ Distinguish the differences between psychoanalysis, group therapy, family therapy, behavior therapy, play therapy, drug therapy, and psychodrama.

_____ Borrow films for your class from the county or state mental health association. What key concepts are stressed?

_____ Discuss the problems and prejudices which a person discharged from a mental hospital may have to overcome.

_____ Make a list of the organizations and facilities concerned with mental health in your community.

_____ Collect quotations and poems by philosophers and poets about friendship, and then try to develop your own definition of friendship.

_____ Make a friendship card with your favorite poem or quotation.

_____ Visit a mental health center that deals with problems of adolescence.

_____ Role play assertive, nonassertive, and aggressive behavior.

_____ Make a bulletin board that depicts the various mental health careers.

_____ Keep a diary for a week, recording the various emotions that you experience. Chart the frequency and the types of emotions experienced.

_____ Write a paper describing your uniqueness.

_____ Rate your decision-making skills, describing the influence of family, friends, and church.

_____ Describe the different types of mental illnesses.

_____ Watch a television show and record the different problems depicted and the coping skills used.

_____ Find out the number of your local suicide prevention hotline.

_____ Write a paper describing your personality.

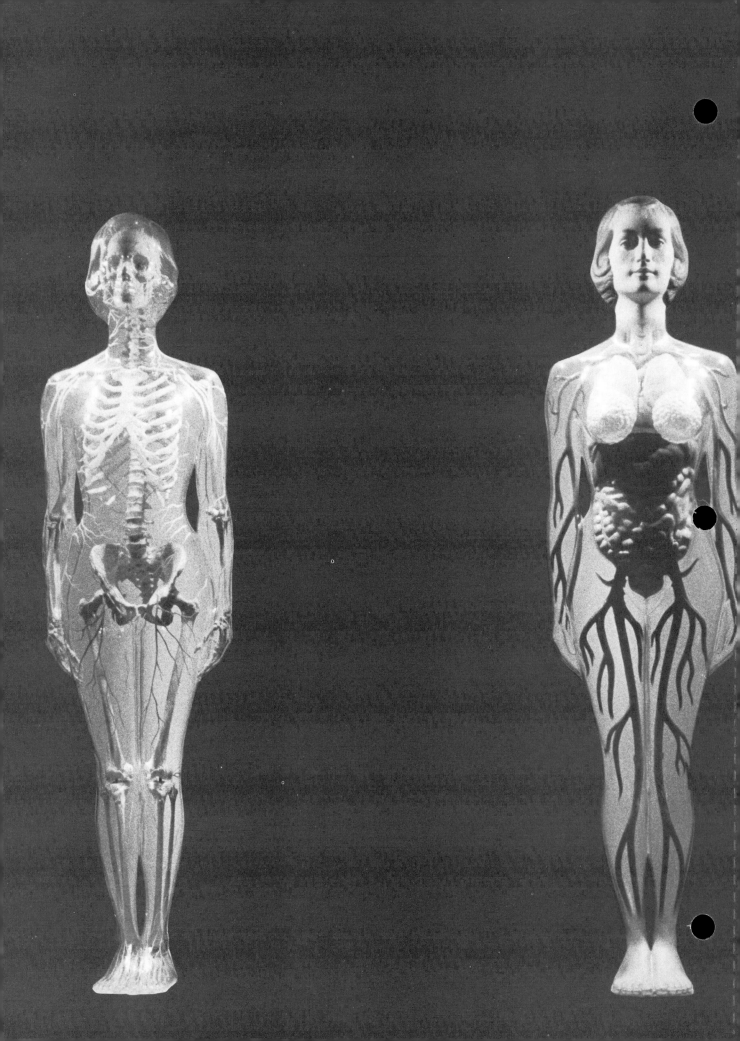

12

Teaching about the Human Body

A basic understanding of the human body facilitates learning about the care and positive health behavior needed to live optimally. This chapter includes an outline of Suggested Topics for Teaching About The Human Body, Three Detailed Lessons that have been used with middle and secondary school students, and additional Selected Learning Activities.

The first lesson, **Many Parts Make a Whole,** provides the student with background information about each body system. Each of the following systems is carefully reviewed: Skeletal System, Muscular System, Nervous System, Circulatory and Lymphatic System, Respiratory System, Digestive System, Urinary System, Endocrine System, and Reproductive System.

The second lesson, **We've All Got Rhythm,** familiarizes the student with *circadian* rhythm, the twenty-four hour period of activity and rest for most living organisms. The student personalizes the information and becomes aware of his own inner timing. Some of the areas of personal awareness include: hunger contractions, thirst, the chill of dropping body temperatures, the quality of fresh vigor, fatigue, mood changes, mental alertness, urine excretion, increased sensitivity to smell, increased sensitivity to light, increased sensitivity to sound, and increased taste sensitivity.

A discussion of the human body would not be complete without a look to the future. The third lesson, **New Frontiers,** discusses medical research as well as raising pertinent questions about values. Such controversial topics as "in vitro fertilization," the test tube baby, and "cloning," the production of a genetically duplicate individual from the biological information contained in a single body cell, are discussed.

Suggested Topics

The Human Body

I. Characteristics of Living Organisms
II. Cells and Body Structure
   A. Structure and Function of Cells
   B. Tissues
   C. Organs

Photo by Bob Coyle

D. Systems—Structure, Function, Diseases and Disorders
   1. Skeletal System
   2. Muscular System
   3. Nervous/Sensory System
   4. Circulatory System
   5. Lymphatic System
   6. Respiratory System
   7. Digestive Systen
   8. Excretory System
   9. Endocrine System
   10. Reproductive System
III. Interdependence of Body Systems
IV. Improving Appearance and General Health
   A. Proper Nourishment
   B. Need for Exercise and Rest
   C. Improving Posture
   D. Reducing Stress
   E. Breaking Unhealthy Habits
   F. Care of Skin, Hair, and Nails
   G. Care of Teeth and Gums
   H. Care of Eyes and Ears
V. Funny Things the Body Does (e.g., Discuss what causes blushing; dimples; yawning; "goosebumps"; hair to turn gray, etc.)
VI. Human Biological Rhythms
VII. Relationship Between Weather and Health
VIII. New Frontiers
   A. Nucleic-Acid "Engineering"/Cloning
   B. Growing New Limbs
   C. Blood Research
   D. Artificial Organs
   E. New Drugs

Lesson Plans

The Human Body
Many Parts Make a Whole

Objectives

1. Each student will research one body part and summarize the information in "first person" form.

2. Each student, portraying a particular body part, will participate in a group skit that will be presented to a younger class.

3. Given an outline of the human body and some of its organs, the student will be able to label correctly at least twelve of its parts and identify the system to which each part belongs.

4. Given an outline of the human body and some of its endocrine glands, the student will be able to correctly label at least six different endocrine glands and predict the influence of their secretions on basic bodily functions.

5. The student will be able to give three examples illustrating the interrelationships that exist between body parts.

6. As part of a small group, the student will assist in the development of an original game or learning activity that evaluates student knowledge of a particular body part or system.

Sources

1. Reprint Editor, *The Reader's Digest,* Pleasantville, New York, 10570.

2. John J. Burt, Linda B. Meeks, Sharon M. Pottebaum. *Toward A Healthy Lifestyle Through Elementary Health Education.* Belmont, California: Wadsworth Publishing Company, Inc., 1980.

3. Edward B. Johns, Wilfred C. Sutton, Lloyd E. Webster (deceased). *Health For Effective Living.* New York: McGraw-Hill Book Company, Fifth Edition, 1970.

4. Text by Samuel Smith; Edited by M. F. Ashley Montagu and Ernest F. Kerby. *Atlas of Human Anatomy.* New York: Barnes and Noble, Inc., Sixth Edition, 1961.

Content and Procedures

Since "I Am Joe's Heart" by J. D. Ratcliff first appeared in the *Reader's Digest* (April, 1967), over thirty organs, endocrine glands, and various body parts have had an opportunity to tell their stories. Write to the *Reader's Digest*[1] for a complete set of these informative articles, available at a nominal charge.

Body Organ Skits

Ask each student to select one *Reader's Digest* article as the basis of an individual research project. The students may wish to consult additional resources before summarizing their human body information in "first person" form.

Let the students then determine how they want to present their information to a younger class. A series of skits around such topics as "The Body Revealed," "The Transparent Person," or "The Gift of Life" can be performed with the students dressed in black tights and leotards. Brightly colored body parts cut out of construction paper could be attached over their appropriate locations in the body, or each student might choose to wear "sandwich boards" made out of large pieces of poster board. The front board might be a large illustration of the organ or gland, while the back board spells out its proper name. A more ambitious project would be to enlist the aid of an art teacher and construct huge papier-mache organs that could be worn. Additional props may be carried, e.g., large wood beads strung together with string to represent the vertebrae that constitute the spine; real animal bones; real teeth; different kinds of pumps (turkey baster, water gun) to simulate the action of the heart; beef organs; model breathing apparatus;[2] and objects to touch, smell, or taste. Each "body part" should be given no more than one minute to describe its importance and relationship with other body parts.

Keeping in mind the concept that a "human being functions as a total organism,"[3] (p. 00) with all parts working together in harmony, the students may wish to appear together as body systems. The organs representing the digestive system, as well as the "teeth" and "tongue" may appropriately line up and pass an item of food from one body part to another, after describing their specific functions. The "nose" may pass a balloon (representing air) to the "windpipe" (trachea), and "lungs." This sequence leads nicely into the circulatory system, where the balloon continues to be passed by the "bloodstream" to the "heart," and onto other waiting parts.

After independent study and group rehearsals of the skits, all students should be aware of the following information.

The Skeletal System

The adult skeletal system consists of some 206 bones, cartilage, and numerous ligaments that provide support, a firm framework, and give shape to the body. "They protect vital organs, such as the heart, brain, and lungs, from injury as well as facilitate bodily movements by acting in cooperation with numerous muscles attached to bones by tendons."[4](p. 00) The red bone marrow manufactures blood cells, while the skeleton stores nearly all of the body's calcium supply. Most disorders of the skeletal system come in the form of dislocations, cracks, and fractures. Joints are subject to rheumatoid arthritis, osteoarthritis, infections, and other types of inflammation.

The Muscular System

The muscular system is composed of 656 *skeletal* muscles (2 single, 327 pairs)[4] that are voluntary in action and control body posture, vocalization by tongue and lips, swallowing, and the movement of other body parts. The involuntary action of *smooth* muscles is present in the walls of the digestive tract as they propel food materials through body passageways; expel materials from the body; constrict or dilate body openings (e.g., the pupil of the eye) and contract or expand blood vessels. *Cardiac* muscle tissue is normally involuntary and found only in the walls of the heart. Common muscle disorders include cramps, spasms, and sprains. In tetanus, the muscles are locked in a sustained contraction. During an epileptic seizure the muscles contract and relax, resulting in jerking movements. Muscular dystrophy is a progressive, inherited disorder that results in the destruction of muscle fibers.

The Nervous System

The primary function of the nervous system is to ensure the coordination of the millions of cells that comprise the human body. The *central* nervous system, consisting of the brain and spinal cord, is concerned with consciousness, memory, learning, feeling, and reactions to messages received by the sense organs. The *peripheral* nervous system includes twelve cranial nerves, 31 pairs of spinal nerves, and the autonomic nervous system. The autonomic (involuntary) nervous system is not a separate entity but a grouping of special nerve components that travel within certain spinal and cranial nerves and innervate smooth muscles, cardiac muscles and glands. The nervous system may be damaged through injuries, such as a sharp blow to the head, irradiation, and poisoning. By using a machine called an *electroencephalograph*, which records electrical impulses generated by the brain, a physician is aided in the diagnosis of such conditions as epilepsy, tumors, infections, and brain hemorrhages.

The Circulatory and Lymphatic Systems

Although most people only think of blood, blood vessels, and the heart, when considering the workings of the circulatory system, there are other body fluids (synovial fluid in joint cavities, aqueous humor of the eye, cerebrospinal fluid in the brain, lymph fluids, etc.) that are necessary as well. The *heart* is a muscular organ composed of four chambers and four valves. Its purpose is to pump blood rich in oxygen and nutrients through a vast network of blood vessels to all living body cells as well as assist in the removal of wastes.

Lymph fluids, however, are not pumped through various lymph ducts. "They are propelled by differences in capillary pressure, muscle action, intestinal movements, and other sources of pressure . . . Lymph ducts resemble veins but have numerous valves and glands (nodes) which filter the lymph, clearing it of bacteria, arresting carbon particles and malignant cells, and manufacture white cells."[4] The spleen, tonsils, and thymus constitute the chief lymphoid organs. Many disorders of the circulatory system are well known. They include high blood pressure, heart defects, and heart disease. See chapter thirteen for additional information.

The Respiratory System

The circulatory system is dependent upon the respiratory system to supply it with the oxygen needed to sustain life. Air from the external environment enters through the nose or mouth, and passes through the pharynx, larynx, trachea, and right and left bronchi, before reaching the alveoli or tiny air sacs of the lungs. The process of diffusion enables an exchange of gases between the blood and lungs to take place. The diaphragm and chest muscles also assist the breathing process by increasing and decreasing air pressure in the lungs. Since the entire respiratory tract represents a direct link with the outside world, it is not surprising that most of its disorders are the result of airborne infections and irritants. Head colds may lead to sinus and ear infections. Laryngitis, tuberculosis, emphysema, pleurisy, and various tumors are other problems associated with this system.

The Digestive System

The organs and accessory glands which comprise the digestive system enable both man and animal to make life out of life. Food enters this system through the mouth, a vestibule formed by the cheeks, lips, teeth, and gums. It is here that food particles are pushed around by the tongue, broken into smaller pieces by the teeth, moistened by the salivary glands, and bound together with mucin to form a *bolus* for swallowing. The bolus is then propelled from the mouth through the pharynx and esophagus to the stomach. The stomach is a J-shaped, temporary storage bin that churns food and gastric juices into a mixture known as *chyme*. Little by little, food leaves the stomach and is pushed into the small intestine, where bile, pancreatic juice, and intestinal secretions further the digestion process. Churning continues another several hours before the digested food proteins and carbohydrates are absorbed by the blood and carried throughout the body. Excess carbohydrate is converted to glycogen and stored in the liver along with other important substances. In addition, the liver operates like a detoxication center for the body, secretes bile, breaks down old red blood cells, and is essential in the manufacture of pro-clotting prothrombin and fibrinogen, and anticlotting heparin.

Remaining foodstuffs are pushed into the large intestine, where water is absorbed and bacteria aid in the decomposition process. After 24 hours or more, a series of contractions push the final waste products through the rectum and out the anus. Disorders of the digestive system include dental problems, internal hemorrhage, infections of the appendix and gall bladder, peptic ulcers, colitis, and cirrhosis of the liver.

The Urinary System

Liquid waste materials are eliminated from the body through the pores in the skin, by breathing, and through the urinary system. Urine (95% water) flows through a small tube (*ureter*) from each bean-shaped kidney, into a muscular bag called the *urinary bladder*. When the bladder is filled, nerves stimulate muscles to expel the urine through the *urethra*. In the male, the urethra extends through the penis and carries both urine and semen. In the female, the urethra is much shorter and serves only as an excretory duct. Disorders of the urinary system include infections, various kidney diseases, kidney stones, and in men, disorders of the prostate gland, which may enlarge and impede the flow of urine.

The Endocrine System

There is a close interaction between the endocrine glands and the central nervous system, as they work together to control the complex activities carried out by the human body. The following endocrine glands secrete hormones ("exciters" or "messengers") directly into the bloodstream to control distant organs.

Glands	Hormones	Action
Pituitary (located at the base of the brain)	hormones have been identified, including TSH, ACTH, FSH, and ICSH	These hormones regulate growth; thyroid activity; adrenal cortex activity; the maturation of sex cells; increase the sex hormone secretions of the body; stimulate the growth of breast tissue and milk production; contract blood vessels; etc.
Thyroid (located in the neck, over the windpipe)	Thyroxin	Regulates body metabolism. Influences growth, development of teeth, and stimulates the nervous system.
Parathyroids (4) (located behind the thyroid gland)	Parathormone	**Aid in maintaining normal functioning of the nerves and muscles by controlling the amounts of calcium and phosphorus in the blood.**
Adrenals (2) (located above each kidney) Cortex-outer portion: Medulla-central core:	Many steroids Adrenalin and Noradrenalin	Many regulatory functions including metabolism of sugar and fat; regulation of salt and water balance; The cortex also secretes sex hormones. These hormones increase the rate and power of the heart; raise blood pressure; and relax smooth muscles.
Pancreas (Islets of Langerhans-located behind the stomach)	Insulin Glucagon	Regulates carbohydrate metabolism. (Failure of the pancreas to secrete adequate insulin causes diabetes).
Ovaries (2) (located in female abdominal cavity) Ovarian follicle: Corpus luteum:	Estrogens Progesterone	Estrogen and Progesterone regulate the development and functioning of female accessory sex organs and secondary sex characteristics. Prepares uterus for implantation; inhibits uterine contractions.

Glands	Hormones	Action
Testis (2) (located in male sac called the scrotum, outside abdominal cavity)	Testosterone	Essential for the growth and enlargement of the entire male reproductive system; a deeper voice; development of pubic, facial, and other body hair; growth of muscles; and development of sex drive.
Pineal Body (located in the mid-brain)	Unknown	The Pineal body reaches its maximum size in childhood; Tumors of the pineal in prepubertal children produce accelerated sexual development.[4]
Thymus (located deep in the neck)	Unknown	This gland decreases in size after puberty. Important in the development of immune response in newborn. Its removal during early childhood has been associated with an increased susceptibility to acute infectious diseases at a later time.
Duodenal Mucosa (upper part of small intestine)	Secretin Pancreozymin Cholecystokinin Enterogasterone	These hormones play an important role in the activities of the pancreas, liver, gallbladder, and stomach; increase flow of bile; Enterogasterone reduces stomach acid and has been called the "anti-ulcer" hormone.
Placenta (a structure formed in the uterus during pregnancy to nourish the fetus)	Chorionic gonadotrophin Estrogens Progesterone	Chorionic gonadotrophin appears in the blood and urine of pregnant women; causes corpus luteum to develop and persist; during pregnancy, the placenta supplements the endocrine functions of the ovaries

The over or under secretion of an endocrine gland can result in many serious disorders, including goiter, cretinism (Thyroid); dwarfism, gigantism (Pituitary); tetany (Parathyroid); Addison's disease, Cushing's syndrome (Adrenal Cortex); Diabetes (Pancreas—Islets of Langerhans); and failure to mature sexually (Ovaries and Testes).

The Reproductive System

Although the chief function of the reproductive system is perpetuation of the species, this system exerts a tremendous lifelong influence over the individual due to the hormones produced by the ovaries and testes.

The principal male reproductive organs manufacture male sex cells, provide means of intercourse, secrete seminal fluid, and convey spermatozoa to the reproductive organs of the female. These organs include: (1) two *testes* (produce spermatozoa as well as testosterone) that are enclosed in a sac called the *scrotum,* located outside the abdominal cavity; (2) a *duct system,* including the *epididymis, ductus deferens* or vas deferens, *ejaculatory ducts,* and *urethra,* which permit sperm cells to travel to the outside; (3) accessory glands, including two *seminal vesicles,* a *prostate,* gland, and two *bulbo-urethral* (cowpers) gland, which contribute to the formation of seminal fluid that nourishes and carries the sperm cells; and (4) the *penis,* a male organ for intercourse and urination.

The principal female reproductive organs manufacture female sex cells, and are primarily concerned with fertilization and embryonic development, menstruation, and pregnancy. These organs include: (1) two *ovaries* (produce ova and secrete hormones); (2) two *Fallopian* (or uterine) *tubes,* through which ova pass on their way from the ovaries to the uterus. Fertilization usually occurs in the upper third of the fallopian tube; (3) the *uterus* (womb) is a hollow muscular pouch located in the pelvic cavity between the bladder and the rectum. If an ovum is fertilized it implants itself in the lining of the uterus and develops into a full term baby. If fertilization does not occur, the lining of the uterus dies and is expelled as menstrual flow. The uterus develops a new lining, and bleeding stops about five days after the onset of menstruation; (4) the *vagina* is a 3 to 4 inch muscular tube extending from the cervix (neck) of the uterus to the external genitalia. It serves as the female organ of intercourse, a passageway for arriving male sperm, a canal through which a baby is born, and a passageway for the menstrual flow; (5) The *external genitalia,* or vulva, consist of the *mons veneris* (fatty cushion over front surface of the pubic bone), *labia majora* (large heavy folds of skin surrounding the external opening of the vagina), *labia minora* (two smaller folds of skin between the labia majora), *clitoris* (a small erectile structure between the labia minora that contains many sensory nerve endings and serves as a receptor and transmittor of sexual stimuli), *vestibule* of the vagina, and vestibular glands including *Bartholin's glands.*

Diseases and disorders of the male reproductive system include crytorchism (failure of the testes to descend into the scrotum during embryonic development, thereby causing sterility); enlargement of the prostate gland, leading to painful urination; and inflammation of the urethral lining or seminal vesicle. The female may be bothered by vaginitis (inflammation of the vagina); tumors affecting the uterus, ovaries, or breasts; a dropped uterus; and ovarian cysts. Either sex may become sterile (unable to produce offspring) or contract a venereal disease, such as Gonorrhea, Syphilis, or Chancroid.

Materials

1. Reprints of "I Am Joe's (or Jane's) . . . articles from *The Reader's Digest.*

2. Outline of the human body and some of its organs (included on page 439)

3. Outline of the human body and some of its endocrine glands (Included on page 440).

Evaluation

1. Answers to Objective 3:
(1)	Brain or Cerebrum	—Nervous System
(2)	Spinal Cord	—Nervous System
(3)	Trachea (Windpipe)	—Respiratory System
(4)	Lung	—Respiratory System
(5)	Heart	—Circulatory System (a muscle)
(6)	Diaphragm	—Respiratory System (but also a muscle)
(7)	Liver	—Digestive System
(8)	Gall Bladder	—Digestive System

(9)	Stomach	—Digestive System
(10)	Kidney	—Excretory System
(11)	Pancreas	—Endocrine System
(12)	Large Intestine	—Digestive System
(13)	Small Intestine	—Digestive System
(14)	Appendix	—Digestive System
(15)	Rectum	—Excretory System

2. Answers to Objective 4:

(1)	Pineal Body	—Unknown
(2)	Pituitary	—Regulates growth, thyroid activity and maturation of sex cells, etc.
(3)	Parathyroids	—Assist in normal functioning of the nerves and muscles.
(4)	Thyroid	—Regulates body metabolism, influences growth and development of teeth, etc.
(5)	Thymus	—Helps to provide immunity from infectious diseases in young children.
(6)	Adrenals	—Aids in metabolism of sugar and fat; regulation of salt and water balance, etc.
(7)	Pancreas	—Regulates carbohydrate metabolism.
(8)	Testes	—Regulate growth and development of male reproductive system, including sex drive.
(9)	Ovaries	—Regulate growth and development of female sex organs and characteristics.

3. Crossword puzzles, original plays, buzz boards, etc. can be developed to evaluate student knowledge of a particular body part or system. Teachers may also wish to use the *Brain Maze* in *Current Health*- The Continuing Guide to Health Education; Vol. 2, #7, March 1976, Curriculum Innovations, Inc. and the game, "Fertilization: A Game of Chance,"[2] from Chapter 8B, Unit 8, *Toward A Healthy Lifestyle Through Elementary Health Education.*

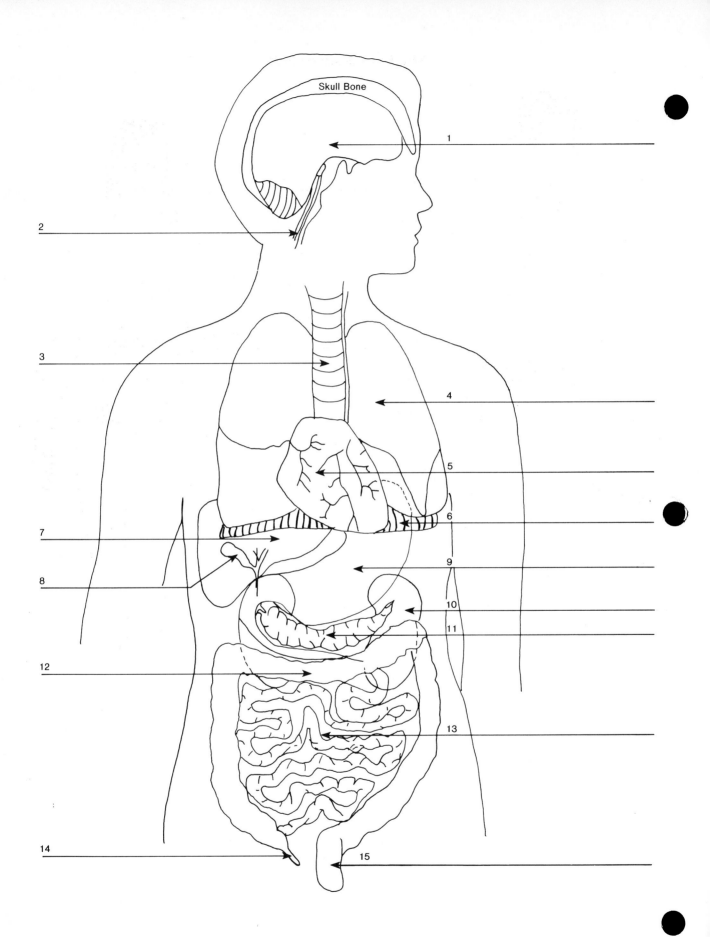

Skull Bone

1

2

3

4

5

6

7

8

9

10

11

12

13

14

15

The Endocrine Glands

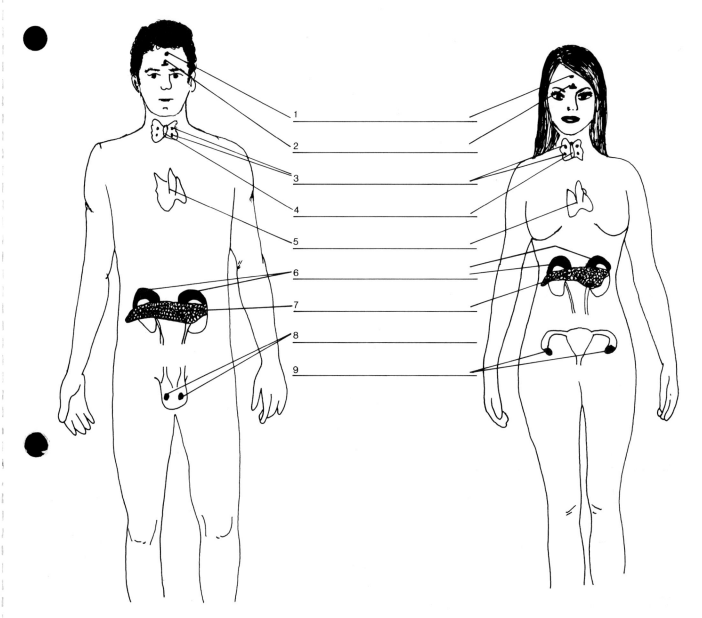

1 _____

2 _____

3 _____

4 _____

5 _____

6 _____

7 _____

8 _____

9 _____

Objectives

1. The student will be able to orally define "circadian rhythm" as approximately the twenty-four hour period of activity and rest for most living organisms.

2. After completing this lesson the student will be able to list at least five circadian cycles not listed during pre-testing.

3. Through introspection and keeping records, the student will begin to develop an awareness of his own inner timing, i.e. hunger contractions, thirst, sleep pattern, urination pattern, and times of peak performance.

Sources

1. Lennart Nilsson, and others. *Behold Man-* A Photographic Journey of Discovery Inside the Body. Boston: Little, Brown and Company. 1973. (English Translation Copyright, 1974).

2. Gay Gaer Luce. *Body Time: Physiological Rhythms and Social Stress.* New York: Pantheon Books, a division of Random House, Inc. 1971. (Bantam Books, Inc., New York: 1973).

3. Lawrence Monroe. "Psychological and Physiological Differences Between Good and Poor Sleepers," *Journal of Abnormal Psychology,* 72:255-264, 1967.

4. Gay Gaer Luce. *Biological Rhythms In Human & Animal Physiology.* New York: Dover Publications, Inc., 1971.

5. Robert Henkin, J.R. Gill, and F.C. Bartter. "Studies on Taste Thresholds in Normal Man and in Patients With Adrenal Cortical Insufficiency," *Journal of Clinical Investigation,* 42:727-735, May 1963.

6. Robert Henkin. "Auditory Detection and Perception in Normal Man and in Patients With Adrenal Cortical Insufficiency," *Journal of Clinical Investigation,* 47:1269-1280, June 1968.

Content and Procedures

"The human body is marvelous. It can move freely, act deliberately, and survive under the most variable conditions."[1] (p.8) It is always changing, responding to invisible rhythms and subtle changes in the environment. During the last twenty years a tremendous amount of scientific research has focused on biological rhythms or time cycles. The results of a survey by Gay Gaer Luce of over 650 scientific investigations indicates that "intermeshed cycles of timing may be the glue that holds us together,"[2] yet how many of us know much about our own biological time cycles and realize that we have a built-in time structure? As a pretest, see if you can list at least five biological time cycles or rhythms that occur within you naturally, on a regular basis:

1.

2.

3.

4.

5.

Do you know how the invisible rhythms of gravity, electromagnetic fields, light intensity, air pressure, and sound influence your health?

"We traverse the life cycle from birth to maturity, aging, and death. We observe the round of seasons, the ceaseless alternation of day and night. We are touched by inner cycles of sleepiness and hunger, yet our self-image is as fixed as a photograph. We expect consistent feeling and behavior in family and friends. We aspire to undeviating performance at work, and measure our state of health against some static norm. . . . All of this hinders us from feeling our rhythmic nature."[2] (Preface)

Circadian Rhythms

Most living organisms show a *circadian* ("about a day") rhythm of activity and rest. You have probably seen films of plant life using time-lapse photography, that have captured the rhythm of leaves lifting and dropping, opening and closing, every 24 hours. Meanwhile, some of the following circadian cycles are silently repeating themselves within our own bodies:

Body Temperature

Body temperature drops one or two degrees during the night and is highest in late afternoon, regardless of whether the individual lies still, exercises, or changes the time of his meals.

1. What are your favorite hours of the day?

   They usually occur in the afternoon or evening for a person who is active by day and sleeps by night, and are likely to coincide with the circadian high temperature point. The circadian low temperature point is when people do not perform as well on tasks requiring close attention or muscle coordination.

2. Do you usually bound out of bed in the morning or drag around for an hour or two before coming to life? _____
   Lawrence Monroe, at the University of Chicago, has reported that a good sleeper's temperature tends to rise before he awakens in the morning and reaches "normal" about the time he gets up. The temperature of "night-people" does not seem to rise so early and is still rising long after the person is up and awake. It neither drops as low, nor rises before awakening.[3]

3. Try slightly changing the hours when you go to bed and wake up. Did you feel better or worse the next day?

Urine Excretion

In 1890, a German researcher named Lahr experimented on himself by staying in bed and taking fluids around the clock. He reported that his urine flow remained rhythmic, dropping to its lowest point during the eight hours when he would ordinarily have been asleep. Greater amounts of urine are excreted in the morning and midday.

1. Keep a record of the times you urinate for seven days, to see whether you can determine your daily pattern of urination.

2. Compare your findings with the rest of the class. Are the patterns similar? Other studies have shown that the kidney itself functions differently at different hours, and the many constituents of urine each rise and fall in concentration rhythmically, but reach their peaks at different hours. For example, potassium and sodium are generally excreted in greatest quantities around midday and afternoon. "Although we may be unaware of the changing chemistry of our urine, it indicates a history of changing emotions and glandular responses to the day's events."[4] (p. 47).

Blood and Hormones

The speed at which blood coagulates, as well as many properties of the blood, seem to fluctuate in a circadian manner. Blood rhythms may also affect our immunity to infection. "Gamma globulin is the fraction of blood serum containing most of the immune antibodies to viruses, bacteria, and other foreign proteins."[2] (p. 129). Animal studies in 1966 by Lawrence Scheving and his associates indicated that animals have their highest levels of gamma globulin during the last six hours of their circadian activity period. This may mean that humans are more immune to infections at the end of the day than late at night, and by staying up late at parties or inverting our sleep schedule by east-west travel, we are exposing ourselves to viruses and infections when we are most vulnerable.[2] (p. 130).

The male hormone, testosterone, reaches a high level during the morning hours, and insulin, blood glucose, and amino acids, also seem to follow a daily rhythm. "Protein eaten at 8:00 a.m. rapidaly raises the amino acid levels in the blood, but the same meal at 8:00 p.m. does not. Some researchers conjecture that foods may be more efficiently utilized early in the day, indicating that a dieter may be well advised to have a hearty breakfast as his main meal of the day."[4] (p. 146). Nevertheless, most people prefer a large midday or evening meal. Perhaps this has something to do with blood levels of hormones that create a rhythm of taste and smell acuity each day.

1. What time of day does food taste best to you?

    _____

2. Keep a record for one week of the times when your sense of smell seems especially good. Can you determine a rhythm of high smell acuity?

3. Can you tolerate more noise in the morning or evening? _____

4. Can you identify certain times of the day when lights may seem irritatingly bright?

    _____

5. Compare your findings with the rest of the class.

An interesting group of experiments in the 1960's by Dr. Robert Henkin and several endocrinologists at the National Institute of Health in Bethesda suggests that adrenal hormones affect our taste, smell, and hearing senstitivities.[5,6]

Subsequent experiments revealed a definite circadian rhythm of adrenal hormones that cause daily fluctuations in sensory acuity and performance in normal people. If a person usually goes to sleep around 11:00 p.m., his sensory acuity is highest around 3:00 a.m., before suddenly dropping. People ordinarily do not listen to music or eat snacks at this time of lowest steroid levels; however, steroid levels drop again in the afternoon, leading to a high point of sensory acuity around 5:00 to 7:00 p.m. At this time, people can do things that require keen detection of taste, smell, or hearing, but not requiring discrimination.[4] (p. 55).

Some Other Circadian Rhythms

There are 24-hour rhythms in liver enzymes; in the biochemicals of the brain and the spinal cord; in the division of cells (skin cells divide mostly between midnight and 4:00 a.m., when a person normally is asleep); and throughout the nervous and endocrine systems. The circadian rhythm of activity and rest is well known, as are the four repeated cycles that occur about every 85–110 minutes during sleep itself. Dreams are almost always remembered if one is awakened during Stage I. This is a period of rapid eye movement (REM), accompanied by irregular pulse and breathing, a complete slackening of skeletal muscles, and changes in brain temperature. During this period there is also abnormal nighttime secretions of gastric acid in people with peptic ulcers, and all males, from infancy to old age, have penile erections around or during this period. Sleep deepens through Stages II and III, until Stage IV, or Delta sleep is reached. Stage IV usually occurs early in the night and is when sleepwalking, bedwetting, and nightmares, most often occur. Stage IV sleep can be enhanced by daily exercise and appears to play a physiological and restorative role that is essential to well-being. The pulse rate and respiration rate also have a circadian rhythm, rising to a peak by day and falling to a low point during sleep.

Monthly, Seasonal, and Annual Cycles

We are influenced by more than daily biological cycles. Depending on where a woman is in her menstrual cycle, monthly hormonal tides influence her physiology, emotional responses, and performance. During the week just preceding the menses, premenstrual complaints seem to be universal among women of diverse cultures, and this is the time of month that women are most likely to be admitted to psychiatric wards. Men also seem to exhibit a few signs of monthly change, including cyclic fluctuations in behavior. Both sexes secrete something known as "summer hormone," a thyroid product that helps to reduce body heat; and animal studies indicate that there are probably many other seasonal and annual changes that are reflected in our metabolism and behavior, waiting to be discovered.

"Biorhythms"

In 1887, Whilhelm Fliess published his formula for the use of biological rhythms in *The Rhythm of Life: Foundations of an Exact Biology*. He asserted that every individual has a male component (strength, endurance, courage) keyed to a cycle of 23 days, and a female cycle (not menstrual, but of sensitivity, intuition, love, and other feelings) of 28 days. They supposedly determine our physical and mental ups and downs and even the day of our death. In the 1930's, a teacher at Innsbruck added a 33-day creativity cycle of mental acumen and power.[4] (p. 8).

Although Fliess' formula reveals a "blatantly unsophisticated understanding of simple mathematics,"[4] (p. 8) new books on "biorhythms" still appear regularly and promise to help the reader chart his own cycles of physical or emotional vulnerability and strength in advance.

While it may indeed be possible for people to forecast their rhythms by keeping very detailed diaries concerning feelings and sensations at different hours of the day for months and years, it is not so easy as a simple formula. There is no denying, however, that biological rhythms do exist and that "they play a formative role in our personalities and the timing of important life events, such as birth or death, and that they bias our response to danger, ability to wake, and health."[2] (p. 23)

Evaluation

Students can begin to develop an awareness of their own inner timing by spending one day recording the following rhythms on an hour-by-hour basis:

1. hunger contractions;
2. thirst;
3. the chill of dropping body temperature;
4. the quality of fresh vigor;
5. fatigue;

6. mood changes;
7. mental alertness;
8. urine excretion;
9. increased sensitivity to smell;
10. increased sensitivity to light;
11. increased sensitivity to sound;
12. increased taste sensitivity.

The Human Body
New Frontiers

Objectives

1. Each student will research one "new frontier" or medical advance currently being made and summarize the information for inclusion in a classroom scrapbook.

2. After completing this lesson the student will be able to briefly describe at least five new areas of medical research.

3. The student will be able to define the terms *"in vitro* fertilization" and "cloning."

4. By participating in small group discussion, the student will be able to clarify his feelings regarding *in vitro* fertilization and cloning.

5. (optional) The student will begin keeping a personal, day-by-day weather calendar in an effort to develop his body awareness.

Sources

1. William J. Sweeney III, MD. "New Arrival: The Test-Tube Baby," *Family Health*, December, 1978, pp. 22–24.

2. Ted Howard, Jeremy Rifkin. *Who Should Play God?* New York: Dell Publishing Company, Inc., 1977.

3. Joshua Lederberg. "Experimental Genetics and Human Evolution," *Bulletin of the Atomic Scientists,* October, 1966, p. 10.

4. Stephen Rosen. *Future Facts.* New York: Simon and Schuster, 1976.

5. H.E. Landsberg. *Weather and Health*—An Introduction to Biometeorology. New York: Anchor Books, Doubleday and Company, Inc., 1969.

6. Theodore Irwin. *How Weather and Climate Affect You* (533) 1976. Available from Public Affairs Committee, Inc., 381 Park Avenue South, New York, N.Y. 1016 (504).

Content and Procedures

What better place to begin than with the beginning of life when pondering the future of health and medicine? Dr. Sidney Fox of the University of Miami, has already narrowed the gap between amino acids and the first living cell. In fact, some of his assembled materials containing chains of amino acids have even self-reproduced. Theoretically, nucleic-acid "engineering" will make it possible to replicate almost any living substance in the test tube. Already people are beginning to wonder about the social, moral, and legal issues involved.

Consider the publicity generated by the birth of Louise Brown, July 25, 1978, in Oldham, England. Hailed as the world's first test-tube baby, in reality, she was out of her mother's uterus for only two and a half days before being reimplanted. However, the fact that some physicians now possess the knowledge and skills enabling them to simulate conditions in the Fallopian tubes, where fertilization usually occurs, and successfully unite a sperm with an egg without gross deformities resulting, raises some questions:

1. Do you think it should be illegal for women with blocked Fallopian tubes (thereby making natural fertilization impossible) to have one of their eggs fertilized outside of their bodies (in vitro fertilization) and then replanted?
2. Should this procedure be limited only to married couples?
3. Should this procedure be limited to couples who cannot conceive in any other way after standard testing, treatment, and counseling?
4. Should in vitro fertilization with donor sperm be permitted?
5. If a woman has a malfunctioning uterus do you think she should be able to have another woman carry her fertilized egg?
6. Should *in vitro* fertilization with a donor egg be permitted for women without ovaries?[1]

Cloning

The book, *Who Should Play God?* discusses cloning, the artificial creation of life, and what it means for the future of the human race. Cloning is "the production of genetically duplicate individuals from the biological information contained in a single body cell. . . . Since all of the chromosomes that make up a new individual are inherited from just one parent, the end product is a genetic duplicate of the original."[2] (p. 117) Many researchers believe that within our lifetimes, carbon-copy human beings will be among us.

1. Would you like a clone made of yourself? One researcher suggests that a clone could be grown and kept in storage against the day you have a medical problem and need an organ transplant, with no concern for graft rejection.[3]

2. How do you think it would feel to be a clone or duplicate of some other individual?

3. Are you like Dr. Elof A. Carlson of UCLA who would like to see cloning turned on the dead "to bring back individuals (e.g. historical personalities) of identical genotype?"

Some scientists predict that body-cell banks will become more significant in the future than sperm or ova banks. If you were killed in an accident, one of your body cells could be removed from the bank and a twin of you could be developed. Immortality could thus be achieved in the biological sense. It is also theorized that extraordinary powers of telepathic communication might exist between clones. Nobel Prize winner J.B.S. Haldane suggests a state-supported retirement at the age of fifty-five, so that you could then raise and train your own clone to assume its place in society. On the other hand, Robert T. Francoeur, author of *Utopian Motherhood,* asks, "Xeroxing of people? It shouldn't be done in the labs, even once, with humans."

Growing New Limbs

Dr. Robert O. Becker, an orthopedist in New York, is experimenting with low-amplitude electrical currents as a technique for inducing partial regeneration in higher animals. Someday amputees may benefit from his work. It also appears that electromagnetic stimulation may promote healing in a variety of organs, such as a damaged portion of heart muscle; the rapid healing of skin ulcers and burns; for promoting healing of bone fractures; and for producing anesthesia.[4] (p. 12).

Blood Research

Dr. Arland Carsten and a team of research scientists in Upton, New York have developed a way to grow human blood cells in a chamber that is implanted in the abdominal cavity of a living mouse. By providing a window on the intricacies of blood formation in health and disease, the diffusion chamber has led to "significant findings on the metabolic causes of at least one type of leukemia" and will provide "a way to investigate the effects of experimental drugs on blood diseases without having to use human patients as guinea pigs."[4] (p. 14).

In a somewhat different vein, research by Dr. Leland C. Clark, Jr. at the University of Cincinnati College of Medicine, may someday make it possible to temporarily substitute man-made liquids for a few hours in emergency transfusions. Scientists are also working on a blood test to detect gonorrhea, a venereal disease that has reached epidemic proportions in recent years, and are testing the effectiveness of a gonorrhea vaccine that was recently developed in Ottawa, Ontario.

Aids for the Heart

Heart patients will soon have unusual freedom to move around thanks to the biobelt that can monitor a patient's heartbeat and body temperature at great distances. Work is also progressing on the development of a totally implantable nuclear-powered artificial heart, which may later be replaced by growing a replica of the original heart. Heart patients will also benefit from a new pocket-size device that will provide early warning of an attack and enable them to transmit their heart rhythms over the telephone to their doctor for analysis.

Artificial Pancreas

Do you know someone who has diabetes? A glucose sensor disk implanted under the skin or in the abdominal cavity to measure blood sugar levels in the body and to provide a dose of insulin if the level is too high, will soon provide relief to many people who suffer from diabetes.

Measuring Body Temperature

Can you name three ways for measuring body temperature? Oral thermometers, rectal thermometers, and placing a thermometer under the armpit have been the usual ways to determine body temperature. Recently however, a swallowable "pill" temperature transmitter has been developed that will provide a precise measurement of body temperature fluctuation and be useful in studies of biological cycles and critically ill hospital patients. The device will be retained by the body for about three days.

Other Discoveries

Future Facts[4] reveals information about the following topics and can be a valuable aid in providing topics for discussion and further research:

1. Measuring the magnetic fields around the heart, brain, muscles, and lungs.

2. Use of the "hoverbed" for treatment of large-area burn patients.

3. Skinlike membrane that accelerates the growth of new skin and reduces the duration of burn therapy.

4. Time-Release Drugs . . .

5. Artificial teeth that can be permanently implanted.

6. Capping teeth with a ceramic material by laser to make them permanently decay-resistant.

7. New materials for bone repair.

8. Electrically induced sleep, anesthesia, and relief from headaches.

9. Drugs to retard aging.

10. Future vaccines for viruses.

Biometeorology

Do you believe there is any significant relationship between symptoms of disease and the weather? When 160 internists were asked this same question 92% answered affirmatively.

The study of biometeorology is a relatively new branch of medical science that investigates the relationship between weather and health.[5,6] Medical scientists "believe that clouds, winds, humidity, barometric pressure, heat, cold, and other variables . . . may exert a subtle, pervasive impact on health, behavior, efficiency, and disposition."[6] (p. 2) Someday weather announcers may issue warnings such as "strong, cold winds coming up; people with heart trouble should stay indoors . . . . The weather will be overcast and foggy—expect to be in a foul mood. . . . Barometer is falling, humidity will be high; watch out if you have arthritis. . . . Dazzling sunshine due today; if you're prone to migraines, take precautions. . . . Storm clouds moving in from the west tonight; don't be surprised if you have a nightmare."[6] (p. 1)

Make a personal weather calendar and learn your reactions to environmental conditions. Such a record should be kept day-by-day for a year or so in order to develop an awareness of the days when perhaps you should perform just routine tasks. Try to follow the rules recommended by medical climatologists for weather-conditioning yourself.[6] (pp. 26–27)

Evaluation

The method to be used for evaluation is clearly stated in the behavioral objectives.

Selected Learning Activities

Teaching about the Human Body

_____ Discuss whether the senses of smell, taste, and touch will be of use to men and women in outer space. What are some sensations which astronauts may not experience?

_____ Make a list of common insects that have more specialized senses than humans and identify which sense is their best one.

_____ Invite the school nurse to demonstrate the slide method of blood typing.

_____ Purchase a copy of "The Wonderful Human Machine" from the American Medical Association (Order department, 535 N. Dearborn Street, Chicago, Illinois 60610), for use as a classroom resource. Use an opaque projector to enlarge and project the illustrations.

_____ Contact your local chapter of the American Cancer Society to obtain the teacher's guide—"Take Joy." This guide includes the six systems of the body on overhead transparency and six spirit duplicating masters that will make at least 200 excellent copies. There is also a film by the same name.

_____ Have students work in groups to produce discovery packs for different parts of the body. If models of the human body are available, audio-tapes can be made to highlight special features of the model, describe what to look for, and list relevant vocabulary words that should be looked up and defined in a workbook. When the discovery packs are completed, they should be made available to other students for independent study.

_____ Develop a nonverbal skit which describes the functions of the different body systems.

_____ Make a word search using at least two words from each of the different body systems.

_____ Play "Body Concentration" by making sets of cards that match and then playing to match the cards just as you do in the card game of concentration.

_____ Describe at least one preventive practice for each body system. Select one and make a poster for the classroom.

_____ Trace the body. Make the organs out of construction paper. Place the organs in their proper location on the traced outline of the body.

_____ Draw a picture of the heart on the floor using chalk. Trace the flow of blood.

_____ Identify a practice and a behavior which will enhance the functioning of each body system and make this into a chart.

_____ Make a mobile of one of the body systems.

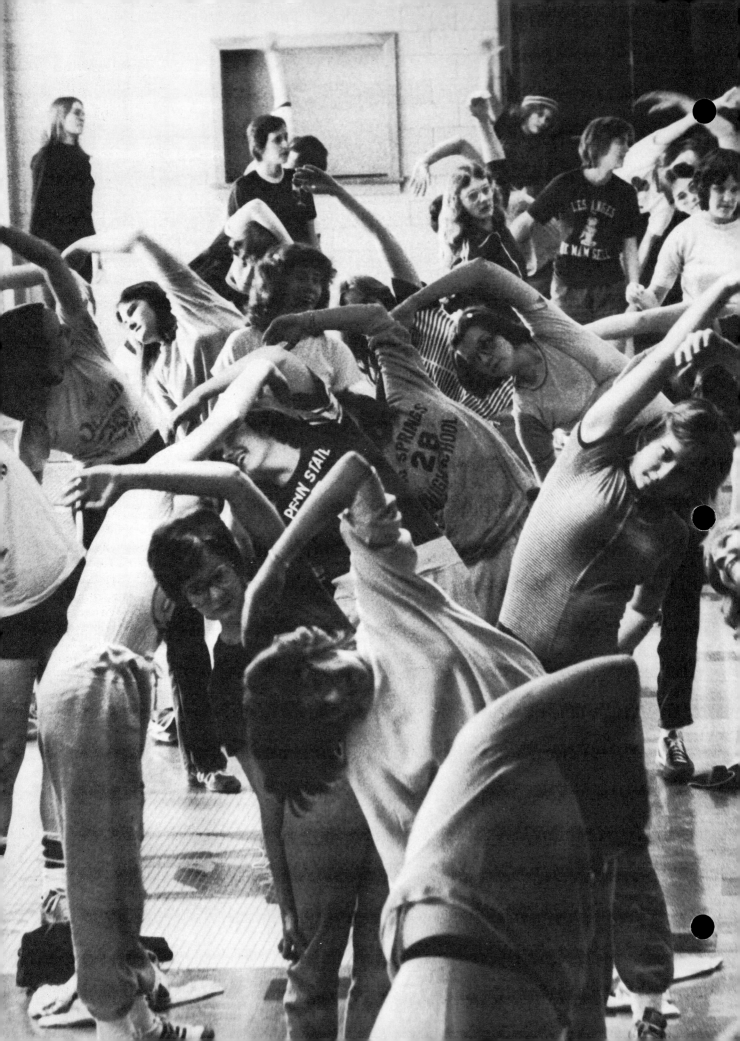

13

Teaching about Cardiovascular Fitness and Health

Approximately six out of ten people in the United States will die from cardiovascular diseases. Many more will be impaired and not live optimally. The middle and secondary student can accept responsibility for life style decisions that will affect cardiovascular health. This chapter includes an outline of Suggested Learning Activities, Three Detailed Sample Lessons designed to promote knowledge and effective decision making, and additional Selected Learning Activities.

The first lesson, **The Heart—Its Structure and Function,** familiarizes the student with the different parts of the heart. The student learns to trace the flow of blood through the cardiopulmonary system. A review of anatomy and physiology is an important prerequisite to the follow-up lessons.

The second lesson, **Coronary Disease Risk Factors,** examines cardiovascular risks and the role of decision-making in reducing risks. Nine risk factors are examined—heredity, stress, cigarette smoking, age, exercise, sex, obesity, diet, and hypertension. The student plays Risko to determine personal risk factors and then can relate the lesson to a life time plan of risk reduction.

To illustrate the importance of assuming personal responsibility for the reduction of cardiovascular risk a lesson is included on **Coronary Disease— Prevention Through Exercise.** The student learns to compute heart rate and examines the value of exercise. The lesson provides the essential background information for the student to examine a personal exercise plan for reducing the risk of cardiovascular disease.

Suggested Topics

Cardiovascular Fitness and Health

I. The Structure and Function of the Cardiovascular System
   A. The flow of blood within the heart
   B. The structure of the heart
   C. The vascular system
II. Diseases of The Heart
   A. Atherosclerosis
   B. Arteriosclerosis
   C. Angina pectoris
   D. Heart attack

Photo by David S. Strickler

III. Risk Factors of Coronary Heart Disease
   A. Age and sex
   B. High density and low density lipoproteins
   C. Hypertension
   D. Diabetes
   E. Diet
   F. Exercise
   G. Obesity
   H. Cigarette smoking
   I. Stress
   J. Heredity
IV. Diseases of The Vascular System
   A. Stroke
   B. Aneurysms
   C. Varicose veins
   D. Phlebitis
V. Treatment of Cardiovascular Diseases
   A. Reducing risk-taking behavior
   B. Drug therapy and hypertension
   C. Antibiotics and heart infections
   D. Coronary bypass
   E. The use of pacemakers and heart valves
   F. Heart transplants
VI. Cardiovascular Fitness
   A. Cardiovascular endurance—its physiological results
   B. Anaerobic exercises
   C. Aerobic conditioning
   D. The jogging phenomenon
   E. Evaluating the value of exercise
VII. Fitness and Food Intake
   A. Caloric Intake
   B. Energy expenditure
VIII. Obesity and Fitness
   A. Distinguishing between overweight and obese
   B. The prevalence of obesity
   C. Regulating weight through exercise
   D. Genetic causes of overeating

Lesson Plans

Cardiovascular Fitness and Health
The Heart—Its Structure and Function

Objectives

1. The student will be able to identify the different parts of the heart.

2. The student will be able to demonstrate the flow blood pursues in the cardiopulmonary system.

Sources

Jolem Ross and Robert A. O'Rourke,
*Understanding the Heart and Its
Diseases,* New York: McGraw-Hill Book
Company, 1976.

Content and Procedures

To better understand the role of exercise and heart disease on the cardiopulmonary system, the student must understand the structure and method of function of the heart muscle.

The Heart at Work

The heart is the size of an average sized grapefruit weighing approximately 11 ounces. It continuously circulates blood through a vascular network which, when laid end to end as a single line would extend for 60,000 miles, or two and one half times the earth's circumference. It pumps enough blood so that it can fill a 75 gallon tank in one hour. The work done by the heart in a 12 hour period can perform a task, the equivalent of raising a 925 ton weight one foot. In a lifetime (approximately 70 years) it pumps 18 million barrels of blood.

This muscle lies in the central portion of the chest directly behind the breastbone. It is tilted so that its lower portion is shifted to the left. Between the heart and its protective encasing sac which is composed of connective tissue is a layer of fluid called the *pericardium*. This layer minimizes the beating heart's friction on the outer surface.

The heart is composed of two main pumping chambers known as *ventricles*. The right ventricle and left ventricle are separated by a thick muscular wall. Each ventricle is connected to its own antechamber called the *atrium* (also known as auricle). The atrium serves as a collecting point for blood and holds it for delivery to the ventricles for each heartbeat. The *superior vena cava* and *inferior vena cava*, the two largest veins in the body, deliver blood low in oxygen and high in carbon dioxide to the right atrium. Blood then travels to the right ventricle to the pulmonary artery to the lungs where carbon dioxide is discharged and oxygen is taken up.

Aerated blood returns from the lungs via the pulmonary vein and reenters the heart through the left atrium. It then travels into the left ventricle which, in turn, pumps blood out through the aorta and into most parts of the body.

Follow the Flow

To have the class gain insight in the direction of the flow of blood, the teacher can have the class actually "walk through" the path blood takes in the heart.

Using masking tape, the teacher can outline a heart on the floor. The picture on the following page can serve as a model.

1. The class can be divided into two teams and at the teacher's discretion, he can divide the heart into point zones. For example, the left ventricle can be worth three points, the right atrium, one point etc.

2. Using an eraser, one student from each team will throw the eraser which will land in a specified point value.

3. To receive points, the student must walk through the path of blood flow, naming each part of the heart it passes as well as what happens between the exchange of gases.

4. The team which gains the largest number of points will be declared the winner.

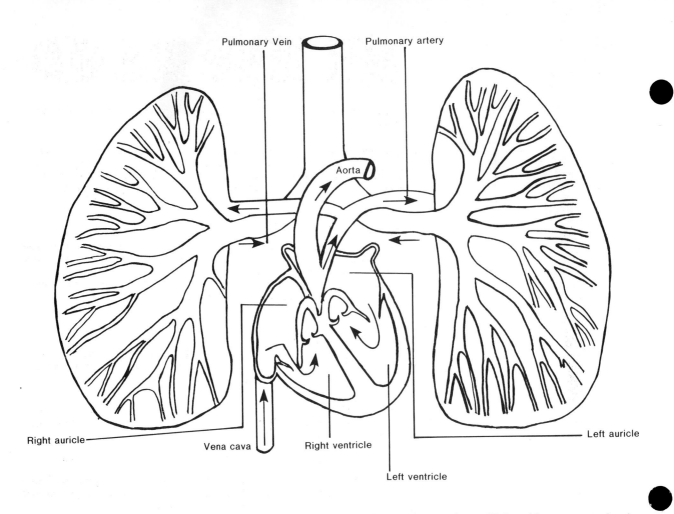

Pulmonary Vein   Pulmonary artery

Aorta

Right auricle
Vena cava   Right ventricle
Left ventricle
Left auricle

Evaluation

After walking around the heart, the teacher will be able to ascertain the percentage of correct answers given by the students.

Ask the students to list, in sequence, the path of blood within each chamber of the heart.

Cardiovascular Fitness and Health
Coronary Disease Risk Factors

Objectives

1. The student will be able to identify nine risk factors related to cardiovascular disease.

2. By playing the game RISKO, the student will be able to estimate his chances of suffering a heart attack.

Sources

1. Michigan Heart Association game, Risko, Detroit, Michigan, 48227.

2. Ross, Jolem and O'Rourke, Robert A., *Understanding the Heart and Its Diseases,* New York: McGraw-Hill Book Co., 1976.

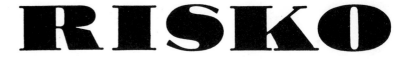

RISKO

The purpose of this game is to give you an estimate of your chances of suffering heart attack.

The game is played by making squares which — from left to right — represent an increase in your RISK FACTORS. These are medical conditions and habits associated with an increased danger of heart attack. *Not all risk factors are measurable enough to be included in this game; see back of sheet for other RISK FACTORS.*

RULES:

Study each **RISK FACTOR AND its row. Find the box applicable to you and circle the large number in it. For example, if you are 37, circle the number in the box labeled 31-40.**
After checking out all the rows, add the circled numbers. **This total — your score — is an estimate of your risk.**

IF YOU SCORE:

6-11 — **Risk well below average**
12-17 — **Risk below average**
18-24 — **Risk generally average**

25-31 — **Risk moderate**
32-40 — **Risk at a dangerous level**
41-62 — **Danger urgent. See your doctor now.**

HEREDITY:

Count parents, grand-parents, brothers, and sisters who have had heart attack and/or stroke.

TOBACCO SMOKING:

If you inhale deeply and smoke a cigarette way down, add one to your classification. Do NOT subtract because you think you do not inhale or smoke only a half inch on a cigarette.

EXERCISE:

Lower your score one point if you exercise regularly and frequently.

CHOLESTEROL OR SATURATED FAT INTAKE LEVEL:

A cholesterol blood level is best. If you can't get one from your doctor, then estimate honestly the percentage of solid fats you eat. These are usually of animal origin — lard, cream, butter, and beef and lamb fat. If you eat much of this, your cholesterol level probably will be high. The U.S. average, 40%, is too high for good health.

BLOOD PRESSURE:

If you have no recent reading but have passed an insurance or industrial examination chances are you are 140 or less.

SEX:

This line takes into account the fact that men have from 6 to 10 times more heart attacks than women of child bearing age.

AGE	10 to 20	21 to 30	31 to 40	41 to 50	51 to 60	61 to 70 and over
HEREDITY	No known history of heart disease	1 relative with cardiovascular disease Over 60	2 relatives with cardiovascular disease Over 60	1 relative with cardiovascular disease Under 60	2 relatives with cardiovascular disease Under 60	3 relatives with cardiovascular disease Under 60
WEIGHT	More than 5 lbs. below standard weight	−5 to +5 lbs. standard weight	6-20 lbs. over weight	21-35 lbs. over weight	36-50 lbs. over weight	51-65 lbs. over weight
TOBACCO SMOKING	Non-user	Cigar and/or pipe	10 cigarettes or less a day	20 cigarettes a day	30 cigarettes a day	40 cigarettes a day or more
EXERCISE	Intensive occupational and recreational exertion	Moderate occupational and recreational exertion	Sedentary work and intense recreational exertion	Sedentary occupational and moderate recreational exertion	Sedentary work and light recreational exertion	Complete lack of all exercise
CHOLES-TEROL OR FAT % IN DIET	Cholesterol below 180 mg.% Diet contains no animal or solid fats	Cholesterol 181-205 mg.% Diet contains 10% animal or solid fats	Cholesterol 206-230 mg.% Diet contains 20% animal or solid fats	Cholesterol 231-255 mg.% Diet contains 30% animal or solid fats	Cholesterol 256-280 mg.% Diet contains 40% animal or solid fats	Cholesterol 281-300 mg.% Diet contains 50% animal or solid fats
BLOOD PRESSURE	100 upper reading	120 upper reading	140 upper reading	160 upper reading	180 upper reading	200 or over upper reading
SEX	Female under 40	Female 40-50	Female over 50	Male	Stocky male	Bald stocky male

© MICHIGAN HEART ASSOCIATION

Content and Procedures

Cardiovascular Disease

Six out of every ten people in the United States will die from cardiovascular diseases. While heart disease often develops early in life, its impact is not noted until one has gotten up in years or has suffered overt signs and symptoms of cardiovascular damage. Unfortunately, young people fail to recognize the severity of cardiovascular diseases since these phenomena are usually labeled as an "old person's concern." To recognize the impact of cardiovascular disease, the student must be aware that he is susceptible to the disease and that this disease can afflict him.

In this lesson, we will focus upon the most common cardiovascular disease—coronary disease.

Risk Factors

There are nine risk factors related to heart disease. Before estimating our own chances of being stricken by a heart attack, it is important that we understand the different risk factors. These factors are:

1. *Heredity*—If a family history of heart disease exists, the chances of your susceptibility are increased. However, this does not mean you will have a heart attack.

2. *Stress*—In their book *Type A Behavior,* Drs. Rosenman and Friedman indicate that a relationship exists between emotional stress and coronary disease. While stress is omnipresent in everyone, one's ability to relieve this will be a factor in promoting or preventing heart disease.

3. *Cigarette smoking*—As the number of cigarettes consumed daily increase, so do the chances of getting a heart attack. The heavy smoker (at least one pack per day) has three times the chance of suffering a heart attack than the nonsmoker. For every cigarette smoked, the resting heart rate will jump approximately 20 beats per minute. In essence, the heart is made to work harder than it would if no cigarette were smoked.

4. *Age*—While the chances of a heart attack increase with age, the fact remains that healthy lifestyle patterns developed at a young age will make old age easier to come by.

5. *Exercise*—Attitudes about exercise have changed over the past several years. Now more than ever before, people are concerned about cardiovascular fitness through exercise—witness the 20 million Americans who jog regularly. While it has not been proven statistically that running will improve cardiovascular fitness or prolong life, the medical profession appears to support the results of aerobic conditioning.

6. *Sex*—While one does not have control over the determination of sex, it is a fact that premenopausal women do have a lower incidence of heart disease. However, after menopause, the incidences between male and female balance.

7. *Obesity*—The relationship between obesity and heart disease is a debated issue. While obesity in itself may not cause heart disease, it does effect other body actions which in turn, can promote an unhealthy heart. For example, obese people will have higher blood pressure and higher serum lipid levels than persons of normal weight. These conditions are factors which can promote coronary disease.

8. *Diet*—The types of food a person eats can be a factor in heart disease. When fats are broken down in the liver, cholesterol is produced. Foods high in cholesterol, such as some animal meats, shellfish, eggs and cheese can raise the cholesterol count in the body to higher than the normal range of 120–250 mg. While some studies show that chances of heart disease increase with high cholesterol levels, controversy exists within the medical realm as to whether or not this is valid.

   Triglycerides, another type of lipid, is thought to be more significant than cholesterol in the role played in heart disease. A reduction in sugar consumed can decrease the triglyceride level.

9. *Hypertension*—Hypertension or high blood pressure is considered a serious predisposing factor to coronary disease. Blood pressure is the force blood exerts upon the walls in which it is contained. Through the use of medication and the reduction of salt intake, high blood pressure can be lowered.

Types of Heart Disease

The afore mentioned risk factors can influence the development of heart disease. Among the most common types of heart disease are:

Atherosclerosis—This is a progressive build-up of fatty materials in the walls of the arteries. The narrowing of the coronary arteries, due to the build-up of lipids can reduce the flow of blood to the heart muscle. Often this can lead to a *heart attack* or myocardial infarct.

Heart Attack—The heart attack is the leading cause of death in the U.S. In a heart attack, the coronary artery becomes closed or a blood clot lodges and blocks the passage of blood to the heart. When this occurs, the heart muscle is deprived of oxygen and can be severely damaged.

Angina Pectoris—Although this is not a disease of the heart, it is a symptom of reduced oxygen flow to this area. A person who has angina can feel pain, pressure or tightness under the breast bone. This pain can be felt down the left shoulder and arm.

Materials

At this point, the students will be familiar with the risk factors involved in coronary heart disease. To help the student understand how he stands with regard to suffering a heart attack, the following game, RISKO can be played.

Evaluation

1. Students can be asked to submit their score on RISKO as well as their method of computing that score.

2. Students can be given a quiz and asked to list and describe the nine risk factors of coronary heart disease.

Cardiovascular Fitness and Health
Coronary Disease Prevention through Exercise

Objectives

1. The student will be able to identify the effect exercise can have on heart performance.

2. The student will be able to evaluate the impact of selected exercises upon physical fitness.

3. The student will be able to compute his resting heart rate and discuss the implications of low heart rate to heart health.

Sources

Kenneth Cooper, *The New Aerobics*, New York: Bantam Books, 1970.

Content and Procedures

The Condition of Your Heart

The heart is a magnificent engine that keeps the body going. Unlike other body organs, the heart tissue is all muscle. The condition of this muscle is dependent upon how well it is supplied with blood. However, heart muscle differs from other body muscles in that it cannot be exercised like these other muscles. The condition of the heart muscle will depend on how enlarged its connecting blood vessels are—that is, are the blood vessels large healthy supply routes for blood?

Another factor that indicates heart health is the resting heart rate. A conditioned person develops a conditioned heart and a conditioned heart will have a lower resting heart rate than an unconditioned heart.

A conditioned person who exercises regularly may have a resting heart rate of about 60 beats per minute. A person who is not conditioned and does not exercise may have a resting heart rate of 80 or more beats per minute.

At this point, the student can be asked to compute the differences between the number of heartbeats per day between a person who has a resting heart rate of 60 beats per minute and a person who has a resting heart rate of 80 beats per minute.

60 beats/minute x 60 minutes = 3600 beats/hour
3600 beats/hour x 24 hours = 86,400 beats/day

80 beats/minute x 60 minutes = 4800 beats/hour
4800 beats/hour x 24 hours = 115,200 beats/day

$$
\begin{array}{rl}
115,200 = & 80 \text{ beats per minute} \\
- \underline{86,400} = & 60 \text{ beats per minute} \\
28,800 = & \text{beats per day more for the person with a resting heart} \\
& \text{rate of 80 beats per minute.}
\end{array}
$$

What are some assumptions we can make about the differences in heart health between a conditioned and unconditioned person?

Now figure out how many times per day your heart will beat. With the teacher as timer, place your index finger over your pulse for one minute and compute your 24 hour heart rate.

The teacher needs to explain the fact that during different parts of the day, heart rate will vary.

A lower heart rate indicates a person is conserving energy and that during activity, the heart has built-in protection against beating too fast.

Aerobic Exercise

One way of lowering the resting rate and improving heart condition is through *aerobic* exercise, popularized in 1968 by Dr. Kenneth Cooper. Aerobic exercise causes the body to use maximum amounts of oxygen (aerobic capacity) over a given period of time. In order to receive a training effect, a person must be capable of sustaining exercise that increases the heartbeat rate to about 140 beats per minute.

The maximum heart rate for students your age is about 200 beats per minute.

According to Dr. Kenneth Cooper, one's present state of fitness can be evaluated by the "12 Minute Test." Below are charts which the student can use to determine his or her fitness level.

12 Minute Test for Secondary School Males

Distance in miles covered in 12 minutes—walking and/or running	Category
less than 1.0	Very Poor
1.0 —1.24	Poor
1.25—1.49	Fair
1.50—1.74	Good
1.75 or more	Excellent

12 Minute Test for Secondary School Females

Distance in Miles Covered in 12 minutes—walking and/or running	Category
less than .95	Very Poor
.95 —1.14	Poor
1.15—1.34	Fair
1.35—1.64	Good
1.65 or more	Excellent

The teacher can ask the student to determine his or her fitness level. Since each mileage-increment is in quarters, the student can get an accurate measurement by running and or walking on a quarter mile track.

Different aerobic activities can promote good physical fitness. Among these activities can be running/jogging, swimming, cycling, walking, running in place (stationary running), and individual, dual and team exercises.

Students can be assigned a log to maintain. At teacher designated intervals, the student will report his progress per week. The chart below can be used for self-reporting data.

The teacher can make a master chart with each student's name and the number of points scored per week and post this on the bulletin board. Each week the student can submit his or her log.

Student Progress Chart Week I		
Day	Activity	Distance and/or Duration
Mon.		
Tues.		
Wed.		
Thurs.		
Fri.		
Sat.		
Sun.		

Evaluation

1. The student can be asked to identify aerobic exercises and how these exercises can improve physical condition.

2. The teacher can monitor student's physical condition based upon weekly logs.

Selected Learning Activities

Cardiovascular Fitness and Health

_____ Write a one page paper on the value of exercise.

_____ Demonstrate one exercise for strengthening arm muscles, leg muscles, abdominal muscles, and back muscles.

_____ Demonstrate two exercises for strengthening cardiovascular-respiratory endurance.

_____ Demonstrate one exercise for increasing your agility.

_____ Differentiate between isometric exercise, aerobic exercise, jogging, and weight lifting.

_____ Collect advertisements for equipment that claims to increase physical fitness and well being. (sauna baths, spot reducing vibrators, belts, etc.) Investigate the validity of the claims made.

_____ Compare the exercise programs, facilities, equipment, and cost of various commercial fitness clubs in your community.

_____ Write to the American Heart Association, National Center, 7320 Greenville Ave., Dallas, Texas 75231 for a copy of "Putting Your Heart Into the Curriculum." This is an excellent compilation of demonstrations, experiments, strategies, and audiovisuals concerned with cardiovascular health.

_____ Chart blood pressures of different persons, asking them whether they experience changes in pressure related to different aspects of life style.

_____ Write a research paper on heart transplants.

_____ Invite a cardiologist to come to class to discuss the various equipment used to assess and to monitor the heart.

_____ Make a "Be Good to Your Heart" poster.

_____ Trace the role of circulatory problems in your family, putting them on a family tree. Discuss the implications of your heredity and your behavior.

_____ Visit a laboratory or blood bank.

_____ Utilize some of the blood typing experiments available from the local Red Cross.

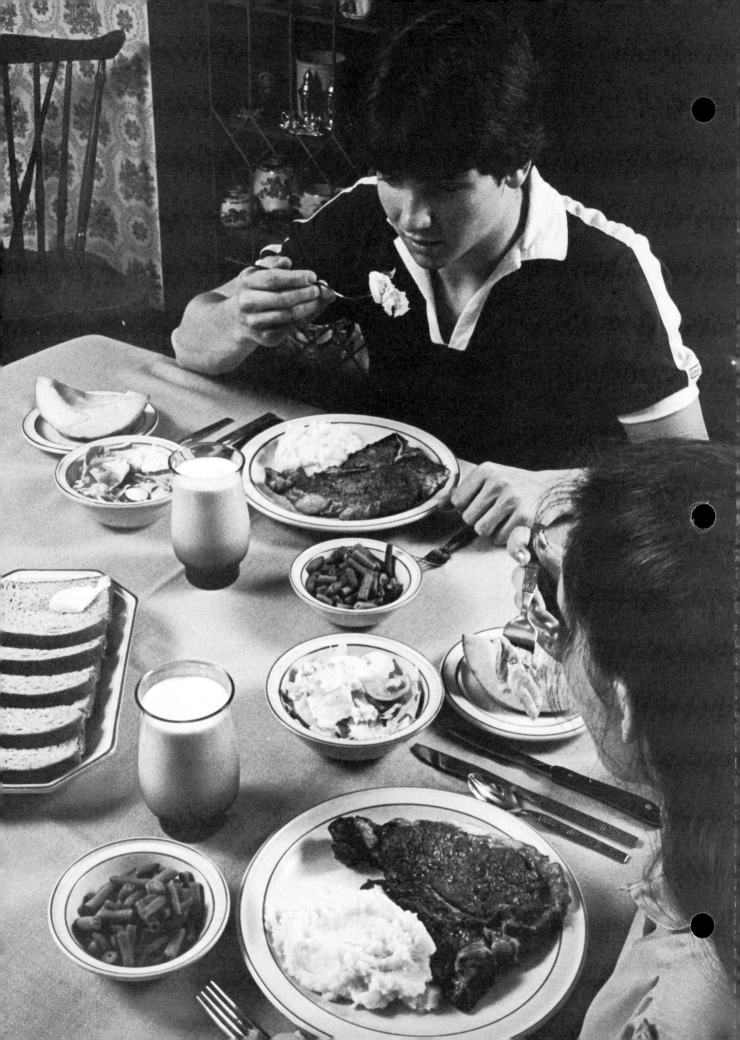

Teaching about Nutrition and Weight Control

A current emphasis on the energy crises and the shortage of fuel in our country might be accompanied with an examination of human fuel and human energy. Are we wasteful with human fuel—food? Are we getting the most human mileage by using fuel in the right proportions? Are we getting a top performance from the types of foods we select?

The importance of nutrition is critical during the adolescent years. In this chapter, you will find Suggested Topics for Teaching About Nutrition and Weight Control, Three Detailed Sample Lessons that examine nutritional needs, values, and attitudes, and additional Selected Learning Activities.

The first lesson, **Nutritional Needs: Womb to Tomb,** examines each of the seven stages of life giving an overview of nutritional needs. A sequential study of nutritional needs helps the student examine changing needs throughout the life cycle. Hopefully, this develops an appreciation for the needs of the entire family and for planning adequate diet.

The second lesson, **Weight Problems in Adolescence,** enables the student to personalize information about nutrition assessing body image and examining ideal weight. The adolescent is particularly prone to what media has to say about desired weight, attractiveness, and sex appeal. Whether you are overweight, underweight, or at an ideal weight, this lesson should promote choices which will alleviate weight problems in adolescence.

The third lesson, **Foods, Fads, and Fallacies,** highlights responsible consumer health. Through examining three basic types of food fads, the student will have the knowledge needed to make better selections at the grocery store. The student will be able to compare the prices, content, and claims made for several basic food items in both health food stores and supermarkets.

Suggested Topics

Nutrition and Weight Control

I. The Basic Nutrients in Food
   A. Protein
   B. Carbohydrates
   C. Fats

Photo by Bob Coyle

D. Vitamins
   1. Water Soluble
   2. Fat Soluble
E. Minerals
F. Water

II. Effects of Nutrition on Growth and Development
  A. Teeth and Gums
  B. Eyes
  C. Bone Structure
  D. Body Development

III. Diseases and Conditions Often Related to Poor Nutrition
(e.g. Anemia; Beriberi; Cretinism; Dryness and Scaliness of Skin; Fatigue; Goiter; Heart Disease; Mental Retardation; Night Blindness; Pellagra; Rickets; Scurvy; Xerophthalmia)

IV. Personal Eating Habits
  A. Breakfast-Skipping
  B. Family Eating Patterns
  C. Snacking
  D. Overeating
  E. Undereating
  F. Vending Machines/Fast Food Chains
  G. Peer Group Influence
  H. Ethnic Foods
  I. Mass Media Influence

V. Weight Control
  A. Defining overweight/obesity/malnutrition
  B. Physical Effects of Overweight/Underweight
  C. Emotional Effects of Overweight/Underweight
  D. Relationship of Infant Eating Habits to Adult Weight
  E. Effectiveness of Various Weight Control Plans

VI. Food Fads and Fallacies
  A. Fad Diets
  B. Food Fallacies
  C. Food Quackery
  D. "Health Foods"

VII. Food Processing and Methods of Preparation
  A. Preserving Nutrients During Cooking
  B. Proper Food Storage and Handling Techniques
  C. Nutrient Additives
  (e.g., artificial sweetners, flavoring agents, food coloring agents, emulsifiers, stabilizers, etc.)
  D. Preservation Methods
   1. Canning
   2. Freeze-Drying
   3. Freezing
   4. Irradiation
   5. Oven Drying
   6. Pasteurization
   7. Salting
   8. Smoking

VIII. Food-Related Careers
(e.g., Baker; Cook; Dietitian; Farmer; Food Service Operator; Grocery Store Manager; Home Economist; Nutrition Educator; Public Health Nutritionist; Research Nutritionist, etc.)

IX. World Food Supply

Lesson Plans

Nutrition

Nutritional Needs: Womb to Tomb

Objectives

1. The student will describe three important functions of nutrients.

2. The student will list the seven special stages of life discussed in class and a special nutritional requirement for each of these stages.

3. The student will write one paragraph describing a major change in infant feeding practices that has occurred during this century and explain why he/she feels it is good or bad.

4. The student will collect and categorize five breakfast recipes for at least three different lifestyles.

5. The student will rank in order ten qualities that may affect their food choices, beginning with #1 as the most important.

6. Using food comparison cards from the National Dairy Council, the student will select at least ten foods that would satisfy the need for additional calories during the later months of pregnancy and at the same time provide good quality protein, mineral elements and vitamins.

7. The student will describe at least four problems that often contribute to inadequate nutrition in elderly people.

Sources

1. Dr. Jean Mayer. "Dr. Jean Mayer's Common-Sense Guide To Nutrition," *Family Health*, April, 1973.

2. *A-B-C's of Good Nutrition* (a Scriptographic booklet), Channing L. Bete Co., Inc., Greenfield, Mass., 1971.

3. Judith Ramsey and seven noted nutritionists. "The Seven Ages of Nutrition," *Family Health*, July, 1970, pp. 31-34.

4. National Dairy Council. "Current Concepts in Infant Nutrition," *Dairy Council Digest*, Rosemont, Illinois, March-April, 1976, p. 10.

5. Antoinette Hatfield and Peggy Stanton. "Menu Magic is Child's Play," *Family Health*, February, 1974 pp. 28-29, 48-50.

6. S. B. Caghan. "The Adolescent Process and the Problem of Nutrition," *American Journal of Nursing*, October, 1975, pp. 1728-1730.

7. C. Young, "Adolescents and Their Nutrition," *Medical Care of the Adolescent*, 3rd Edition, Edited by J. Gallagher and others. New York. Appleton-Century-Crofts. 1976, pp. 15-24.

8. U.S. Center For Disease Control. *Ten State Nutrition Survey, 1968-1970*, (DHEW Publication # (HSM) 72-8134: 72-8133) Washington, D.C., U.S. Government Printing Office. 1972. Vol. 1, pp. 1-12: Vol. 5, pp. v81-v85.

9. Carolyn T. Torre. "Nutritional Needs of Adolescents," *The American Journal of Maternal Child Nursing*, March/April 1977, pp. 118-127.

10. National Dairy Council. "Nutrition and Athletic Performance," *Dairy Council Digest*, Rosemont, Illinois, March-April, 1975, pp. 7-10.

11. David Costill Ph.D. "Sports Nutrition: The Role of Carbohydrates," *Nutrition News*, Rosemont, Illinois, National Dairy Council, February, 1978, pp. 1-4.

What Is Nutrition

Nutrition starts the moment a microscopic wiggly sperm cell pushes its way into a much larger egg cell, joins forces with it, and a human being begins to exist. Nutrition exerts a profound influence on the growing embryo, who must depend on the mother for adequate sustenance. If the mother is not healthy and well nourished, she may fail to furnish the embryo with the nutrients needed to prevent deformities, stillbirths, mental retardation, and other possible troubles which can develop in later life.

But just what is *nutrition?* As the noted Harvard nutritionist Dr. Jean Mayer says, "It is a science dealing with the effects of food on the body."[1] (p22) "It's the food you eat and how your body uses it to live, to grow, to keep healthy and to get the energy for work and play."[2] (p.2)

The consumption of an adequate amount of essential nutrients in our daily diet is necessary if our body is to: grow, repair and maintain itself; regulate its own inner processes; and provide body warmth and energy. This is important for people of any age; however, as we grow older and our activity decreases, we need fewer calories to retain the weight that is best for us. Beginning with infancy, can you think of "Seven Ages of Nutrition,"[3] or stages of life, that have special nutritional requirements?

1. *Infancy*

Breast milk or infant formula provides nearly all of the essential nutrients and calories that a baby needs, although breast milk is easier to digest and contains certain antibodies that may protect the infant against specific viral infections. Many commercially prepared formulas supply vitamins C and D, plus iron, which babies definitely need, however, breast milk also contains sufficient vitamin C if the mother's diet is rich in citrus fruits and certain vegetables. A vitamin or mineral supplement may be prescribed if one or more of the essential nutrients are not present in adequate amounts.

Activities: A major change in infant feeding practices that has occurred during this century is the decline in breast feeding and the corresponding increase in bottle feeding. Why do you think this has happened? Research the advantages and disadvantages of both practices. Call your local La Leche League for information regarding the advantages of breast feeding. Speakers are available in many cities and educational literature can be obtained by writing to La Leche League International, 9616 Minneapolis Street, Franklin Park, Illinois, 60131.

Another trend in infant nutrition is the feeding of solids to infants at an increasingly earlier age. Why do you think this happens? How does this practice contribute to iron-deficiency anemia? (Iron-deficiency anemia "is considered the most prevalent nutritional disorder among infants and children in the United States, particularly those between six and 24 months of age[4]). Throughout the world, the incidence of iron-deficiency anemia is highest among this age group. How can this disorder be eliminated?

Compare the labels of foods commonly fed to infants during the first year of life with respect to iron content, salt content, sugar content, etc.

2. *Childhood*

Good eating habits should already have been established at home before the child enters school. This is done by serving a variety of appetizing, well-balanced meals and snacks. Children have greater needs for some nutrients than adults because of their rapid growth and high activity, but also have a limited stomach capacity. Therefore the foods eaten must be chosen for their nutritional value. Milk, for calcium, riboflavin, and vitamin D . . . meat and fish, for protein, iron, and niacin . . . citrus fruits for vitamin C . . . potatoes, enriched breads and cereals for vitamin B₁ and carbohydrates . . . and vegetables for vitamin A, are all important. (See figure 14.1: *Nutrients For Health*). Children have a greater need for breakfast than most adults do, and need a variety of foods whenever they are hungry.

Activities: How do you get children to eat what they need rather than what they want? After reading "Menu Magic is Child's Play,"[5] ask the students to try creating their own brightly colored plates of food using magazine pictures of food, construction paper, crayons, or actual food. It may even be possible to invite a class of elementary age students over for lunch.

If it is possible for students to prepare the food at school or bring a small plate of food that has been prepared at home, photograph the artistically prepared food and share the results with parents during a parent-teacher meeting. Since children always love a milkshake out of the blender, ask each student to create a healthful concoction of his/her own, and compile the recipes into a booklet of "Delectable Drinks."

3. *Adolescence*

The teen years are a period characterized by rapid, recognizable changes in the individual's physical makeup. Ironically, the accelerated growth during puberty creates increased nutritional needs at a time when meeting these needs is difficult because of internal and external factors. Among these factors are a desire to express a developing sense of self and independence through adhering to extreme or fad diets, incomplete knowledge of the effect of present food intake on future health, and insufficient time to prepare or eat nutritious foods.[6,7]

The unfortunate consequence of such behavior is reflected in a study finding that adolescents, ages 10–16, had the most unsatisfactory nutritional status of any other age group.[8] The Ten-State Nutrition Survey revealed deficiencies in the intakes of Vitamin A, riboflavin, calcium and iron by adolescents, when compared with their recommended allowances.[8] Such inadequacies are accentuated in situations that demand extra nutrients, as in adolescent pregnancy. Three of the most frequently mentioned problems arising from young people's improper eating habits are iron deficiency anemia, dental caries, and obesity.[9]

Activities: Begin a classroom discussion with the following questions: Do you eat a variety of fresh fruits and vegetables daily? Do you avoid "fast foods"? Do you eat breakfast every day? The many adolescents who answer "no" to these three questions usually fit very nicely into a dietary pattern contributing to nutritional deficiencies. Discuss why many adolescents miss breakfast. (The meal is not prepared for them; they are not hungry in the morning; they are trying to lose weight; they don't get up early enough to take time to eat breakfast, etc.)

Encourage several volunteers to read the following articles that appeared in *Family Health* magazine, prepare and eat some of the suggested breakfast recipes, and then share the experience with the rest of the class.

"Get-Up-And-Go Breakfasts," April, 1973
"Break Out of the Breakfast Rut," September, 1972
"The Take-Along Breakfast," September, 1976
"Hearty, Headstart Breakfasts & Brunches," Sept. 1977.

Collect and categorize breakfast recipes for the following lifestyles: "On the Run," "Hard-Working," "Country-Style," "Weight Watching," and "Sophisticated."

Guide to Good Eating...

A Recommended Daily Pattern

The recommended daily pattern provides the foundation for a nutritious, healthful diet.

The recommended servings from the Four Food Groups for adults supply about 1200 Calories. The chart below gives recommendations for the number and size of servings for several categories of people.

Food Group	Recommended Number of Servings				
	Child	Teenager	Adult	Pregnant Woman	Lactating Woman
Milk — 1 cup milk, yogurt, OR **Calcium Equivalent:** 1½ slices (1½ oz) cheddar cheese* / 1 cup pudding / 1¾ cups ice cream / 2 cups cottage cheese*	3	4	2	4	4
Meat — 2 ounces cooked lean meat, fish, poultry, OR **Protein Equivalent:** 2 eggs / 2 slices (2 oz) cheddar cheese* / ½ cup cottage cheese* / 1 cup dried beans, peas / 4 tbsp peanut butter	2	2	2	3	2
Fruit-Vegetable — ½ cup cooked or juice / 1 cup raw / Portion commonly served such as a medium-size apple or banana	4	4	4	4	4
Grain, whole grain, fortified, enriched — 1 slice bread / 1 cup ready-to-eat cereal / ½ cup cooked cereal / pasta, grits	4	4	4	4	4

*Count cheese as serving of milk OR meat, not both simultaneously.

"Others" complement but do not replace foods from the Four Food Groups. Amounts should be determined by individual caloric needs.

Nutrients for Health

Nutrients are chemical substances obtained from foods during digestion. They are needed to build and maintain body cells, regulate body processes, and supply energy.

About 50 nutrients, including water, are needed daily for optimum health. If one obtains the proper amount of the 10 "leader" nutrients in the daily diet, the other 40 or so nutrients will likely be consumed in amounts sufficient to meet body needs.

One's diet should include a variety of foods because no *single* food supplies all the 50 nutrients, and because many nutrients work together.

When a nutrient is added or a nutritional claim is made, nutrition labeling regulations require listing the 10 leader nutrients on food packages. These nutrients appear in the chart below with food sources and some major physiological functions.

Nutrient	Important Sources of Nutrient	Some major physiological functions		
		Provide energy	Build and maintain body cells	Regulate body processes
Protein	Meat, Poultry, Fish / Dried Beans and Peas / Egg / Cheese / Milk	Supplies 4 Calories per gram.	Constitutes part of the structure of every cell, such as muscle, blood, and bone; supports growth and maintains healthy body cells.	Constitutes part of enzymes, some hormones and body fluids, and antibodies that increase resistance to infection.
Carbohydrate	Cereal / Potatoes / Dried Beans / Corn / Bread / Sugar	Supplies 4 Calories per gram. / Major source of energy for central nervous system.	Supplies energy so protein can be used for growth and maintenance of body cells.	Unrefined products supply fiber—complex carbohydrates in fruits, vegetables, and whole grains—for regular elimination. Assists in fat utilization.
Fat	Shortening, Oil / Butter, Margarine / Salad Dressing / Sausages	Supplies 9 Calories per gram.	Constitutes part of the structure of every cell. Supplies essential fatty acids.	Provides and carries fat-soluble vitamins (A, D, E, and K).
Vitamin A (Retinol)	Liver / Carrots / Sweet Potatoes / Greens / Butter, Margarine		Assists formation and maintenance of skin and mucous membranes that line body cavities and tracts, such as nasal passages and intestinal tract, thus increasing resistance to infection.	Functions in visual processes and forms visual purple, thus promoting healthy eye tissues and eye adaptation in dim light.
Vitamin C (Ascorbic Acid)	Broccoli / Orange / Grapefruit / Papaya / Mango / Strawberries		Forms cementing substances, such as collagen, that hold body cells together, thus strengthening blood vessels, hastening healing of wounds and bones, and increasing resistance to infection.	Aids utilization of iron.
Thiamin (B$_1$)	Lean Pork / Nuts / Fortified Cereal Products	Aids in utilization of energy.		Functions as part of a coenzyme to promote the utilization of carbohydrate. Promotes normal appetite. Contributes to normal functioning of nervous system.
Riboflavin (B$_2$)	Liver / Milk / Yogurt / Cottage Cheese	Aids in utilization of energy.		Functions as part of a coenzyme in the production of energy within body cells. Promotes healthy skin, eyes, and clear vision.
Niacin	Liver / Meat, Poultry, Fish / Peanuts / Fortified Cereal Products	Aids in utilization of energy.		Functions as part of a coenzyme in fat synthesis, tissue respiration, and utilization of carbohydrate. Promotes healthy skin, nerves, and digestive tract. Aids digestion and fosters normal appetite.
Calcium	Milk, Yogurt / Cheese / Sardines and Salmon with Bones / Collard, Kale, Mustard, and Turnip Greens		Combines with other minerals within a protein framework to give structure and strength to bones and teeth.	Assists in blood clotting. Functions in normal muscle contraction and relaxation, and normal nerve transmission.
Iron	Enriched Farina / Prune Juice / Liver / Dried Beans and Peas / Red Meat	Aids in utilization of energy.	Combines with protein to form hemoglobin, the red substance in blood that carries oxygen to and carbon dioxide from the cells. Prevents nutritional anemia and its accompanying fatigue. Increases resistance to infection.	Functions as part of enzymes involved in tissue respiration.

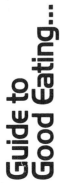

Figure 14.1. Nutrition

Create an environment where the students feel free to talk about their snacking behaviors—both good and bad—by playing the record, "I'm Just A Junk Food Junkie."

Permit the students to explore issues surrounding snacking: Do they think snacks are good for them? Does having an allowance affect their eating behavior? Where and when are snacks consumed? Are nutritious foods more or less expensive than junk foods?

Distribute calorie and food composition charts so the students can investigate the contribution of snack foods to their diets.

The following activities were suggested during a Nutrition Education workshop by the Ohio Department of Education: Beginning with your most favorite food, rank order the ten foods that you like best.

		A	B	C	D	E	F	G
1.								
2.								
3.								
4.								
5.								
6.								
7.								
8.								
9.								
10.								

In column A, place a checkmark next to the foods you would not want to give up for even one week.

In column B, place a checkmark adjacent to the foods you have eaten within the last month.

In column C, place a checkmark next to the foods that would have been on your "best-liked" list ten years ago.

In column D, place a checkmark next to the foods you think will be on your "best-liked" list five years from now.

In column E, place a checkmark next to the foods you feel are "nutritious".

In column F, place a checkmark next to the foods you listed that would be disliked next to most other people.

In column G, place a checkmark adjacent to the foods you would encourage other people to try.

Our country, with its diverse ethnic mix, has a particularly wide range of food preferences. Compile a booklet of special ethnic recipes that are prepared for religious or other holidays.

Rank order the following qualities that may affect your choice of foods, beginning with #1 as most important to you:

A. Nutrient Content   _____

B. Number of Calories   _____

C. Cost   _____

D. Taste   _____

E. Texture   _____

F. Presence of Food Additives/Preservatives   _____

G. Ease of Preparation   _____

H. Amount and Type of Fat   _____

I. Amount of Cholesterol   _____

J. Amount of Sugar   _____

4. *Athletes*

What effect does participation in sports have on an adolescent's nutritional needs? Athletes need proteins, carbohydrates, fats, minerals, vitamins, and water, just like their more sedentary peers, although in different quantities, due to greater energy expenditures. Depending upon the strenuousness of a sport, an athlete may burn anywhere from 3,000 to more than 5,000 calories a day.

> "Contrary to popular opinion, a high-protein diet is not physiologically necessary for the athlete since even heavy exercise is not accompanied by significant protein catabolism. In fact, protein is an expensive and rather inefficient source of energy. On the other hand, high carbohydrate diets are reported to increase work capacity, particularly during strenuous exercise, by providing greater energy per liter of oxygen consumed than either fat or protein and by contributing to glycogen reserves."[9,10,11]

While some research suggests that athletes also need increased levels of vitamins C and B complex, most investigators do not advocate vitamin supplementation.[9,10] They do recommend an adequate intake of salt and water. Salt requirements are usually met by a varied diet and modestly salting foods at meals. Water lost in perspiration needs to be replaced daily so that the body can dissipate heat and maintain its proper temperature.

Activities: Research the number of calories that are burned up by daily participation in various sports.

Find out if your coaches suggest special diets for their athletes. If so, how are they different from an ordinary nutritious diet?

Although the sports community gave tremendous publicity to some isotonic solutions such as *Gatorade, Sportade,* and *Bike Half Time Punch,* which were introduced in the 1960's, "there is yet no conclusive evidence of their physiological advantage over water, saline solutions, or glucose syrup drinks in improving performance."[10] How do you feel about these products?

How do you feel about the drastic weight loss regimen frequently undertaken by wrestlers prior to a match in order to qualify for the lowest possible weight class? Research the reasons why the American Medical Association condemns the still common practice of total starvation alternated with semi-starvation and dehydration.

Jean Mayer and other researchers have stated that food faddism and ignorance are more prominent in the area of athletics than in any other sphere of nutrition. Why might this be true? What are some nutritional misconceptions relative to athletes' diets?

5. *Pregnancy*

Pregnancy is another instance where a wide variety of foods rich in protein, vitamins, and minerals is especially important, since the mother is nourishing the child through her own body. Enough fats, carbohydrates, and starches should be eaten to meet energy requirements, but a large weight gain early in the pregnancy should be avoided. Although physicians disagree as to the amount of weight a woman can safely gain, the government's Committee on Maternal Nutrition is presently recommending an average gain of 24 pounds.

Pregnant women are advised to avoid fatty, hard-to-digest foods and highly seasoned dishes. Too much salt can lead to water retention, swelling, and more serious problems for both the mother and fetus. Medications, including vitamins, should only be taken on the advice of an obstetrician. When vitamins are prescribed, they are intended only as a safeguard and not as a substitute for wholesome foods.

Activities: Discuss why the development of good food habits and the maintenance of an appropriate body weight for one's height and frame is important to establish before pregnancy.

How does nutrition relate to the fact that maternal and infant complications occur about twice as frequently among early teen-age mothers as among mature women?

Using food comparison cards from the National Dairy Council, ask the students to select foods that would satisfy the need for additional calories during the later months of pregnancy and at the same time provide good quality protein, vitamins and minerals. Plan a day's meals for a woman in her 8th month of pregnancy.

Investigate the possible dangers, if any, that could result from a diet during pregnancy that was deficient in the following nutrients: Protein, carbohydrates, calcium, iron, vitamin A, vitamin D, vitamin K, and vitamin B_1 (Thiamine).

6. *Middle Age*

According to Dr. William E. Connor, the middle-aged American's usual diet might be suitable if the person was stalking prey, defending against marauders, planting and reaping crops, and tending the herd and the brood.[3] However, it is much more common to find today's middle-aged person doing a lot of sitting, rarely exercising, and eating an excess amount of fats, sugars, and starches which are not burned up.

In the interest of longevity, it is especially necessary for people in this age group to cut down drastically on foods containing cholesterol; to exchange a diet high in saturated fat, including fatty meats, for a diet high in polyunsaturated fats, including fish; develop a cooking style that includes a lot of baking and broiling instead of frying; and to reduce the amount of salt that they consume.

Activities: Contact your local chapter of the American Heart Association for pamphlets about the ill effects of obesity, cholesterol, and high blood pressure. Ask for a listing of foods that are low in cholesterol and high in polyunsaturates.

Develop a skit showing "Mr. Cholesterol" at the dinner table with "Mr. and Mrs. Middle-Aged America." "Sammy Salt," "Suzy Sugar," and "Fried Fats," may also be present, while "Corn Oil," and various fruits, vegetables, poultry, fish, and cereal are looking through the window discussing how they can get in and save "Mr. and Mrs. Middle-Aged America" from possible harm. It may be possible to arrange an evening presentation of this play for parents, along with a short talk by a Nutritionist or Home Economist, and the distribution of helpful pamphlets.

Read the *Family Health* article, "The Men At the Top—How They Keep Fit," (December, 1973), then interview several individuals holding top jobs in your community and learn how they make keeping fit an integral part of their daily schedules.

7. *Old Age*

Can you name five special problems that often contribute to inadequate nutrition in elderly people?

1. The elderly person on a retirement pension often cannot afford a well-balanced diet.

2. Poor teeth or improperly fitting dentures may make eating uncomfortable.

3. Diminishing senses of taste and smell, as well as difficulties in swallowing, may reduce the pleasure of eating.

4. A person living alone often does not prepare proper meals and may find meal time especially lonely.

5. Physical problems may make regular grocery shopping difficult or impossible.

6. Biochemical and physiological changes often predispose older individuals to depression and indirectly contribute to lack of appetite.

7. While some elderly individuals eat too little, others eat excessively (especially sweets) as an apparent substitution for the loss of other satisfactions.

Elderly people need a varied, well-balanced diet, but fewer calories. Too often their diet is high in carbohydrates, which are cheaper and require less preparation than other foods, while low in proteins, vitamins A and C, and iron.

Activities: Learn more about some of the experimental food programs that have been set up in an attempt to deal with the nutritional problems of the aged. For instance, the meals-on-wheels project delivers appetizing hot meals to elderly persons who are confined to their homes. Another program provides reasonably priced meals and an opportunity for socializing in a high school cafeteria at hours when the students are in classes. A third program provides personal assistance in food shopping and preparation. What is being done in your community?

Materials

1. Articles from *Family Health* magazine listed under content and procedures.

2. Various brands of common baby foods with labels intact.

3. Magazine pictures of food, construction paper, and scissors.

4. The record, "I'm Just A Junk Food Junkie."

5. Food comparison cards from the local chapter of the National Dairy Council.

Evaluation

In addition to being able to complete the behavioral objectives, the student should be able to complete the following activities:

1. Keeping in mind that young children have a smaller stomach capacity than adults, but need many nutrients for growth and energy, plan five snacks that combine one or more foods from the breads and cereal group, fruits and vegetables group, and are a good source of protein.

2. Suggest at least two ways for making breakfast time more pleasant for the members of your family.

3. Complete the following sentences:

A. A nutritious food is _____.

B. Snacking is _____.

C. Breakfast is _____.

D. Nutrition education involves _____.

E. Food affects my health _____.

F. The food I eat affects my appearance _____.

G. I eat too much _____.

H. I eat too little _____.

I. Foods that are new or strange to me are _____.

Nutrition
Weight Problems in Adolescence

Objectives

1. After discussing television programs, commercials, and paintings as media that graphically promote varying ideas of beauty and ideal weight, the student will be able to give or show three examples depicting individuals considered too thin, and three examples of individuals considered too fat, by the standards of most Americans today.

2. The students will each write one paragraph describing their body—how they feel about it, and how well they take care of it.

3. The student will determine if he or she is overweight, normal weight, or underweight, through the use of visual inspection, scales and weight charts, and by taking the pinch test.

4. Following class discussion and assigned readings, the student will list and explain at least three psychological disadvantages and five physical disadvantages, that can result from being overweight.

5. The student will describe two problems often faced by extremely underweight individuals and explain why there may be very little that a physician can do to help "fatten up" these people.

6. The student will be able to suggest at least five medically approved ways for helping an overweight adolescent.

7. After completing this lesson, the student will demonstrate his/her knowledge of diet and nutrition by accurately completing the "Are You Puzzled About Nutrition?" crossword puzzle.

Sources

1. "Is Your Weight Your Fate?" *Current Health,* Highwood, Illinois: Curriculum Innovations, December, 1975, p.4.

2. Dr. Jean Mayer. "Fat Babies Grow into Fat People," *Family Health,* March, 1973, p. 24.

3. National Dairy Council. "Current Concepts of Obesity," *Dairy Council Digest:* Rosemont, Illinois, July–August, 1975.

4. Carolyn T. Torre. "Nutritional Needs of Adolescents," *The American Journal of Maternal Child Nursing,* March–April, 1977.

5. Robert H. Kirk and Michael H. Hamrick. *Focus on Health and Nutrition:* National Dairy Council, Rosemont, Illinois, 1977.

6. Pauline S. Powers, M.D. "Weight Problems in Adolescence," *Primary Care,* Vol. 3, #2, June, 1976.

7. National Dairy Council. "What's New in Weight Control?" *Dairy Council Digest:* Rosemont, Illinois, March–April, 1978.

8. Jack D. Osman. *Thin From Within,* New York, N.Y., Hart Publishing Company, Inc., 1976.

Content and Procedures

What Is Ideal Weight

How can a person determine his or her ideal weight? Ideas about ideal weight vary from generation to generation and culture to culture. Obesity is often looked upon as a mark of distinction in societies where food is scarce, because it indicates that the person has enough money to eat well. "Some Polynesian cultures consider it a sign of distinction and beauty to be so well-nourished as to become fat. Other cultures take adolescent girls to "fattening houses," where they become obese before being offered in marriage to the adolescent males."[1] On the other hand, when food is abundant, as it is for most Americans, and was among the Greeks and Romans, there is often a distaste for fatness.

Today's mass media encourages the "thin is in" image by much of its programming while interposing commercials for high calorie, sugar-laden foods. Art work is another medium which has graphically promoted varying ideas of beauty and ideal weight. Ask students to locate photographs of various examples of artwork that depict beautiful women of another era that would be considered either very thin or fat today. (Peter Rubens, a 17th century artist, painted many voluptuous women; American women in the 1920's were depicted as being extremely thin.)

As in most areas, moderation is probably the key word, since there are definite psychological and biological dangers in being too fat . . . or too thin.

Answer Some Questions

Take several minutes to answer the following questions:

1. Describe your body—how you feel about it, and how well you take care of it.

2. Do you consider yourself to be short _____, medium _____, or tall _____?

3. Do you consider yourself to be overweight ____, normal weight ____, or underweight ____?

4. Do you have enough energy to enjoy the things you do and do the things you enjoy? _____

5. Do you feel healthy most of the time? _____

6. Do you consider your overall body condition to be good _____, fair _____, or poor _____?

7. How would you like to take better care of your body?

Ideal weight is often considered to be the weight at which you feel and look your best. You can learn whether you are overweight or underweight in many different ways: Give yourself a long, honest look in the mirror sometime after you have stepped out of the shower. Do you see bulges, flabby upper arms and thighs, a double chin, or protruding abdomen? Does your face appear thin and drawn? Do your ribs protrude? Are your back, thighs, and buttocks adequately covered with muscles?

When you put on clothes are there bulges where they shouldn't be? Do you have trouble closing your zipper? Do you avoid wearing certain clothing because it isn't comfortable any more or hangs like a loose sack on you?

What do your scales tell you, especially when compared to weight charts designed by the National Dairy Council or life insurance companies? Weight charts are usually based on desirable weights for your sex, age, height, and body frame. Insurance companies define ideal weight as the weight at which one will live the longest.

The Pinch Test

If you still aren't sure, take the pinch test. This is a way of estimating how much fat is stored under your skin. Pinch the skin at the back of your upper arm or over your lowest rib where it extends under your armpit. If the skinfold thickness is more than one inch, then you probably have too much fat over your entire body. If the fold of skin just below your bottom rib is less than one-quarter of an inch thick, it means that you need to gain weight. Physicians sometimes use *calipers,* instruments that look like a big pair of tongs, to measure body fat. Either overweight or underweight can be the result of *malnutrition,* although in a number of studies stretching over 20 years, Dr. Jean Mayer showed that the big difference between most overweight children and adolescents and their thin contemporaries was "not that the overweight youngsters eat more, but that they exercise far less than other children who are of normal weight."[2]

A number of nutritionists and pediatricians are also concerned that overfeeding infants results in the production of a greater number of fat cells that greedily sop up nutrients from the blood of the individual for their entire life. This leads to overeating and excessive fat.[2,3]

Problems with Excess Body Weight

Why do you think there is so much concern over excess body weight?

Psychological Disadvantages

Since so many people believe that extra pounds detract from good appearance, it is not surprising that obese adolescents often suffer from a "defective body image, low self-esteem, depression, and social isolation."[4] Adolescence is a time for comparing assets and inadequacies. Hopefully, most people emerge from this period with positive feelings about themselves, however chronically overweight individuals often find themselves the object of jokes, the last ones chosen for teams, uninvited to social gatherings, and even unable to find properly fitting clothes.[1] It is no wonder that they become even more self-conscious and withdrawn. Such frustration leads to more overeating and increased vulnerability to biological problems.

Physical Disadvantages

Serious health problems can arise from overweight or be aggravated by it. They include dangers to the heart and circulatory system (diets high in saturated fats and cholesterol seem to contribute to atherosclerosis, a leading cause of heart attack and stroke); increased vulnerability to gall bladder disorders (due to hardened accumulations of cholesterol, enzymes, and proteins); gout (obesity is often accompanied by an increase in uric acid, a primary factor in the development of gout); liver disease; heightened risk of acquiring diabetes, hypertension, and hypothyroidism. Overweight also increases surgical risk and ones chances of susceptibility to an infectious disease. While overweight is usually associated with decreased physical activity, mobility may be further impaired by osteoarthritis, a disorder characterized by a wearing down of cartilage in the joints. Stand up and look at the size of your knee joint. Now imagine that you are 60 pounds heavier. Has your knee joint increased in size? No, but the amount of stress and weight placed on the knee and hip joints has increased.

For these reasons, Michael Irwin, M.D. is probably correct when he says: "The longer the belt line, the shorter the life line." It might also be appropriate to add that the *quality* of life often diminishes as well.

Ask students to role play problems related to overweight and obesity, as well as to give suggestions for correcting the problems. Debate overweight as a cause and an effect of emotional imbalance.

While the effects of obesity are pretty grim, being underweight also has its problems. Extremely thin people are often very self-conscious about their appearance and try to find special clothes to cover their protruding bones. They may lack energy and be more susceptible to infections. Underweight individuals receive little sympathy from most people and may become desperate to alter their body image. In fact, Dr. Jean Mayer has found that the overweight are less likely to kill themselves than their thinner brethren.

Since research shows that there seems to be a genetic determination of thinness, probably a lack of adipose cells to collect fat, there is often very little that can be done to help "fatten up" the very thin individual. These people are generally *ectomorphs,* meaning that they have a thin, elongated skeleton, narrow hands and feet, and long fingers and toes. Extremely thin people often have sudden and complete feelings of satiety, where they will gag if given another mouthful of their favorite dish.

Some slightly overweight individuals set a weight goal and achieve it by following a sensible diet, however, they then set a new and lower goal. The "death spiral" may continue into starvation if the victim develops a condition called *Anorexia Nervosa.* Although rare, its most common victims are teenage girls. Like obesity, "there are marked eating disorders, pronounced endocrine and metabolic changes, abnormalities in activity levels, anatomical and cytological changes, and usually psychological disturbances."[6] Since the underlying cause is mental, rather than physical, psychotherapy is recommended to help improve the victim's self-confidence.

How to Deal with Overweight

What can be done for the overweight individual? Carolyn Torre believes that the paramount goal when working with obese adolescents is to help them to like and accept themselves rather than to significantly reduce their intake of calories, since this may throw growing adolescents into negative nitrogen balance. However, she does suggest the elimination of high carbohydrate foods in order to prevent further gain in weight. Other recommendations include eating small portions of nutritious foods more than three times a day; always beginning the day with a high-protein breakfast; and making exercise an integral part of the obesity treatment plan. Since obesity tends to follow a family pattern, dietary counseling is recommended for the entire family, as well as special counseling tailored to the individual needs and circumstances of the young person involved.[4]

Some of the treatment methods for those with excess body fat include (a) dietary management, (b) exercise, (c) drug treatment, (d) surgical treatment, and (e) behavior modification. Less commonly employed methods include jaw wiring, acupuncture, and hypnosis. Evidence seems to indicate that the most effective approach to weight reduction and maintenance is a combination program consisting of nutritionally sound dietary management, regular exercise, and behavior modification directed at the first two components.[7]

Additional Classroom Activities

Additional classroom activities include appointing committees to study various methods for losing weight and reporting their findings to the class. Ask students to investigate the various organizations in your community which meet to discuss weight control and weigh their members (e.g., Weight Watchers and T.O.P.S.). Write to the Cling Peach Advisory Board, One California Street, San Francisco, California, 94111, for their "Join the Trim Team!" kit of free materials to aid in the teaching of weight control. These materials are based on behavior modification techniques and include six lessons, six sample handout sheets, six 23x35 inch posters, and menus—including recipes and low-calorie meal suggestions. Ask the class what effects they think stress has on their individual nutritional habits. Select some of the values clarification exercises found in Osman's book, *Thin From Within,*[8] for use with your students.

Materials

1. Art books

2. Kit of free materials from the Cling Peach Advisory Board.

3. Handouts incorporating activities from Jack Osman's book, *Thin From Within.*

4. "Are You Puzzled About Nutrition?" crossword puzzle from *Current Health* magazine, December, 1977, Curriculum Innovations, Highwood, Illinois 60040.

Evaluation

1. The methods to be used for evaluation of objectives one through six are clearly stated in the behavioral objectives.

2. A nutrition crossword puzzle is included in this lesson with the permission of Curriculum Innovations, Inc. The answers to this puzzle are given below: *Across:* 4. diet; 5. fad; 7. adipose; 9. iodine; 10. ill; 11. fiber; 12. intestine; 13. obese; 15. scale; 18. sugar; 19. chart; 20. calorie; 21. jaw; 22. caliper. *Down:* 1. fat; 2. niacin; 3. pounds; 6. diabetes; 8. glands; 9. iron; 14. energy; 16. calcium; 17. organic; 18. skinfold (Pinch test).

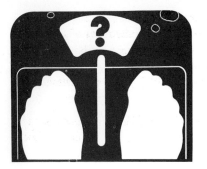

Are You Puzzled about Nutrition?

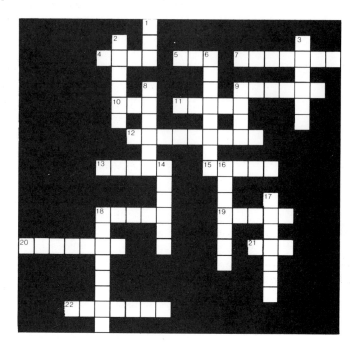

Across

4. What you eat is your _____
5. Beware of this type of diet
7. Fat tissue
9. A mineral found in iodized salt
10. One suffering from anorexia nervosa may become very _____
11. Fruits and vegetables are a good source of this
12. Part of this may be removed surgically to lose weight
13. Considerably overweight
15. Seldom lies about your weight
18. A source of immediate energy
19. This tells you what you should weigh
20. Each one counts
21. Some wire this closed to lose weight
22. Instrument to measure skin thickness

Down

1. Not chubby but _____
2. The vitamin found in whole grain cereal
3. Many would like these to melt away
6. This desease is four times more common among the overweight
8. Many overweight people blame their _____
9. A mineral frequently missing in teen's diet
14. Inadequate intake of nutrients may result in a lack of this
16. This mineral is a bone builder
17. Natural fertilizers are used on these foods
18. Name of test that measures skin thickness

Reprinted with permission from *Current Health*—The Continuing Guide to Health Education; Vol. 4, #4, December, 1977, Curriculum Innovations, Inc., 501 Lake Forest Avenue, Highwood, Illinois, 60040.

Nutrition
Foods, Fads, and Fallacies *

Objectives

1. The student will corectly match the terms carnivorous, herbivorous, omnivorous, entomophageous, and anthropophagus with foods that typify these types of diets.

2. After class discussion and viewing the filmstrip, "Food Fads: You Bet Your Life," the student will be able to read an advertisement about a "miracle" food or diet and assess its probable worth, as well as identify any implied threats, thoughts started but never finished, and any false premises on which arguments are then built.

Foods, Fads, and Fallacies is also the name of an excellent four-part filmstrip series and Teacher's Guide produced by Walt Disney Educational Media Company, that examines food myths, past and present, and the effect they have on our lives.

3. The student will be able to give an example for each of the three basic types of food fads, namely: (1) those in which special virtues of a particular food are exaggerated and purported to cure specific diseases, (2) those in which certain foods are eliminated from the diet due to the belief that harmful constituents are present, and (3) those in which emphasis is placed on "natural" foods.[4]

4. The student will list at least five different vitamins that are necessary to human health and opposite each vitamin listed, write the name of a food that contains that vitamin.

5. The student will compare the prices, content, and claims made for several basic food items found in both health food stores and supermarkets.

Sources

1. Ayerst Series on Gastrology. "Food, The Stomach, and Geography." (#6 in a series), *M.D.*, March, 1971. (Ayerst Laboratories, New York, N.Y. 10017)

2. Gwen Schultz. "Food Taboos," *Today's Health,* February, 1964, pp. 28–32.

3. Dr. Jean Mayer. "Pills, Potions, and Promises—The Cruel Hoax of Food Fads," *Family Health,* June, 1974.

4. National Dairy Council. "Food Fadism" *Dairy Council Digest,* Rosemont, Illinois, January-February, 1973.

5. Eleanor Young, E. Brennan and G. Irving. "Perspectives on Fast Foods," *Public Health Currents.* Ross Laboratories, 625 Cleveland Avenue, Columbus, Ohio 43216, Vol. 19, #1, Jan.-Feb. 1979.

Content and Procedures

Pretest

"For most of the world's inhabitants, two-thirds of whom suffer from malnutrition, utilizable food is that which can be grown, gathered, or hunted in one's own geographical setting."[1] As a pre-test, ask students to match the following people with the foods they are likely to consume:

_____ 1. Arctic Eskimo

_____ 2. Native along border of Kalahari Desert in Africa

_____ 3. Samoan

_____ 4. Australian Aborigine

_____ 5. African

A. Plants, Tubers, and Roots.

B. Cockchafer grubs, woodlice, caterpillars and ants.

C. Seal, Walrus, Narwhal, and Polar Bear.

D. Starch soup, flying fish, taro dumplings, raw bonito, baked sea turtle and roast pig.

E. Animals, birds, fish, and reptiles—but large caterpillars are their delicacy.

(Answers: 1-C; 2-A; 3-D; 4-E; 5-B)

A prisoner of geography, the Eskimo is a *carnivore* (kár'-ni-vors) or flesh-eater, out of necessity. In fact, the word "Eskimo" means "eaters of raw meat" and the Eskimo can easily consume four to eight pounds of meat daily.

Natives who live along the borders of the Kalahari Desert in Africa are almost entirely *herbivorous* (her-biv'-o-rus) or vegetarians. The desert provides a great number of tubers and roots but few animals. This type of diet may also be found in the lush tropics. Where a wide variety of foods are readily obtainable the people are usually *omnivorous,* (om-niv' o-rus) meaning that they eat all kinds of food.

In areas where most protein sources are rare but insects are abundant, many of the people are *entomophageous,* (en-to-moph'-a-gus). Some forms of insects are highly nutritious, such as termites. For example, one hundred grams of fried termites yields 561 calories, and is quite high in protein. Locusts and grasshoppers are other rich sources of protein in Africa, and are eaten toasted, fried, or boiled. When ground, dried, and salted, they will keep for months.

Nutritional Influences

Although the eating of insects, walrus, or shark stomach may seem strange to us, it does not necessarily represent food faddism. Advertising has a tremendous influence on our eating habits. (Have students monitor the advertisements in print and on television for one week and report their findings. What kind of eating habits does the food industry promote? Discuss how the overeater is influenced by advertising.) Our nutritional choices are also influenced by our heritage, culture, religion, and place on earth. People will eat what they can grow most easily; for this reason, the Japanese eat more rice, while Mexicans eat more corn. Ask the students to name all of the hygienic or religious restrictions or prohibitions with which they are familiar. (e.g., Pork taboo in the Middle East; Beef taboo in the United States. Probably the most universal food taboo is the eating of flesh of other human beings, although cannibalism (anthropophagy) is still practiced in interior New Guinea, as it was in other places until recently.) [1,2]

What Is a Food Faddist?

While our food choices may be different, a well-balanced diet is still possible for all. The food faddist is *not a person* whose diet is "different" *but one* who believes that certain "magic" substances (e.g., megavitamins, lecithin, wheat germ or honey) will solve all his/her problems. These substances are discussed by Dr. Jean Mayer in his informative article "Pills, Potions, and Promises—The Cruel Hoax of Food Fads,"[3] as well as rules for helping to spot a fad or faddist.

Activities

Show filmstrip #1, "I Eat What I Like, Regardless."[5] Discuss why there is a growing emphasis on fast foods and convenience foods. Interested students may wish to read, "Perspectives on Fast Foods,"[6] which includes nutritional analyses of fast foods. Ask students to make a list of all the food products and devices they can think of which are sold on the promise that they will keep a person young or "young-looking." Discuss why this is an important value to many people.

Show filmstrip #2, "Food Fads: You Bet Your Life,"[5] after the students have listed all the "miracle" diets they can recall. Ask each student to list all the vitamins that research has so far shown as necessary to human health on the left column of a sheet of paper. Opposite each vitamin listed, have the student write the name of a food that contains that vitamin.

Since October 1, 1973, dosages of vitamins A and D that exceed certain levels have only been sold by prescription. (These vitamins have proven alarmingly toxic when taken in large, unneeded quantities.) Since January 1, 1975, pills and capsules containing more than 150% of the government established Recommended Daily Allowance for any vitamin have been labeled and sold as drugs rather than as dietary supplements. These actions have disturbed many believers in vitamins. Have the students discuss whether they think the government should or should not restrict the people's right to take vitamins and supplements as they wish. Should these products be more expensive and harder to obtain? Interested students may wish to read the articles, "The Verdict On Vitamins," by Dodi Schultz, *Today's Health,* January, 1974 and "Vitamins Are Vital," *Current Health,* October, 1975.

After devising a basic food shopping list, have some students visit an "organic" or health food store and price the items there. Have other students price the items in a local supermarket. Compare the results. It may also be possible to compare the contents and claims for each food item. Interested students may wish to read the article, "Health Foods Versus Traditional Foods: A Comparison," by H. Appledorf, W. B. Wheeler, and J. A. Koburger, *Journal of Milk Food Technology,* April, 1973 (Volume 36:242).

Before showing filmstrip #3, "Is 'Natural' Healthy?"[5] ask students the following questions: (Teacher's Guide)[5]

1. Why do farmers use fertilizers in growing crops?

2. What is the difference between a pesticide and an herbicide? Why do farmers use these substances?

3. List all the additives you can think of. Explain why additives are used in food processing.

4. List ten processed foods that are commonly used in your home.

5. What led to the development of pasterurized milk?

Ask students if they think there is such a thing as a "perfect diet," before showing the filmstrip, "Is There A Perfect Diet?"[5] Discuss the advantages and disadvantages of a vegetarian diet. Obtain a vegetarian cookbook and list the protein sources that substitute for meat.

Materials

1. Filmstrips—*Foods, Fads, and Fallacies,* Walt Disney Educational Media Company.

2. Various diet advertisements.

Evaluation

The following short quiz may be used to evaluate objective #1.

Select the term that best describes the type of diet being eaten in the following examples. . . .

_____ 1. "I am having a spinach souffle, eggplant casserole, and a soybean patty for lunch."

_____ 2. "I will probably only have Arctic hare or white whale for my meal since no vegetables grow where I live."

_____ 3. "By eating the heart of my human victim, I hope to gain his courage." (Uncommon diet)

_____ 4. "I ate roast beef, mashed potatoes, and green beans for dinner tonight"

_____ 5. "Boiled locusts are OK for dinner, but I sure hope Mom gives me a large caterpillar for dessert."

A. Antropophagus

B. Carnivorous

C. Entomophageous

D. Herbivorous

E. Omnivorous

To evaluate objective #2, prepare descriptions of "new, miracle" diets such as "Calories Don't Count!" or "The Miracle of Vitamin P" and ask students to (1) assess their probable worth; (2) identify any implied threats; (3) identify any thoughts begun but never concluded; and (4) identify any false premises on which arguments are built.

Student knowledge may also be evaluated by requiring a two page essay on one of the following topics:

1. Nutrition education is the best means of offsetting the false propaganda of food faddists.[4]

2. Traditional ways of presenting nutrition education are ineffective.

3. A belief in fad diets and bizarre food supplements as a barrier against disease or aging is misleading and can be fatal.

Selected Learning Activities

Nutrition and Weight Control

_____ Design posters about nutrition for display in the lunchroom and in the classroom.

_____ Survey students as to their favorite and least liked foods. Develop menus that combine foods that are both nutritious and well liked.

_____ Invite a dermatologist to speak about the role nutrition plays in maintaining a good complexion.

_____ Compare the appearance, cost, flavor, and nutrients for particular food items that may be purchased fresh, canned, or frozen. How do these items compare at different times of the year?

_____ Plan a special holiday meal that is similar to the traditional meal but lower in calories.

_____ Research surgical procedures that have been used to help people lose weight.

_____ List the current fad diets, giving at least one advantage and one disadvantage of each.

_____ Check with the local library and your local bookstore for a list of diet books. What is on the cover? What is the appeal? What different kinds of diets are there?

_____ Design a daily, healthy nutrition log.

_____ Discuss the nutritional value of the different fast food chains that you and your friends frequent. Develop a nutritional rating scale. What is the most nutritious fast food chain? the least?

_____ Bring a nutritious snack to class and share at least two facts about the class with your classmates.

_____ Prepare a foreign food either at home or in class. How does this food serve the nutritional needs of its country?

_____ Have a class discussion on "Thin Is In."

_____ Make a mobile depicting the four basic food groups.

_____ Make a list of "junk" foods found in your school building and in your home.

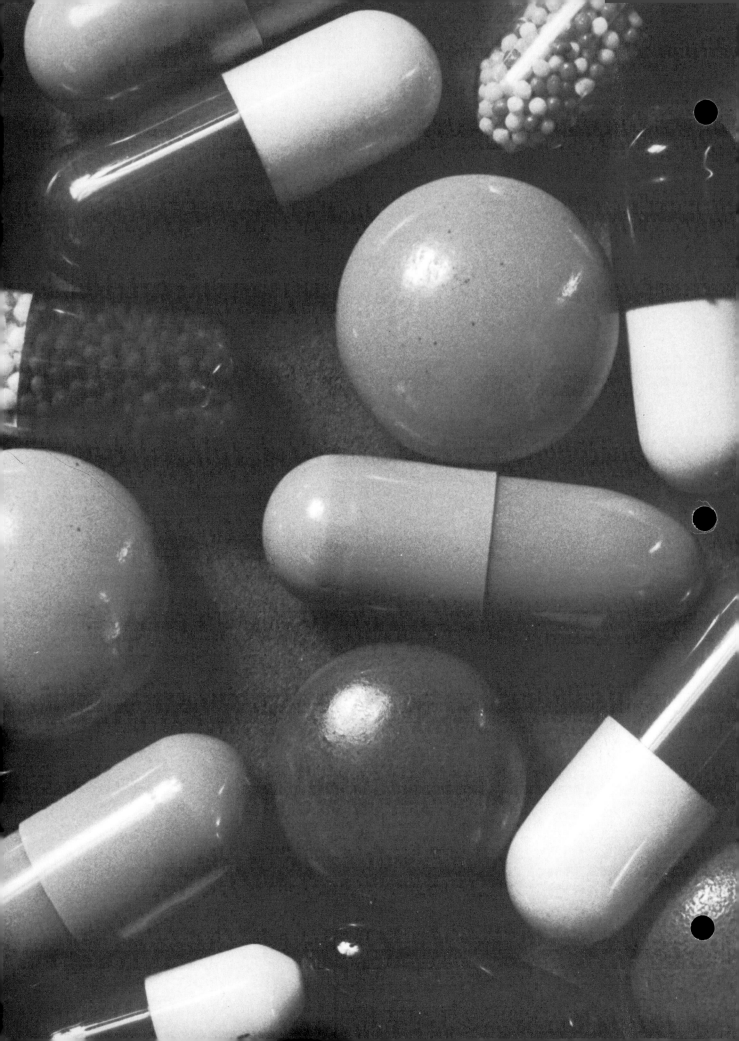

15

Teaching about Drugs
Use and Abuse

Americans are known to be a drug-taking society. The reasons for drug usage are as varied as the resulting influences of these drugs on the body. In a health education curriculum dedicated to the selection of behavior from a variety of alternatives, and to accountability, a unit on the use and abuse of drugs is essential.

The Suggested Topics for Teaching About Drugs: Use and Abuse, and the additional Selected Learning Activities, can be expanded to meet the needs of your particular community. We recommend that you develop additional lessons that reflect the type of drug usage in your community and the types of treatment programs available. The Three Detailed Sample Lessons included reflect three of the topics which we feel are important for middle and secondary students. Another topic, Tobacco, is covered in the next chapter.

The first lesson, **Alcohol,** examines the effects of alcohol on the body. The student should be able to describe the relationship between the amount of alcohol consumed and the degree of intoxication. An Alcohol Myth Response Sheet is included for classroom usage. The teacher may also want to invite a guest speaker to class to discuss state and local liquor laws.

A lesson on **Over-the-Counter Drugs** helps the student examine the drugs found in the home and to evaluate reasons for use of these drugs. Many drugs which are typically found in the medicine cabinet are heavily promoted on television and in magazine ads. The student not only learns about over-the-counter drugs but also examines responsible consumer behavior.

The third lesson on **Prescription Drugs** differentiates between brand name and generic name prescription drugs. The student is able to define prescription drugs and will be able to identify the need for making some drugs available only by prescription.

Suggested Topics

Drugs: Use and Abuse

I. Defining Drugs
   A. Psychoactive drugs
   B. Legal vs illegal drugs

Photo by James L. Ballard

II. Drug Abuse
  A. Illegal drugs
  B. Over-the-counter and prescription drugs
III. Drug Hazards
  A. Drug habit
  B. Drug tolerance
  C. Drug addiction
IV. Causes of Drug Abuse
  A. Social factors
  B. Addictive substances in drugs
  C. Psychological factors
V. Depressants
  A. Barbiturates
  B. Opiates
  C. Alcohol
VI. Stimulants
  A. Caffeine
  B. Amphetamines
  C. Nicotine
VII. Hallucinogens
  A. Marijuana
  B. LSD
  C. PCP
VIII. Tranquilizers
  A. Types of tranquilizers
  B. The widespread use of tranquilizers
IX. Treatment of Drug Abuse
  A. Residential therapeutic communities
  B. Chemical treatment
  C. Counseling
  D. Self-help groups
X. Economic Factors Related to Drug Use and Abuse
  A. Occupational considerations
  B. Safety and work
XI. Physiological Impact of Drugs
  A. Negative effects on the body
  B. Positive effects on the body
XII. Drugs and Society
  A. Societal problems
  B. Control of drug use in the future on society
  C. Positive affects of drugs on society
XIII. Mental Health and Drugs
  A. Development of self-esteem
  B. Dealing with peer pressure
  C. Alternate ways of getting high without the use of drugs

Lesson Plans

Drugs: Use and Abuse
Alcohol

Objectives

1. The student will identify the physiological effects of alcohol on the body.

2. The student will identify the relationship between the amount of alcohol consumed and the degree of intoxication.

Source

1. Joel Fort, *Alcohol: Our Biggest Drug Problem.* New York: McGraw-Hill Book Company, 1973.

2. Charles R. Carroll, *Alcohol: Use, Nonuse, and Abuse*, Dubuque: Wm. C. Brown Company Publishers, 1975.

Content and Procedures

A depressant is a drug that slows down or reduces cellular, and consequently, body functions. The most used and abused depressant in the United States today is alcohol. It is this drug which is considered the most prevalent and potentially dangerous mood-modifying representative of the *psychotropics* (affecting the mind or mental activity). Unlike most other drugs, alcohol plays many different roles in our society. In addition to its economic impact—its manufacture, use and sale, *most* Americans find alcohol to be a pleasant and enjoyable part of social gatherings, celebrations, dinners and parties. Unlike the other drugs such as opiates, marijuana and other hallucinogens, alcohol is accepted in our society and is a legal drug. It only becomes a problem of illegality under certain circumstances. Driving while intoxicated, being a public nuisance while under the influence, and manufacturing and distributing alcoholic beverages without imposing taxes are examples. It is the many problems created by alcohol that cause today's consumer to be alarmed—problems such as 25,000 alcohol-related highway deaths, nine million alcoholic Americans, and a high incidence of cirrhosis of the liver among people who drink.

The Effects of Alcohol

When talking about alcohol, it should be understood that an alcoholic beverage may be wine, beer, whiskey, rum, cordials or brandy. The effect alcohol will have on the user depends on several variables. Many people tend to think of alcohol as a stimulant, since its initial effects may cause one to get "up." However, pharmacologically, alcohol is an anesthetic, a tranquilizer, a depressant to the brain and central nervous system.

Body size is one variable that determines what the effects of alcohol will be. Since the liver oxidizes alcohol (breaks it down chemically), it is safe to assume that a person with a large liver will more readily be able to endure the effects of the alcohol than a person who has consumed the same amount but has less body weight. In essence, the smaller the person, the more he will be affected by a similar quantity of alcohol consumed by a larger person. An intoxicating effect is assumed when alcohol reaches the brain and is not able to be oxidized by the liver. Since alcohol is not digested like food but is absorbed into the bloodstream, partly through the stomach and partly through the small intestine, its effects do not take too long to surface.

Proof

The *proof* of an alcoholic beverage also determines its physiological effects. The word *proof* indicates the concentration of alcohol in a beverage. Alcohol content is determined by dividing the proof number in half. Thus, if a bottle of whiskey is 90-proof, its alcohol content is 45 percent. The higher the *proof* of alcohol, the greater are its intoxicating powers. The different forms of alcoholic beverages vary in their concentration of alcohol. Beer and ale which are made from cereal grains contain three to six percent alcohol; wine, made from the juice of grapes is 10–14 percent; adding alcohol to wines which in turn produce sherry, vermouth, and muscatel, bring their alcohol content up to 18–24 percent; gin, whiskey, brandy and rum, made from fermented mixtures (the growth of yeast in sugar and water solution to produce alcohol) of cereal grains or fruits contain 40 to 50 percent alcohol. Contrary to the belief of many, mixing drinks will not cause a person to get "higher" than if the same drink were continually consumed. You've probably heard people say: "Don't drink scotch after having had a glass of wine—you will really get high or sick. Drink another glass of wine if you're going to have anything at all." Statements of this nature are misleading. The one single determinant in this case is the *alcohol content,* and not the mixing of different substances which produces an effect.

The amount of food present in the stomach is another factor which will determine the effect an alcoholic beverage will have on the individual. Food can slow the absorbtion of alcohol into the bloodstream by as much as 50 percent. The presence of fatty foods along with certain proteins such as milk and cheese will also protect the drinker from becoming intoxicated quickly.

The rapidity with which alcohol is consumed also plays a role in its ability to produce intoxicating effects. As long as the liver is able to completely oxidize the amount of alcohol consumed, none of the effects of "being under the influence" will be manifested. As a result, slow drinking and small doses will not have as great an effect as if one were to ingest a drink the same as they would water.

Blood Alcohol Level

It is the *blood alcohol level* (the amount of alcohol which is carried from the blood to the brain) which will indicate *how* intoxicated a person will be. A blood alcohol level of 0.01 to 0.02 percent (one part to two parts per 10,000) will have little noticeable effect on an individual; 0.03 to 0.10 percent will cause definite impairment including lightheadedness, sense of well-being and a release of some personal inhibitions; a blood alcohol level of 0.10 percent to 0.15 percent will cause an impairment in vision, hearing, judgment and motor skills. This is the level which most states consider as "driving under the influence"—which many times will cause immediate revocation of one's drivers license.

Relationship Between Type and Amount of Alcoholic Beverages Consumed and the Estimated Potential Blood Alcohol Concentration

Beverage	Amount	Time Frame Consumed Within	Alcohol Concentration in blood
beer	2	15 minutes	.03%
cocktail	1	15 minutes	.03%
highball	1	15 minutes	.03%
beer	4	30 minutes	.06%
cocktail	2	30 minutes	.06%
highball	2	30 minutes	.06%
beer	6	one hour	.09%
cocktail	3	one hour	.09%
highball	3	one hour	.09%
beer	8	two hours	.12%
cocktail	4	two hours	.12%
highball	4	two hours	.12%
beer	10	three hours	.15%
cocktail	5	three hours	.15%
highball	5	three hours	.15%

If the alcohol concentration reaches 0.20 percent, the drinker will demonstrate the obvious signs of drunkenness—difficulty in walking and speaking, and often he may exhibit antisocial behavior. Concentrations above 0.40 percent will produce a coma; 0.60 to 0.70 percent, death. Fortunately, the latter rarely occurs, since the drinker will lose consciousness at the 0.40 level, or vomit due to the irritating effects of alcohol on the stomach lining, thereby preventing further absorption of a fatal dose. The following page contains a chart which indicated the relationship between the type and amount of alcoholic beverages consumed and the estimated potential blood alcohol concentration.

Often we hear of people "taking a nip" when they feel the need to warm up. This has a converse effect on remaining warm. Taking a drink of alcohol causes blood vessels near the skin to dilate. Although this vasodilation of the blood vessels creates a warm feeling, the body is actually losing heat more rapidly, thereby causing a decrease in the body temperature.

Alcohol creates other physiological effects. Since it is known to constrict the coronary arteries, the chance of developing a heart related problem is increased.

Alcohol and the Digestive System

Alcohol can also effect the tissues lining the stomach and throat, usually producing a burning sensation in these areas. Even in small amounts, alcohol will cause a secretion of digestive juices in the stomach, thereby creating a sensation of hunger. Over long term use, constant irritation of the stomach lining because of alcohol's ability to cause the stomach to produce gastric juices may cause *gastritis*—a chronic inflammation of the stomach lining.

Cirrhosis of the Liver

Cirrhosis of the liver is eight times more common among alcoholics than among nonalcoholics. This condition may be brought about by heavy consumption of alcohol, which in turn destroys healthy liver tissues, and these are then displaced by fat or scar tissues. Eventually the functioning of the liver is impaired and the individual may suffer from weight loss, digestive and circulatory ailments. With over 9 million alcoholics, it should be no surprise that cirrhosis is one of the ten leading causes of death in the United States.

Under certain circumstances, alcohol can produce confusion, hallucinations, and permanent or temporary psychotic conditions. Since alcohol does share common features with other depressant drugs, physical dependence can be developed. A "hangover" is considered by some to be a form of mild withdrawal. Alcohol addicts are known to have seizures and hallucinations or DT's (delirium tremens) after continued long term use.

Is Alcohol a Food?

One question which often arises is the classification of alcohol as a food. Although alcohol is considered a food because of its caloric value, it contributes absolutely nothing toward good nutrition. It provides no vitamins, minerals, proteins, fats or usable carbohydrates. Beer may be the only exception, and its contribution to good nutrition is insignificant. In addition, alcoholic beverages promote disorders associated with chronic drinking, such as vitamin deficiencies (particularly vitamin B).

Psychological Effects of Alcohol

The psychological effects of alcohol are similar to those of other psychoactive drugs. Signs of intoxication manifest themselves in the form of distorted perception, decreased reaction time, and impairment of the learning, thinking, remembering, and reasoning process. Emotional behavior may also be affected—resulting in anxiety, hostility, tension, and fear.

Studies have shown that a blood alcohol level of 0.01 percent which is considered as having very few noticeable effects will, however, cause the drinker to feel more relaxed, lose some of his rapidity of motor responses, and impair hearing and vision.

Of all the psychotrophic drugs being used today, none has generated as much concern as alcohol. This drug is considered the most used and abused of the mind-altering substances. The physiological effects alcohol has produced led to an abundance of psychosocial health problems—the extent of which has had an impact upon millions of Americans—either directly or indirectly. Only by understanding about the "alcohol problem" can we begin to deal effectively with a useful drug which is man's self-made menace.

The Alcohol Myth Response Sheet

Based upon the information covered, ask students to respond to the following myths related to alcohol.

1. Mixing drinks will get you more drunk than if you consumed the same drink.

2. Drinking brandy will make you warmer if you are outdoors on a cold day.

3. People are friendlier when they drink.

4. Mixing or switching drinks at a party will cause you to become sick.

5. The average alcoholic is a "skid row bum."

6. You can only become an alcoholic if you are over 20 years of age.

To grasp a better understanding of the effects of alcohol on the body, the teacher can use tape to outline a body on the floor. Called "Mr. Booze" (or whatever name you desire), ask the students to walk through the path alcohol takes in the body.

Ask the students to identify the effects of alcohol on the specific parts of the body. The teacher can also discuss the implications of having different body parts affected by alcohol.

1. How do the effects of alcohol relate to automobile accidents?

2. What are the effects of alcohol on the cardio-vascular system?

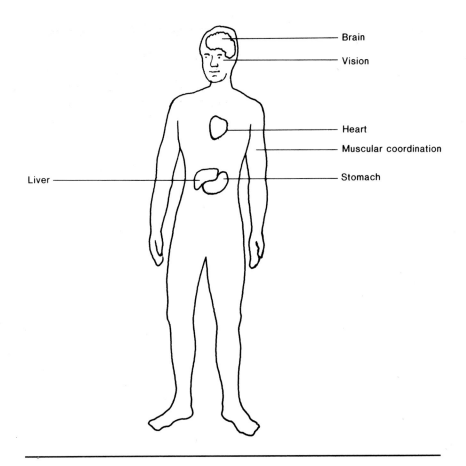

Brain
Vision
Heart
Muscular coordination
Liver
Stomach

Evaluation

1. The completion of the Alcohol Myth Response Sheet will indicate the degree to which information was learned.

2. Have the students describe the effects alcohol has on the following body areas:
   a. brain
   b. liver
   c. vision
   d. muscular system

Drugs: Use and Abuse
Prescription Drugs

Objectives

1. The student will be able to define prescription drugs.

2. The student will identify the need for prescription drugs.

3. The student will differentiate between brand name and generic name prescription drugs.

Source

Warren E. Schaller and Charles R. Carroll, *Health Quackery and the Consumer*, Philadelphia: W. B. Saunders Company, 1976.

A prescription drug is one that is prescribed by a physician and filled by a pharmacist. Generally, prescription drugs are more powerful than OTC's—(over-the-counter) this is why they are prescribed by medical doctors. The physician is the person best qualified to determine the nature of a health problem and therefore, its cure.

The degree to which a prescription drug will be effective depends somewhat on you. Tell the doctor everything related to your malady—signs and symptoms, allergic reactions to past drugs, length of illness, etc.

Symptoms and Reactions

The user of prescription drugs should be careful about adverse symptoms and reactions. Dizziness, rashes, headaches, and nausea should be reported to your physician. Unknowingly, some people may consume alcohol while taking prescriptions. To play it safe, your doctor should be asked before any combination of alcohol and medication is consumed. If you begin to feel better and you have some of the prescription left, complete the medication, since the full dosage may be needed to work effectively.

The Drug Industry

Prescription drugs are widely used. An average of 20 prescriptions are written per family per year. For this reason, it is easy to understand why the drug industry is the most profitable in the United States, showing incomes that are twice the national average for all industries. (Projected world-wide sales for 1975 by the U.S. pharmaceutical industry was 12 billion dollars.) Naturally, the prescription drug market has created accompanying problems. One reason usually given for the increased use of illegal drugs especially amphetamines and barbiturates, is the prices the consumer must pay. A prescription drug may be sold one of two ways: under its *generic* name (its chemical structure) or under its *brand* name (its trademark). Brand name drugs may cost several times more than generic drugs, though the chemical composition may be the same. Doctors will usually write prescriptions using the brand name, thereby requiring a higher price for the consumer. Drug abusers often prefer to obtain psychoactive drugs illegally via the black market since they are less expensive, even when legal prescriptions are available.

Another issue concerning drug prices is advertisement. Drug companies have been against the posting of prices of prescription drugs since they feel their profit would be decreased. However, consumer groups have been active in this area, and in New York prescription drug prices must now be posted in pharmacies. The cost of advertising drugs adds to the cost of prescribed and over-the-counter drugs.

Adverse Reactions

Adverse reactions to prescription drugs are not uncommon. An estimated 1.5 million Americans are admitted into hospitals every year for this reason. Some of these reactions may be due to the body's response to the drug—perhaps an allergic reaction—even when taken as prescribed, or they are attributable to unconscious misuse by the user. If you have adverse reactions, you should consult your physician. All prescription drugs should be labeled with specific instructions which can be easily followed. Drugs should be taken in prescribed dosage, specified manner, and at specific time intervals. You should ask your physician to have the name of the drug (medicine) included on the label.

Failure to adhere to these rules is a major reason for the abuse of prescription drugs. Since the majority of prescription drugs are psychotrophic, it is not uncommon for the consumer to take larger than necessary doses to obtain an euphoric feeling. Though laws have imposed restraints, prescriptions for certain depressants and minor tranquilizers may be refilled up to five times in six months (with authorization by the physician). Thus, it is still possible for the individual to abuse these drugs. Although each prescription is individualized, some abusers may take a friend's prescription to "get high."

While the restrictions on the prescription drug market have been getting tighter and the abuse that existed at one time has been somewhat minimized, drug use and abuse is still an individual choice.

Evaluation

Have students locate a prescription drug in their home or the home of a friend. The student is then required to do the following tasks:

1. Identify the drug by its *brand* name and *generic* name. If you know either one, you will be able to determine the other by asking a pharmacist.

2. Go to three drugstores and ask for the cost of filling this prescription—by its generic and brand name. Complete the information on the chart below.

3. Did you locate any prescriptions that were expired? What did you do?

Brand Name	Price at Store 1	2	3

Generic Name	Price at Store 1	2	3

Objectives

1. The student will be able to define over-the-counter (OTC) drugs.

2. The student will be able to explain the uses of OTC's.

3. The student will be able to identify methods of persuasion as they relate to OTC's.

4. The student will identify the different OTC's in his own home.

Source

Warren E. Scholler and Charles R. Carroll, *Health Quackery and the Consumer,* Philadelphia: W. B. Saunders Company, 1976.

Content and Procedures

How to Buy Drugs

There are three ways drugs are made available to consumers. First, by way of the black market—among these may be amphetamines and barbiturates, stolen from drug companies and physicians offices and illegally purchased and sold from individual to individual. Second, other psychoactive drugs as well as antibiotics may be obtained with a doctor's written approval. These drugs are known as prescription drugs—drugs which are highly individualized and are usually used under the physician's supervision. Third, the widest channel of drug distribution is sold over-the-counter (without a prescription) in drugstores, supermarkets, and discount service centers. More and more consumers utilize the two latter outlets.

Over-the-counter (OTC) Drugs

Over-the-counter (OTC) drugs are used for the relief of discomforts which may be due to headaches, minor aches and pains, and many other common, everyday minor ailments. These drugs are sold without a prescription because the chemicals they contain are considered safe if consumed according to the directions on the package. The principle behind their use is the assumption that the consumer is mature enough to successfully self-treat his illness if he is familiar with its signs and symptoms. An estimated 75 of every 1,000 people will have signs and symptoms of an illness each month and 500 of these people will turn to OTC drugs. Since the OTC drugs may be readily purchased it is important that pertinent information be supplied to prevent their abuse—a concern expressed by doctors and federal agencies, as well as by consumers. Today, federal law requires OTC drug labels to list the name of the product and manufacturer, the names of the active ingredients for safe use, its purpose, and the precautions, warnings, and limitations of its use.

Advertising

Probably the major reason for the wide-spread use of OTC drugs is the advertising compaign which is carried on by drug companies. Over $100 million per year is spent on advertisements for headaches and over $500 million per year is spent by consumers for drugs to cope with this common ailment. Companies employ many different tactics to gain consumer confidence. The "statistical" approach, whereby a company will state that "four out of a group of five people were benefited by our product" is often seen in magazine ads and on TV commercials.

Viewers often interpret this to mean 80 percent of the entire population of the USA when in actuality, only 100 groups of five people may have been tested, and only one group had four people who "benefited."

The "word game" is another method used by advertisers to sell their product. Words such as "faster," "more effective" and "quicker-acting" are often used to describe many OTC drugs. The question one must ask is "Compared to what are they faster, more effective, and quicker acting than?"

Consumers often think that OTC products will relieve an illness, when only the signs and symptoms of that illness are treated. For example, aspirin will treat the signs and symptoms of a headache but not treat the cause of that headache. Or antihistamines might help to dry a runny nose, but there is no cure for the common cold.

Deceptive advertising practices are reviewed by the FTC (Federal Trade Commission). Some drug companies are presently in the courts trying to settle the legal issues arising from FTC regulation. As a result, changes have begun to take place in drug advertisements on TV commercials. There has been a reduction in the use of children in ads for adult drugs, as well as a reduction in the failure to instruct users to follow package instructions. However, studies indicate that drug promotion on television tends to encourage favorable attitudes toward the consumer's inclination to use a particular drug by means of exaggerated claims.

Everyday, television viewers are made aware of how "Bufferin may treat signs and symptoms of a headache," "ExLax can help maintain regularity," "Sominex can help you sleep," "Clearacil may help clear acne" and "Alka Seltzer may help relieve upset stomaches." Statements of this nature have been known to influence consumers to rely upon OTC drugs as a cure-all. Although OTC drugs are relatively harmless in themselves, their overuse and misuse can be instrumental in the development of harmful physical effects.

Aspirin

Aspirin is the second most widely used drug in the world. Second only to alcohol, it is a drug whose impact has already been discussed. Incredible as it may seem, Americans consume 44 million aspirin tablets each day, usually for one of three reasons: it is effective in blocking somatic pain, it can reduce body temperature caused by fever, and it can reduce inflammation and soreness in an injured area. With the positive uses of aspirin come adverse side-effects. Excessive and continuous use is known to cause gastrointestinal bleeding. Although millions use aspirin safely, there are many who experience toxic effects. Children, especially those under age five, have been accidentally poisoned by aspirin. This may be due to self-ingestion (which is made more difficult today with safety caps on bottles), or improper dosage administered by a parent. However, it should be noted that no other drug has the positive uses with relatively low toxicity as aspirin. All brands are just about equal in their effectiveness, therefore, the wise consumer should purchase the aspirin that is least expensive.

In addition to aspirin, several other OTC drugs are abused. The overuse of laxatives can create disorders of the digestive tract—a more serious problem than mild constipation.

Vitamins

Vitamins, though not classified as drugs in our current context, are used by consumers to treat various signs and symptoms of illness. The vitamin C issue has continued since Linus Pauling extolled its effectiveness in preventing colds.

To date, there is no conclusive evidence that this vitamin does what its proponents claim. In fact, large doses are known to irritate the lining of the stomach. The consumption of a daily balanced diet which includes vitamin C eliminates the need for vitamin concentrates.

Cough and Cold Remedies

Cough and cold remedies are among the most used and sometimes abused OTC drugs. Although effective in treating signs and symptoms of a cold, they do not treat the cold itself. Misuse of these remedies are common since they may contain ingredients which may produce psychotrophic effects. Thus, the person who consumes a higher than normal dose of a cough syrup may develop a mild high from the codeine (the cough suppressant found in cough medicine) and impair his psychomotor responses. This may be dangerous in situations such as driving an automobile or standing on a ladder.

Self-Treatment

A problem associated with OTC drugs is over-reliance by the consumer on that particular drug. The person best suited to diagnose an illness is a physician. Self-treatment medications can delay the diagnosis and treatment of an illness or disease, and for that matter, create complications. A person who constantly takes aspirin to treat a frequently recurring headache may actually have a developing tumor. The delay in seeking medical help will allow the condition to get worse. The person who takes a laxative to reduce stomach pain may actually be having an attack of appendicitis, thereby aggravating the condition. These forms of personal "quackery" create much concern about over-the-counter drugs. However, it must be said, that much more education for self-help—(i.e., through health education)—is necessary to improve our quality of life and health.

Evaluation

To determine whether our objectives have been met, the student can be given the following log to complete.

Instructions: To become more familiar with the frequency with which OTC's are found around the household as well as the effects OTC's may have on individuals, you are to complete the following chart and return it to class. Complete this chart with OTC's found in your home.

Name of OTC	How Much Can Be Taken in One Day	# of Days It Can be Taken	Side Effects	Warnings	Place a Check in This Column if You Have Heard This Drug Advertised

The teacher can follow-up with the following questions:

1. Have you ever taken any of the drugs listed?

2. How have you seen these drugs advertised?

3. Do you think these drugs were of help to you or your family?

4. Have you or your family ever gotten sick from the effects of the drug?

Selected Learning Activities

Drugs: Use and Abuse

_____ Develop a bulletin board or large collage depicting the following ideas: Drug abuse is dangerous to your health; drug abuse is expensive; long term use of drugs often results in changed appearance; drug users are more "accident prone;" drug misuse can lead to physical and psychological dependency; drug abuse is illegal; and drug supplies are not dependable.

_____ Discuss the dangers of consuming any type of drug including alcohol if you are pregnant.

_____ Learn how many male and female secondary school students were arrested on drug related charges in your community last year. How do these figures compare with figures from five to ten years ago?

_____ Discuss the ways that people can get "high" without a mind altering substance. Make a poster to show a positive way that you can get "high."

_____ Discuss the role that advertising plays in creating a need for over the counter drugs.

_____ Analyze popular songs for their message about drug usage.

_____ Make a list of all the drugs that you have used in the past year and rank them in order of importance in improving your well being. Which ones could you have done without?

_____ Invite a speaker to explain how various alcoholic beverages are made and the difference between different beverages and different proofs.

_____ Discuss what you would do if you were a parent and your son or daughter was driving with a drunk driver.

_____ Write to the U.S. Department of Transportation, National Highway Traffic Safety Administration, Washington, D.C. 20590 for volume 2 of _Alcohol and Alcohol Safety_—a curriculum manual for senior high level with a teacher's activity guide.

_____ Play drug charades. One person acts out a drug and the rest of the class must guess what it is.

_____ Invite a pharmacist to class to discuss over the counter and prescription drugs. (S)he might also discuss the careers related to pharmacology.

_____ Bring an empty medicine bottle to class. Read the label. Discuss the contraindications and warnings.

_____ Write laws for the use of the following drugs: alcohol, tobacco, marijuana, cocaine, barbiturates.

_____ Make a mobile that depicts at least two safety precautions for the use of prescription drugs.

_____ Role play a party where you are offered a drug and refuse to accept it. How many different ways can you think of to handle this situation?

_____ Examine your medicine cabinet. What kinds of drugs do you have in your home? Are any of your drugs out of date? What classification does each drug fall in? How many are prescription? How many are over-the-counter? How often is each type of drug used?

_____ Play drug trivia for one week. Each day you are to look up one fact about drugs. You ask the class a question about your fact and see if they can guess the correct answer.

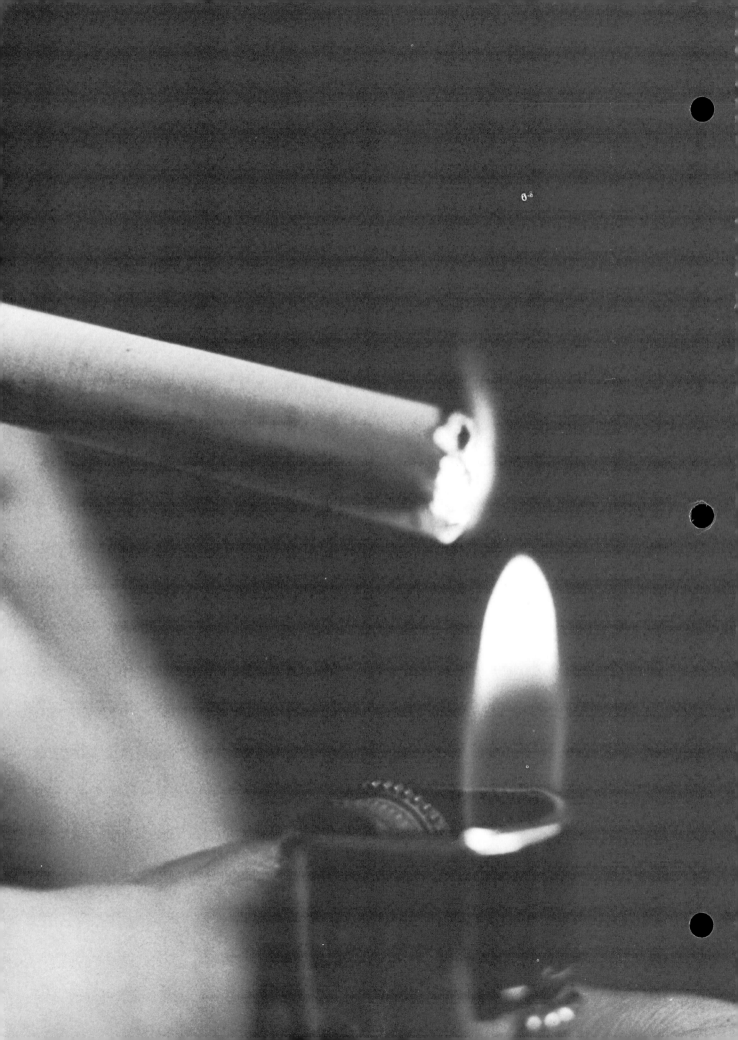

16

Teaching about Tobacco and Health

A Gallup survey released in April, 1979 showed that the percentage of teenage smokers had fallen since 1974 from 16 percent to 12 percent. The decrease in teenage smoking is comforting, yet an alarming statistic still remains. In 1979, Health Education and Welfare Secretary Joseph Califano, Jr. said there were 1.7 million girls and 1.6 million boys between the ages of 12 and 18 who were regular smokers.

This chapter includes an outline of Suggested Topics for Teaching About Tobacco and Health, Three Detailed Sample Lessons geared to reduce the smoking incidence in the middle and secondary school, and additional Selected Learning Activities.

The first lesson, **Tobacco: The Facts,** describes the physiological effects of cigarette smoke on different body sites. The resulting smoking related diseases are also described.

The second lesson, **Smoking: The Other Facts,** amplifies the first lesson. The student examines sidestream and mainstream smoke, the health implications of cigarette smoking to pregnant women, and the economics of the smoking industry.

The third lesson, **To Smoke or Not to Smoke,** examines the reasons why teenagers begin smoking, and then asks each student to examine personal choices. This lesson was developed with the assistance of the Evaluation Committee of the School Health Education Project, the National Center for Health Education.

Suggested Topics

Tobacco and Health

I. Why People Smoke
   A. The media
   B. Peer pressure
   C. Self concept

II. Physiological Effects of Smoking
    A. Lung cancer
    B. Other forms of cancer
    C. Respiratory diseases
    D. Heart disease and circulatory impairment
    E. Smoking and pregnancy
    F. Other problems

III. Components of Cigarette Smoke
    A. Nicotine content
    B. Other toxic chemicals

IV. A Profile of the Smoker
    A. The teenage boy
    B. The teenage girl
    C. Trends in use

V. Smoking Related Issues
    A. Smokers versus nonsmokers rights
    B. Smoking ordinances

VI. Breaking The Habit
    A. Self-help organizations
    B. Individual methods and techniques

VII. The Surgeon General's Report
    A. Prevalence of tobacco use
    B. Second hand smoke and side stream smoke

VIII. Tobacco and the Law
    A. Smoking ordinances
    B. Control of advertisement

Lesson Plans

Tobacco and Health
Tobacco: The Facts

Objectives

1. The student will be able to identify smoking related diseases.

2. The student will be able to describe the physiological effects of cigarette smoke on different body sites.

Sources

1. Various publications from the U.S. Department of Health, Education, and Welfare, (Washington, D.C.: U.S. Government Printing Office: *The Facts about Smoking and Health, 1970; Smoking and Illness, 1969; Facts: Smoking and Health, 1971.*

2. Public Health Service, National Clearinghouse for Smoking and Health, *The Health Consequences of Smoking: A Report to the Surgeon General,* Washington, D.C.: U.S. Government Printing Office, 1972.

Content and Procedures

Contrary to what many believe, cigarettes did not become a major article of consumption until the early 1900's. Up to that time, people used tobacco in the form of cigars, chewing tobacco, and snuff (powdered tobacco which is inhaled through the nose). In 1900 only about 4 billion cigarettes were manufactured in the United States annually. Today, that figure has increased to 620 billion per year. The sudden and astronomic increase has had or will have a direct impact upon the life of almost every person—whether that person be a smoker or nonsmoker. The following lesson will examine the role cigarette smoking plays in the process of developing a healthy lifestyle.

The Basic Facts

The effects of cigarette smoking contribute to over 300,000 deaths each year in the United States.

Cigarette smoking causes harmful effects upon the circulatory and respiratory systems, the body's sense organs and the teeth, just to name a few parts of the body it attacks.

Emphysema

Emphysema is a late effect of a chronic infection or irritation of the alveoli (air sacks) in the lungs. When the alveoli become immobile, difficulty in breathing becomes evident. A person can become out of breath while trying to walk from one side of the room to another, or he may not be able to blow out a match.

The heart may undergo a great deal of strain since it has difficulty obtaining oxygen from the damaged alveoli. This often leads to heart failure.

The damage caused to the alveoli cannot be reversed since these air sacks do not regenerate (grow back).

Although we do not know how to prevent emphysema, we do know that not smoking can avoid damage for many who would otherwise develop this disease which has tripled over the past 11 years.

Chronic Bronchitis

Bronchitis is an inflammation of the lining of the bronchial tubes. The bronchial tubes connect the windpipe to the lungs.

An inflammation of the bronchi causes labored breathing and a heavy mucus or phlegm is coughed up.

Some people suffer *acute bronchitis*—a brief attack with fever, coughing and spitting when they have severe colds.

During *chronic bronchitis,* the coughing and spitting continue for months each year.

Since chronic bronchitis is almost always associated with heavy cigarette smoking, it is often dismissed as "smoker's cough." Without treatment, the effects become more damaging and the person may be susceptible to serious lung diseases or to heart failure. The congested bronchial tubes are known to serve as an ideal breeding place for infections.

To clear up bronchitis, it is necessary to give up the source of the irritation. This usually means stop smoking.

Heart Disease

Premature heart disease is the most critical specific health consequence of cigarette smoking. One-fourth of all heart disease deaths in 1975 were attributed directly to smoking.

Cigarette smokers have between two to three times the risk of death from heart disease than nonsmokers.

Smoking tends to increase cholesterol within the inner walls of the arteries, thus making arteriosclerosis (deposits in the arteries) more severe. This gradually clogs the arteries to the heart. In turn, this increases the likelihood of blood clots.

Since some of the poisonous gases from cigarette smoke displace oxygen, the heart must work harder to pump oxygenated blood throughout the body. This causes undue stress on the heart. An example of this stress can be observed each time a cigarette is smoked. The heart rate will increase 10–20 beats per minute. The activity on the next page can help the student visualize the effects of tobacco smoke on the lungs.

Lung Cancer

Over 3,000 substances have been identified in cigarette smoke—many of which are *carcinogens* (can cause cancer).

The risk of developing lung cancer is 10 times greater for cigarette smokers than for nonsmokers.

Although factors such as air pollution and occupational exposures may also cause lung cancer, cigarette smoking is considered the major instigator.

Cilia are tiny hair-like structures which sweep out dirt and germs before they get to the lungs. Cigarette smoking can paralyze the cilia which in turn can open your lungs to all kinds of infections. Thus, tars can easily enter your lungs, stain them, and cause lung cancer.

The Senses

Smoking can rob your keenness of smell. This may be positive since the smoker cannot smell the stench of stale cigarette smoke that has permeated his clothing, hair, or house.

Smokers' taste buds are not as keen as those of nonsmokers. Since nicotine can cause a numbing effect upon areas of the tongue, smokers will often seek out spicier foods or other "enhancers" to compensate for the lack of taste. Smokers require salt concentrations 12 to 14 times greater than the nonsmoker.

The Tissue Experiment

To enable students to see the tar produced by cigarette smoke, place a tissue over the end of a cigarette.

Compare the accumulations on the tissues for cigarettes with: filters vs non-filters, smoking the whole cigarette vs ½ of a cigarette, and taking five puffs from a cigarette as opposed to ten puffs.

Smoking impairs thinking. We are not saying it damages the brain. Rather, it means one's ability to concentrate can be reduced. An example of this is the fact that smokers have a higher rate of automobile accidents than nonsmokers. Their attention to other cars, rules of the road, and pedestrians is often impaired.

The senses of taste and smell as well as the ability to concentrate will return to normal shortly after the smoking habit is ended.

Your Mouth

Smokers have a higher incidence than nonsmokers of all different types of gum disease.

Tobacco may delay oral wound healing, for example, after tooth extractions.

Smoking is a social handicap since it promotes *halitosis* (offensive bad breath). Often a smoker does not know he has halitosis since his sense of smell quickly adapts to his own unpleasant breath odors.

Smoking plays an important role in fostering cancer of the mouth and throat. Approximately 90% of these types of cancers are associated with tobacco.

Cigarette smoke causes teeth to become stained. This promotes the depositing of calculous material (tartar) around the teeth. In turn, the gums become more susceptible to disease and infection.

Evaluation

Since this section was didactic, the teacher can give an objective examination to determine the amount of information gained.

Essay: Describe how cigarette smoking has an effect on the following:

a. emphysema
b. bronchitis
c. heart disease
d. lung cancer
e. the body's sense organs

Matching: Match the diseases in Column A to the symptoms in Column B.

A	B
1. emphysema	A. continuous coughing
2. chronic bronchitis	B. smokers have three times the risk of this than nonsmokers
3. heart disease	C. irritation of the alveoli
4. lung cancer	D. a brief attack with fever, coughing and spitting
5. acute bronchitis	E. is ten times greater for smokers than nonsmokers.

Tobacco and Health
Smoking: The Other Facts

Objectives

1. Students will be able to differentiate between sidestream smoke and mainstream smoke.

2. Students will examine the health implication of pipe and cigar smoking.

3. Students will identify the implications of cigarette smoking to pregnant mothers.

4. Students will identify factors related to smoking and economics.

Sources

Free pamphlets from the American Lung Association, *Second-Hand Smoke, Cigar and Pipe Smoke*, 1978.

Second-hand Smoke

The majority of our population are nonsmokers. Although one in three adults smoke, there has been a decrease in the number of smokers in this group. Unfortunately, the number of junior and senior high school smokers has steadily increased. While only a few years ago, the majority of teenage smokers were boys, today these figures have leveled, so that girls smoke as frequently as boys.

If you do not smoke, you are susceptible to harm from the cigarette smoke of others. Cigarette smoke contains hazardous compounds such as: tar, nicotine, carbon monoxide, cadmium, nitrogen dioxide, ammonia, benzene, formaldehyde, and hydrogen sulphide. These compounds are inhaled by the nonsmoker when he is in the presence of a smoker.

Tobacco smoke enters the atmosphere from two sources. First, there is *sidestream* smoke. This is the smoke which goes directly into the air from the burning end of the cigarette. Then, there is *mainstream* smoke. This is the smoke which the smoker pulls through the mouth when he or she inhales or puffs.

A cigarette smoker inhales and exhales cigarette smoke (mainstream) eight or nine times with each cigarette. This process uses approximately 24 seconds. However a cigarette burns for 12 minutes. During these 12 minutes of sidestream smoke, the air becomes polluted. The concentrations of pollution become greater with pipe and cigar smoke, since these sources burn for longer periods of time.

Sidestream smoke contains twice as much tar and nicotine and 5 times as much *carbon monoxide* as mainstream smoke. Carbon monoxide is an odorless and colorless gas which robs the blood of oxygen. This, in turn, causes the body cells to starve for its source of life (oxygen). As a result, smoking a cigarette or being in the presence of a smoker can cause an increase in blood pressure and heart beat rate.

Pipe and Cigar Smoking

People who smoke pipes and cigars do not face some of the hazards encountered by cigarette smokers. However, pipes and cigars are responsible for an increase in other hazards.

Because the majority of pipe and cigar smokers do not inhale, their lungs and blood stream are not as bombarded by the harmful particles and noxious (poisonous) gases. Therefore, chronic bronchitis, emphysema and lung cancer are not as common among pipe and cigar smokers as they are among cigarette smokers.

When pipe and cigar smokers *do* inhale, the chances of developing heart and lung diseases are *higher* than for the cigarette smoker. Of course, this is dependent upon how deeply and how often they inhale.

Many cigarette smokers try to reduce the harmful effects of their habit by switching to pipes or cigars. However, they often keep their habit of inhaling. As a result they can perpetuate a habit that is worse than the original one (inhaling pipe and cigar smoke as opposed to cigarette smoke).

Although pipe and cigar smoke is not inhaled, it can enter the throat and windpipe. It can also travel to the upper breathing passages.

Smoke can also be dissolved in the saliva and absorbed by the mucous membranes of the mouth. Upon swallowing, the harmful substances can travel to the digestive tracts. As a result, pipe and cigar smokers have an incidence of some cancers that is as high or in some cases, higher than cigarette smokers. These cancer sites are located in the mouth, throat, larynx (voice box) and stomach.

Pipe smoking seems to be a direct cause of lip cancer—either in combination with cigarettes or by itself.

Many persons—both male and females—smoke little cigars. The hazards are the same as those of big cigars. If the little cigars are inhaled, the smoker will face the same threats which the cigarette smoker faces.

Although the effects of sidestream and mainstream cigar and pipe smoke have not been determined yet, they are probably more harmful than cigarette smoke.

The smoke from cigars and pipes is usually more offensive to nonsmokers than the smoke from cigarettes. The eyes, nose and throat often become irritated.

Smoking and Babies

Since most of you will be mothers and fathers, there are certain facts about smoking and pregnancy that need to be brought out.

Some of the harmful substances in cigarette smoke can pass from the mother's bloodstream to that of her developing fetus. Even if the mother quits smoking before pregnancy, there is evidence that she will still give birth to a below average weight baby.

Since carbon monoxide can force oxygen out of the mother's red blood cells, the supply of oxygen to the baby is decreased.

Some of the facts worth noting about babies born to smoking mothers are:

1. They weigh less than babies born to non-smoking mothers.
2. They have a greater chance of dying before or soon after birth than a baby born to a nonsmoking mother.

You are married and you have just learned your wife is pregnant. She is a pack-a-day smoker and she has no intention of quitting. As the father, you are concerned about the implications for your child. Describe three strategies you would employ to have your wife quit smoking.

1. _____

_____

2. _____

_____

3. _____

_____

Come up with a master list from your class of strategies that can be used to encourage a pregnant woman to stop smoking.

Which do you feel would be most effective and why?

Smoking and Economics

Since smoking makes us more susceptible to respiratory infections and diseases such as cancer and emphysema, the time we lose from work and the expenses for medical bills have a great effect upon our financial stability.

The money people spend for cigarettes accumulates to large sums. Today, many brands are sold for 60¢ per pack. Vending machines charge as much as 75¢ per pack.

A pack-a-day smoker who spends 60¢ per pack will spend $218.40 per year. If this money were put in a savings account which yields 5% per year (the interest rates are slightly higher), at the end of the year, $229.32 would have been saved.

Assuming you can save $229.32 per year, list five things you would do with this money.

1. _____
2. _____
3. _____
4. _____
5. _____

Assuming you can save $1,000 in four years (this figure includes price increases), list five things you would do with this money.

1. _____
2. _____
3. _____
4. _____
5. _____

Smoking and Accidents

Careless smoking is responsible for automobile accidents—dropping a lighted cigarette on the lap or seat, momentary distraction to "light up," reaching for matches or lighters, and coughing.

Home accidents due to smoking can be caused by:

1. falling asleep in bed while holding a lighted cigarette
2. dropping ashes on the carpet
3. disregarding cigarettes in a wastepaper basket.

Smoking and the Government

In 1964, the Surgeon General's Report on Smoking and Health was released. In essence, it said cigarette smoking *is* a serious health hazard. This was confirmed in the 1978 Surgeon General's Report.

Immediately after the Surgeon General's 1964 Report, annual cigarette sales dropped to 505 billion cigarettes from 516 billion a year earlier.

In 1969, sales dropped again due to the growing impact of anti-smoking Public Service Announcements on radio and television.

In 1971, cigarette advertising was banned on radio and T.V., yet sales rose by 1% to 2%. This increased trend continues today. The cigarette companies are making more money than ever before. The major reason is the increase in the number of teenage smokers who take up the habit.

Since 1966, more than 150 bills affecting the cigarette industry have been introduced to Congress but none have been passed since 1970. This is due to the strength of the tobacco lobby, combined with influence from tobacco-state senators and congressmen.

The government has strengthened the warning on cigarette packages to read: "The Surgeon General has determined that cigarette smoking is dangerous to your health."

In the future, the government may require warning labels on cigarette packages to read "Warning: Cigarette Smoking is Dangerous to Your Health and May Cause Death from Cancer, Coronary Heart Disease, Chronic Bronchitis, Pulmonary Emphysema, and Other Diseases."

Other bills call for the prohibition of smoking in certain areas of government and publicly-owned facilities.

Evaluation

1. Ask students to differentiate between sidestream and mainstream smoke.

2. Ask students to write a position paper on the issue of smoking and pregnancy.

Tobacco and Health
To Smoke or Not to Smoke

Objectives

1. The student will examine reasons why people begin to smoke.

2. Students will examine their own decision in choosing to or not to smoke.

Sources

The enclosed exercise adopted from work of the Evaluation Committee of the School Health Education Project, The National Center for Health Education.

Content and Procedures

The number of secondary school student beginning to smoke has been steadily increasing while the number of adult smokers is decreasing. One reason may be the perceived susceptibility of the dangers of smoking, that is, adolescents do not see cigarette smoking as an immediate danger whereas adults may have had friends who died due to lung cancer.

Reasons for Smoking

Among the types of rationale given by teenagers for beginning to smoke are:

1. "It makes me look sexy, (handsome)."

2. "My grandfather is 80 years old and he smokes two packs per day."

3. "By the time I am older, a cure for cancer will be found."

4. "I don't feel any illness from smoking."

Students have their own perceptions of how their smoking behavior is viewed by their peers. Ask for student volunteers to depict the following smoking characters:

1. "Sexy Suzy"
2. "Macho Max"
3. "Social Sally"

Students can act out what they feel will be exhibited by the above smoking characters.

After the exercise, students will complete the following sentence for *each* of the characters:

"I felt that (*name of character*). . . ."

For example, "I felt that "Sexy Suzy" looked anything but sexy", or "I felt that "Social Sally" lit up a cigarette because she was nervous."

The teacher can then ask each student to share their responses.

Decision-making ability is often neglected when discussing cigarette smoking. The exercise on the next page will take students through a process of decision-making and smoking-related behavior.

Evaluation

Through observations and classroom participation, the teacher will determine the extent to which the objectives were met.

Ascertain students' attitudes about smoking by having them repeat the Smoking Survey on pages 286–287. Were there any differences after versus before?

Smoking Survey

You are in a situation in which you can smoke a cigarette without anyone knowing.

Step I
From the statements below check ( ) any of those you would think about in your decision to smoke or not to smoke.
( ) Smoking is fun
( ) My parents don't smoke
( ) Smoking causes cancer
( ) Some of my relatives smoke
( ) It is wrong to smoke
( ) Smoking makes people feel and look older
( ) Cigarette smoke smells bad
( ) Some of my friends smoke
( ) None of my friends smoke
( ) Smoking cuts down your endurance (ability to run or be active for a long time)
( ) It is worth trying once

Step II
In making your decision name the three choices (in order of importance) above you consider to be most important.
1.
2.
3.

Step III
Would you decide to smoke? Yes ( ) No ( ) Maybe ( )

Adapted from: National Center for Health Education, Evaluation Committee, 1980.

Step IV

What do you believe would be the most important result of your decision?

Step V

Finish this sentence: "I made this choice because _____

_____

_____

_____

Selected Learning Activities

Tobacco and Health

_____ Contact the local branch of the American Heart Association, American Cancer Society, and the American Lung Association for pamphlets, posters, and films concerned with cigarette smoking.

_____ Design cartoons depicting the pleasures of NOT smoking.

_____ Collect smoking advertisements from a variety of magazines and divide the pictures into groups according to their psychological appeal. (adventure, feminity, masculinity, love, nature-natural, scientific, good taste, sociability) Rate the advertisements in terms of their appeal and in terms of their content.

_____ Discuss some of the poisonous substances found in tobacco smoke and how they affect the body.

_____ In small groups, plan an anti-smoking campaign to reduce smoking among your fellow students. Share your proposal for a campaign with other groups in the class. Do you feel that the different ideas will be helpful? Will any ideas encourage smoking?

_____ Discuss whether secondary students should be permitted to have a smoking lounge on school property.

_____ Think of as many ways as possible to motivate someone to quit smoking.

_____ Outline the body and put a black star by each organ that is affected by cigarette smoking.

_____ Make ads for television and radio that advertise NOT smoking.

_____ Approve or disapprove of the following statement—"Cigarette Smoking Should Be Banned."

_____ Write a Bill of Rights for Nonsmokers.

_____ Visit local associations to obtain free material. Distribute "Thank you for not smoking" signs in your neighborhood for persons to put on their window or door.

_____ Role play typical situations that students feel the pressure to begin smoking.

_____ Ask one of the coaches to discuss smoking and athletic performance.

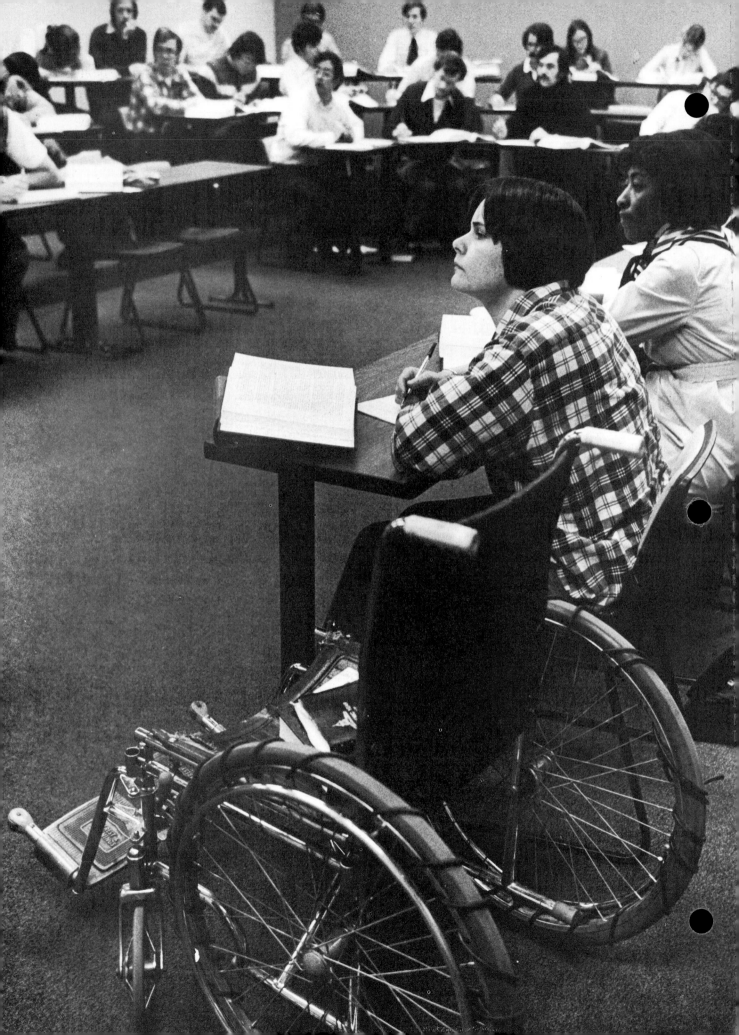

17

Teaching about Diseases and Disorders

The outline of Suggested Topics for Teaching About Diseases and Disorders, The Three Detailed Sample Lessons, and the additional Selected Learning Activities should be helpful in assisting the teacher in developing an informative and creative unit.

The first lesson, **The Nature of Disease,** helps the student understand how diseases are described and categorized. The student develops a disease vocabulary including words such as acute, anticipated, chronic, communicable, congenital, constitutional, contagious, deficiency, degenerative, endemic, epidemic, familial, functional, hereditary, hypokinetic, idiopathic, infectious, malignant, molecular, occupational, pandemic, parasitic, psychosomatic, and venereal. This lesson provides important background for the student.

The second lesson, **Face-to-Face with the Enemy,** deals with the identification of diseases and disorders. In this lesson the student examines environmental elements that may be health hazards. The student also learns the importance of screening devices in the early detection of diseases and disorders.

The third lesson, **Planning for Your Well Being,** further examines procedures for the early detection and prevention of diseases and disorders. The lesson focuses on student assumption of responsibility for the development of a lifestyle that incorporates factors that contribute to longevity.

Suggested Topics

Diseases and Disorders

I. Understanding the Disease Process
   A. Signs of Disease
   B. Describing and Categorizing Diseases
   C. Causes of Disease
   D. Stages of Disease
   E. Resistance/Body Defense Mechanisms
   F. Lifestyle Risk Factors

II. Disease and Society
   A. The Economic Impact of Disease
   B. Methods of Detection
      1. Self Examination
      2. Genetic Tests/Counseling
      3. Screening Tests
      4. Diagnostic Tests By A Physician
   C. Methods of Treatment
      1. Chemotherapy
      2. Changes in Diet
      3. Physical Therapy
      4. Psychotherapy
      5. Surgery
   D. The Impact of Disease Upon the Family
   E. Public and Voluntary Health Agencies
III. Profile of Chronic Illnesses and Disorders
   A. Allergies (e.g., Hay Fever; Asthma; Eczema)
   B. Cancers
   C. Cardiovascular Diseases
   D. Diseases of the Bones, Joints, and Muscles (e.g., Osteoarthritis; Rheumatoid Arthritis; Gout; Muscular Dystrophy)
   E. Disorders of the Digestive System (e.g., Peptic Ulcer; Colitis; Cirrhosis of the Liver)
   F. Disorders of the Nervous System (e.g., Epilepsy; Parkinson's Disease; Multiple Sclerosis; Cerebral Palsy)
   G. Genetic Disorders (e.g., Huntington's Chorea, Sickle Cell Anemia, Tay-Sachs, Cystic Fibrosis; Hemophilia; Down's Syndrome)
   H. Glandular Disorders (e.g., Diabetes; Goiter; Cretinism; Addison's Disease; Cushing's Syndrome)
   I. Kidney Diseases
   J. Respiratory Diseases (e.g., Bronchitis; Emphysema; Pleurisy)

Lesson Plans

Diseases and Disorders
The Nature of Disease

Objectives

1. Given 24 short, descriptive phrases for a particular type of disease, the student will be able through investigation to identify a disease that accurately fulfills the criteria for at least 20 of the descriptions.

2. The student will be able to identify the four *general* factors that have the most influence on his/her health.

3. Given a list of seven habits related to life expectancy, the student will mark all the habits that are a part of his/her lifestyle and explain why they consider the other habits unimportant.

4. Given a list of various diseases, the student will be able to determine whether the diseases are communicable or chronic, and will describe four general criteria that help to distinguish chronic diseases from communicable diseases.

5. The student will be able to describe the natural chain of events that occur following the entrance of a disease-producing agent into a human host and be able to give examples of the type of intervention that may be provided by health professionals at various stages.

6. Using Freidson's system for classifying illness, the student will be able to complete correctly the six categories with examples of illness different than those discussed in class.

Sources

1. Clayton L. Thomas, M.D., Editor. *Taber's Cyclopedic Medical Dictionary*. Philadelphia: F. A. Davis Company, 1977.

2. Donald M. Vickery, M.D. *Lifeplan For Your Health*; Reading, Massachusetts: Addison-Wesley Publishing Company, 1978.

3. David Mechanic. *Medical Sociology*. New York: The Free Press, a division of Macmillan Publishing Company, Inc., 1968.

4. Felix Marti-Ibanez, M.D., Editor. *The Epic of Medicine*. New York: Bramhall House. Copyright 1959 by MD Publications, Inc.

5. Eliot Freidson. *Profession of Medicine*. New York: Harper and Row, Publishers, Inc., 1970.

6. Talcott Parsons. *The Social System*. New York: The Free Press of Glencoe, 1951, pp. 428–447.

Content and Procedures

What do you think of when you hear the word "disease?"

_____

_____

How does the word make you feel?

Diseases may be described in the following ways. . . .[1] See if you can give an example for each category:

		Examples
Acute:	Rapid onset; Relatively short duration.	
Anticipated:	May be predicted to occur in individuals who have certain genetic, biochemical, physical or geographical characteristics.	
Chronic:	Slow onset; Long duration.	
Communicable:	Caused by an organism which is directly or indirectly transmissible from one person to another through a carrier or vector.	
Congenital:	Present at birth; May be due to hereditary factors, prenatal infection, injury, or the effect of a drug the mother took during pregnancy.	
Constitutional:	Due to an individual's hereditary makeup; A disease involving the body as a whole in contrast to one involving specific organs.	
Contagious:	An infectious disease readily transmitted from one person to another.	
Deficiency:	Results from an inadequate intake or absorption of essential dietary factors, e.g. vitamins or minerals.	

Degenerative:	Characteristic of old age; Results from degenerative changes that occur in tissues and organs.
Endemic:	A disease which is present more or less continuously or recurs in a community.
Epidemic:	Attacks a large number of individuals in a community at the same time.
Familial:	A disease which occurs in several individuals of the same family.
Functional:	No anatomical changes can be observed to account for the symptoms present.
Hereditary:	Due to hereditary factors transmitted from parent to offspring.
Hypokinetic:	Physical or mental illness produced by lack of or by insufficient exercise.
Idiopathic:	No causative factor can be identified.
Infectious:	Results from the presence of a pathogenic organism in the body.
Malignant:	Disease in which the progress is extremely rapid and generally threatening or resulting in death within a short time.
Molecular:	A hereditary disease that may be caused by a defective molecule.
Occupational:	Resulting from factors associated with the occupation in which the patient is engaged.
Pandemic:	An epidemic disease which is extremely widespread, involving an entire country, continent, or possibly the entire world.
Parasitic:	Results from the growth and development of parasitic organisms in or upon the body.
Psychosomatic:	Structural changes in or malfunctioning of organs are due to the mind, especially the emotions.
Venereal:	A disease usually acquired through sexual relations—either heterosexual or homosexual.

Four Factors That Influence Health

Do you view disease as the stumbling block in your pursuit of optimum health? What four factors do you think have the most influence on your health?

(1) Lifestyle, (2) Environment, (3) Medical, (4) Heredity. Contrary to popular belief, medical care is not as important to your health and well-being as environment and lifestyle. The effects of heredity are difficult to pinpoint. Even if we knew more about heredity there is not much that can be done about it, short of genetic manipulation. Furthermore, other factors can modify the contribution of heredity. For example, "the risk of a family history of hypertension may be negligible if you are not overweight, have your blood pressure taken yearly, and treat hypertension should it occur."[2]

Health Throughout History

Looking at the nation's health over the last 200 years, Dr. Vickery has divided these two centuries into three periods. (Figure 17.1)

The first and by far the longest period was dominated by the "Age of Environment." When communicable diseases presented the greatest threat to our health, man's efforts in filtering and chlorinating the water supply, pasteurizing milk, and organizing public health campaigns, proved to be very successful.

The discovery of antibiotics in the 1930's and 40's ushered in the "Age of Medicine". Important advances in medical care occurred and the decline in death rate accelerated. Meanwhile, "modern man" was stuffing himself with foods rich in cholesterol and fats. He was sitting around more than usual, becoming dependent on his private automobile and a pack of cigarettes a day.

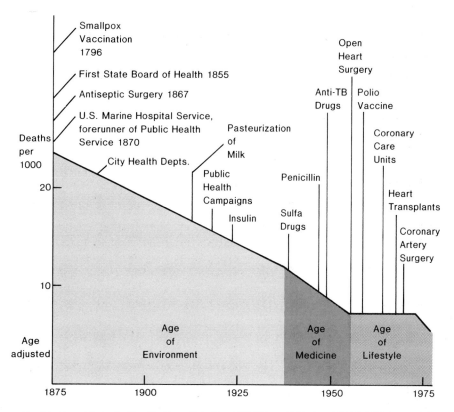

Reprinted from *Lifeplan for Your Health*, p. 18, by Donald M. Vickery, M. D., Copyright (c), 1978, by permission of Addison-Wesley Publishing Company, Reading, Mass.

Figure 17.1.

Suddenly, the "Age of Lifestyle" dawned. The trend of several centuries came to an end in the early 1950's when the death rate stopped declining. For the next 20 years there was no increase in life expectancy despite the advent of high-technology medicine—coronary care units, heart surgery, etc. Man's habits had caught up with him, and no pill or vaccination was available to alleviate his serious health problems. Only hard physical exercise, a reduction of cholesterol and saturated fats, and throwing away the cigarettes during the early 1970's was able to once again stimulate a decline in the death rates.

Health Habits

This is good news, because it means that we have the opportunity to improve our health substantially by adopting habits such as those suggested by Drs. Nedra Belloc and Lester Breslow:

	Yes	No
Do you eat three meals a day, avoiding snacks?	___	___
Do you eat breakfast every day?	___	___
Do you exercise moderately two or three times a week?	___	___
Do you get seven or eight hours sleep every night?	___	___
Are you a nonsmoker?	___	___
Are you of moderate weight?	___	___
Do you avoid drinking alcohol or only drink in moderation?	___	___

It was found that a 45 year-old man who had up to three of these habits had a life expectancy of 21.6 years and could expect to live to about 67. If he had six or seven of these habits, he could expect to live to about 78. The more beneficial lifestyle increased life expectancy by 11 years! Numerous other studies, including Dr. Victor Fuchs comparison of mortality rates between nonsmoking, nondrinking, family-oriented Mormons in Utah with residents in neighboring Nevada, and studies of Mormons and Seventh-Day Adventists, all confirm the importance of lifestyle.

Nevertheless, it is very difficult to prove the existence of cause and effect when dealing with human disease. Only in the realm of communicable diseases is it relatively easy to identify the underlying conditions responsible for one's personal discomfort. When one thinks of alcoholism, schizophrenia, and obesity, the basic roots of the problem become much more ambiguous. When cause and effect has not been proven, the term "risk factors", is often substituted.

Individuals vary considerably in their susceptibility to certain illnesses, and such characteristics as age, sex, race, ethnic background, and occupational status may determine who is at a greater risk for developing a given illness. One's level of resistance to the agents involved will also affect the severity of an illness. We have mentioned how detrimental living habits will contribute to the development of a chronic disease. Many behavior patterns, such as overeating, avoidance of exercise, and cigarette smoking are established before and during early adolescence; these habits often contribute to chronic disease conditions that become apparent during middle age.

Chronic Diseases vs. Communicable Disease

Can you think of four general criteria that help to distinguish chronic diseases from communicable diseases?

1. _____

2. _____

3. _____

4. _____

> Chronic diseases usually develop slowly, while communicable or acute diseases develop rapidly;
>
> Chronic diseases bring about long term disability and pain, unlike most communicable diseases that have symptoms of short duration;
>
> Chronic diseases may cause progressive deterioration of body tissues, as in the case of osteoarthritis, and leave residual impairment;
>
> Communicable diseases are produced when the body is invaded by living microorganisms (pathogens) that can be passed onto other susceptible individuals; knowledge of the specific mode of transmission of a given disease means that an efficient means of control can often be developed;
>
> Chronic diseases usually have more than one cause, and may be related to environmental, hereditary, and lifestyle factors.

Since man came into being, no matter where he has existed, the need for help and relief of pain and discomfort has persisted. He has looked toward "gods", magic, chemicals, and other men for assistance. Some students may be interested in constructing a time-line that graphically highlights man's struggle against disease. Books by Martí-Ibáñez, M. D., including *The Epic of Medicine,*[4] offer a vast amount of medical history and are excellent resources. The time-line may be divided into major periods, i.e. prehistoric and magic medicine; archaic medicine; Greek medicine—including Hippocrates; Roman medicine; Byzantine medicine; Arabian medicine; Renaissance medicine; Baroque medicine; medicine in the Age of Enlightenment (18th century); Nineteenth century medicine; and Twentieth century medicine.[4]

Stages of Disease

As one studies various diseases, it is evident that organically, all diseases pass through certain identifiable stages: (Figure 17.2)

1. Prior to pathogenesis, the individual falls somewhere along a "state of health" continuum. Although no signs of disease are present, the individual may vary in his/her physical, mental, and social well-being. A health hazard appraisal taken at this point could identify potential risks due to age, environment, etc. (Sometimes an abnormal condition exists, but because the condition is so common among a particular group of individuals, it is not defined as an illness condition.) "In short, health and disease, as well as their definitions, are often molded by the social context within which they occur."[3] (pg. 16)

2. Disease begins as a consequence of the interaction between known and unknown environmental conditions, specific agents, and a wide variety of aspects of the host. Genetic factors, nutrition, immunity mechanisms, social roles, stress, personality, climatic and atmospheric conditions are

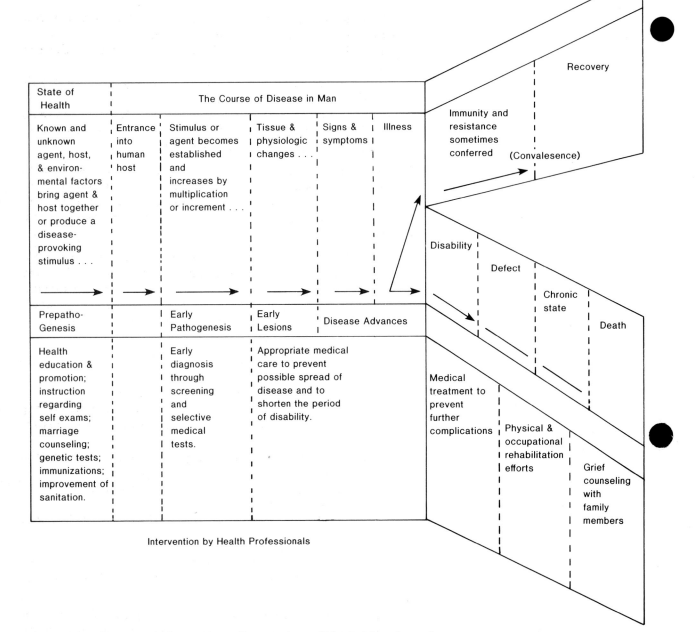

Figure 17.2. The natural history of any disease of man (Adapted from Leavell & Clark, Preventive Medicine for the Doctor in His Community).

all important components that influence whether an individual will contract the disease to which he has been exposed. For example, tuberculosis results from an attack of the tubercle bacillus on the host. Without the bacillus, it is impossible to contract tuberculosis. However, different hosts have varying abilities to withstand the attack, depending on specific physical, social, psychological, and environmental factors. Why do you think researchers should worry about these other factors when the tubercle bacillus provides a method of controlling the disease?

David Mechanic notes four reasons why these larger issues remain important:

    a. Many disease conditions do not easily yield to the assumption of a single necessary cause which can be controlled;

    b. Often when the major cause is isolated, it is extremely difficult to control;

    c. Understanding social factors in disease frequently provides the basis for reform important to health; and

    d. More detailed knowledge of disease processes, in general, provides a more sophisticated perspective on disease problems, and it increases our understanding of both disease and behavior.[3] (p. 273)

3. Early pathogenesis represents the incubation period. During this time the stimulus or agent becomes established and increases by multiplication or increment. Selective biochemical tests may detect the disease or disorder, but the condition is asymptomatic (no symptoms) and the individual usually feels fine.

4. A feeling of well-being may persist despite early tissue and other physiological changes. Periodic health examinations and multiphasic health screening can detect some illnesses; however, this is not the case for most diseases. Dr. Vickery believes there are at least six requirements which must be met before it is worthwhile to attempt to detect a particular disease before it causes symptoms:

    a. The disease must have a significant effect on the quality or quantity of life.

    b. Acceptable methods of treatment must be available.

    c. Disease must have an asymptomatic (no symptoms) period during which detection and treatment significantly reduce disability and/or death.

    d. Treatment in the asymptomatic phase must yield a result superior to that of delaying treatment until symptoms appear.

    e. Tests for detecting the condition in the asymptomatic period must be available at reasonable cost.

    f. The incidence of the condition must be sufficient to justify the cost of screening."[2] (p. 10)

This leaves strong evidence for only three *routine* procedures: blood pressure, self-examination and physician examination of the breast, and Pap smears.[2]

5. The recognition of deviations from personal standards of functioning or the experience of unfavorable changes in one's life situation alerts the person to a problem. . . .Once some deviant signs and symptoms have been recognized, social and cultural ideas about the cause of particular problems become relevant."[3] (p. 22)

6. Depending on the nature of the illness, a person may seek medical expertise. A doctor's conception of the illness is molded by his professional training and clinical experience. The patient's views are influenced by the need to cope with a particular problem and his/her cultural and social understanding of the nature of the problem.[3]

Classifying Illness

Freidson has developed the following system of classifying illness based on the four elements of the sick role postulated by Parsons.[6] To understand Freidson's classification of illnesses, one must distinguish between three kinds of legitimacy although the ideology (if not the actual behavior) of professionals in the health field asserts that no illness is illegitimate. The table distinguishes between minor and serious illness and implies quite different consequences for the individuals involved.

7. Like Figure 17.2, Freidson's table recognizes that some illnesses result in recovery, while other illnesses may be chronic and/or result in defects and disabilities. "In cell 1, stigma somewhat spoils one's regular identity, but does not replace it. In cells 2 and 3, 'illness' or 'impairment' qualifies but does not replace regular roles, the qualification being temporary in cell 2 and permanent in cell 3. The sick role, as Parsons defines it, is only to be found in cell 5 of the table. Stigmatized roles are to be found in cell 4, and, chronic sick or dying roles are to be found in cell 6."[5] It should be understood that movement between categories is quite common, e.g. the first response to perceived illness is likely to be found in cell 2. If the perception of deviance persists and responses to it intensify, the responses may move to cell 5—the sick role—or to other possibilities.

As a given disease progresses through man, various health professionals often intervene. This may happen even before an individual realizes that he/she is ill. Discuss the type of health professionals that may be involved and their possible functions.

Contemporary American Middle Class Societal Reaction To Types of Illness For Which the Individual Is Not Held Responsible. [5]

Imputed Seriousness	Illegitimate (Stigmatized)	Conditionally Legitimate	Unconditionally Legitimate
Minor Deviation	#1: "Stammer" Partial suspension of some ordinary obligations; few or no new privileges; adoption of a few new obligations.	#2: "A Cold" Temporary suspension of few ordinary obligations; temporary enhancement of ordinary privileges. Obligation to get well.	#3: "Pockmarks" No special change in obligations or privileges.
Serious Deviation	#4: "Epilepsy" Suspension of some ordinary obligations; adoption of new obligations; few or no new privileges.	#5: "Pneumonia" Temporary release from ordinary obligations; addition to ordinary privileges. Obligation to cooperate and seek help in treatment.	#6: "Cancer" Permanent suspension of many ordinary obligations; marked addition to privileges.

Materials

1. Resource materials.

Evaluation

1. Twenty-four phrases describing various types of disease are included under content and procedures. Duplicate enough copies for each student in your class, then provide all of them with enough time to study various resources and fill-in a disease that accurately fits the description.

2. Answers for Objective 2 are lifestyle, environment, medical care and heredity.

3. Objective 3 may be fulfilled by using the seven habits suggested by Drs. Nedra Belloc and Lester Breslow. They are included under content.

4. The following diseases may be given to students in order to evaluate their ability at distinguishing chronic illnesses from communicable diseases: (Chronic) Sickle cell anemia, Diabetes, Tay Sachs, Emphysema, Cancer, Cardiovascular disease, Multiple Sclerosis, Arthritis, Epilepsy, Cirrhosis of the Liver, Asthma, Cerebral Palsy, and Muscular Dystrophy.

   (Communicable) Cold, Influenza, Strep throat, Pneumonia, Measles, Mumps, Diphtheria, Chicken pox, Syphilis, Whooping cough, Mononucleosis, and Rabies.

5. Objective five is self-explanatory.

6. Duplicate copies of Freidson's model[5] (see sample) and ask each student to fill in six examples of illness under the category that most accurately reflects the general reaction of contemporary American middle class individuals.

Imputed Seriousness	Illegitimate (Stigmatized)	Conditionally Legitimate	Unconditionally Legitimate
Minor Deviation			
Serious Deviation			

Diseases and Disorders
Face-to-Face with the Enemy
(Identification of Diseases and Disorders)

Objectives

1. Given a list of non-communicable diseases, each student will select, research, and report on a disease which interests him or her.

2. The student will be able to document his report with information gained from at least six different resources.

3. The student will be able to briefly describe three diseases or disorders that are inherited or appear at birth.

4. The student will be able to discuss the far-reaching influence of environment on health and will provide five examples of how the environment may be directly responsible for a specific disease or disorder.

5. The student will be able to briefly describe the importance of the following three screening techniques:
   a. breast-self examination;
   b. Pap test;
   c. blood pressure test.

Sources

1. "The Ten Least Wanted," *Current Health 2*, September, 1977, pp. 3-13.

2. Joseph D. McInerney, Faith M. Hickman, and Manert H. Kennedy. "Human Genetics: A Context for Health Education," *Health Education*, July-August, 1978, pp. 33-35.

3. "Genetics: Blueprint for Life," *Current Health 2*, May, 1977, pp. 3-13.

4. Robert H. A. Haslam and Peter J. Valletutti, Editors. *Medical Problems in the Classroom.* Baltimore: University Park Press, 1975.

5. Donald M. Vickery, M.D. *Lifeplan For Your Health.* Reading, Massachusetts: Addison-Wesley Publishing Company, 1978.

6. Vivian K. Harlin, M. D. "Teaching Breast-Self Examination in the High School," *The Journal of School Health*, April, 1977, pp. 243-247.

7. Herb Jones. "Preventing Cancer with Education," *Health Education*, May-June, 1978, pp. 26-28.

8. Donna Cherniak and Allan Feingold. *VD Handbook* third edition. Montreal Health Press, Inc., P.O. Box 1000, Station G, Montreal, Quebec, H2W2N1, 1977.

Content and Procedures

Incidence of Chronic Illness

Pick up any newspaper and you will probably be able to read about a murder that occurred recently. Maybe you feel a slight bit uneasy when the crime takes place in your neighborhood and the killer has not been apprehended. How would you feel if there was a small band of killers who had grouped together and just announced their grandiose plan to kill more than a million Americans next year? Their unsuspecting victims would include both the rich and poor, young and old, male and female, and assorted cultures and races. As a young, strong, healthy person, would you bet your life that these killers would not kill or maim you? How would you protect yourself? Does the thought of the killer being a disease rather than a human make the possibility of your death seem more remote? Statistically, you probably have more than 50 years of good health ahead of you. But you can strengthen your defenses and use improved diet, habits, and lifestyles as your weapon against these killers.

Activity—Chronic Illness Report

Select a chronic illness or disorder that interests you and investigate its "crime." Use the worksheet, "Profile of a Chronic Illness or Disorder," to formally report your findings and informally share your work with other students.

Activity—Sources of Information

Are you aware of the many resources available to individuals interested in learning more about specific disorders? By using at least six of the ten specific resources described in the worksheet, "Sources of Information," you will not only become better informed, but your work can benefit others. After the disease profile and source worksheets are completed they should be combined in a 3-ring notebook and kept in the classroom or school library as a reference book to be referred to throughout the year. Students may wish to supplement and update the notebook with appropriate materials as they become available.

Activity—Chronic Illness Cards:

After each student has investigated a chronic illness, ask him to write a *brief* description of that disease or disorder on one side of a 3" x 5" notecard in "Who am I?" style. The description may include an early warning sign that indicates the need for a medical examination. These cards may be used in a variety of ways: If the names of the disorders are written on the opposite side of the cards they may be used for review, self-evaluation, or as question cards in a modified "spelling-bee" that pits two teams against each other. You may wish to ask students to prepare *two* index game cards—the question card should describe the particular illness they researched, and the answer card should have the name of the illness written on it. If there are 30 students in your class, there will be 60 playing cards. A group of four students would each be dealt 15 cards, and six students would be given ten cards. The object of the game is to be the first person to run out of cards. This is done by matching descriptive question cards with their corresponding disease. Students may try to exchange either one, two, or three cards at one time with whoever is willing to trade. Since all students will be bartering at once, this activity may get a little noisy! (This game can be simplified by including the name of the disease on the question card.) Another way to use these cards is to attach all the question cards to one side of a bulletin board, then ask each student to draw an answer card and correctly pin it across from the illness described.

Sex-linked Disorders

Unlike many chronic illnesses which are caused either by lifestyle or environmental factors, some diseases and disorders are inherited or appear at birth. Can you think of five *single-gene* disorders that are *sex-linked?*

There are more than 150 known disorders of this type.[3] Since the defect is carried on the X chromosome, a female carrier may appear normal if she has one normal X chromosome that can mask the defective recessive gene. A male is not so fortunate, since his Y chromosome is unable to mask the defective X chromosome. He not only has the abnormality—including baldness, color-blindness, hemophilia, muscular dystrophy (Duchenne type), and immunity deficiencies (see next chapter),—but is a carrier as well.[3] ACTIVITY: A person's eye color is a sex-linked trait. Ask several interested students to illustrate their family gene tree for eye color. (Their parents can probably go back two generations with good accuracy on eye color).[3]

Chromosome Abnormalities

Chromosome abnormalities probably account for one third of all miscarriages that occur.[3] Since many genes are involved, there can be many defects. Down's syndrome (mongolism) is the most common chromosomal disorder and is usually characterized by eyefolds that make the person look oriental; a large tongue; small head; mental retardation; congenital heart disease; and poor muscle tone. The children also seem to be more susceptible to respiratory infections and leukemia.[3,4] Contact the National Foundation of the March of Dimes for the following free publications: "Chromosome 21 and its Association with Down's Syndrome"; "Guide to Human Chromosome Defects, Vol. IV, #4, Birth Defects: Original Article Series"; and "Is My Baby All Right?"—a series of booklets about (1) clubfoot and congenital dislocation of the hip; (2) spina bifida and hydrocephalus; (3) cleft lip and cleft palate; (4) diabetes and other inborn errors of metabolism; (5) minimal brain dysfunction; and (6) chromosome abnormalities and Down's Syndrome.

Did you know that you probably carry between one and ten defective recessive genes? These genes are harmless when counterbalanced by a normal gene, but have a significant chance of combining with another defective recessive gene if you marry a close relative, such as your first cousin, and decide to have children. Certain genetic diseases are also more common within a particular ethnic group or race, e.g. Tay-Sachs is highest among Jewish people with ancestors from central and eastern Europe; Cooley's anemia attacks many Italians, Greeks, and others whose ancestors came from Mediterranean regions; sickle cell anemia is highest among blacks; while cystic fibrosis occurs most often in whites.[3]

Students should be encouraged to identify diseases for which they may have inherited a predisposition, and to learn how they can decrease their risk. For example, although research has shown that smoking dramatically increases an individual's risk of developing lung cancer, there also seems to be a genetic component involved. In other words, if you have relatives who have developed lung cancer, you may be more susceptible to lung cancer than another person who smokes the same amount as you do.[2] If Tay-Sachs disease has killed a blood relative of yours or you are Jewish and have ancestors from central or eastern Europe, consider having a simple blood test to determine if you are a carrier of this gene. Likewise, Blacks should consider having a red blood cell test to determine if they are carriers of the sickle cell trait. Genetic counseling is recommended for people who have genetic disorders or for whom a particular genetic disease may be a problem. See the article, "Genetics: Blueprint For Life,"[3] for more information about genetic counseling and genetics in general.

Knowledge concerning specific elements in the environment that may be hazardous to our health is rapidly increasing. Can you correctly match the following environmental elements with their probable health hazard? (In some instances, more than one answer can be used)

Environmental Health Hazards Quiz

Environmental Elements

_____ 1. Prolonged exposure to asbestos

_____ 2. Increased amounts of solar radiation reaching the earth's surface

_____ 3. Dumping of the chemical, kepone, into the James River in Virginia

_____ 4. Air pollution

_____ 5. Excessive use of X-rays

_____ 6. Prolonged exposure to coal tar, pitch, or creosote

_____ 7. Prolonged exposure to vinyl chloride, an industrial chemical

_____ 8. Prolonged exposure to nickel and chromium compounds

_____ 9. Poor living conditions

_____ 10. Prolonged inhalation of fiberglass, raw cotton dust, and fungi

_____ 11. Eating paint chips from old buildings / excessive exposure to automobile exhaust / production of batteries and rubber tires

_____ 12. Prolonged exposure to excessive noise

Health Hazards
(may be used more than once)

A. Skin Cancer

B. May lead to food poisoning

C. Lung Cancer

D. Angiosarcoma of the liver

E. Plumbism (lead poisoning)

F. Pneumoconioses (lung inhalation diseases)

G. Increased stress

H. Nervous system disorders, including tremors, weakness, and loss of coordination

I. A wide variety of cancers

J. Often contributes to development of tuberculosis

We would be remiss in our discussion of chronic diseases if we did not briefly mention several screening techniques of whose effectiveness there is good evidence:

Breast Self-examination

"A Gallup survey found that three out of four women who had heard about breast self-examination (BSE) did not practice it. These women identified their own ignorance of the technique as their reason for inaction."[6] Effective breast self-examination skills are vital for early detection of breast cancer. Although breast cancer rarely occurs among high school females, the problem is significant when one realizes that one in fifteen women will develop it at some point in her life. Many experts believe that high school is the best time to develop effective BSE skills because health habits are still being established.[6,7]

Most programs designed to increase a student's level of knowledge about breast cancer are directed at girls, however, it is often a boyfriend or husband that first detects a lump. Informed men may also encourage women to begin

BSE and be on the lookout for cancer's danger signals. They may be the first person a woman turns to when she suspects something is wrong. For these reasons, a program about breast cancer and BSE should be available to interested persons of both sexes. Such a program may include (1) an explanation of the program and pre-testing of knowledge and behavior; (2) a brief presentation about cancer conducted by a physician or nurse; (3) showing a film such as "Something Very Special" which presents the issues of breast and uterine cancer; (4) a question and answer period, with the physician or nurse answering previously submitted written questions; (5) administration of the posttest; and (6) an opportunity to work with the Betsy Breast model and for informal discussion. Sample pre-tests may be found in the December 1977 Human Sexuality Supplement to *Current Health 2*, and in the article "Preventing Cancer With Education."[7] Call the local chapter of your American Cancer Society and request their free pamphlet, "How to Examine Your Breasts."

Pap-Test

The "Pap test" is a simple and painless way to test for cancer of the cervix. Body tissues regularly shed a number of cells. These "cast off" cells of the cervix and uterus are collected by the doctor or his/her assistant, and examined under a microscope to see if abnormal cells are present. The "Pap" test can detect possible cancer before symptoms appear and when it is more easily cured. The pretest found in the article "Preventing Cancer With Education",[7] also includes several questions about uterine cancer and the Pap test. An easy-to-understand explanation of what happens during a gynecological examination and illustrations of a speculum (a medical instrument that holds the vaginal walls apart so the vagina and cervix can be inspected) can be found in the *VD Handbook*.[8]

Blood Pressure Test

A blood pressure test is used to detect *hypertension*, a condition where a person's blood pressure remains high for an extended period of time. When this happens, organs such as the heart, kidneys, brain, and arteries can be damaged. After discussing how blood pressure is measured, invite a nurse to demonstrate the proper technique and explain how blood pressure is recorded. If a sphygmomanometer and stethoscope are available to you over a period of several weeks, invite students to record their blood pressure every other day and plot it on a graph. More than one reading is needed to adequately determine a person's average blood pressure because exercise, tension, emotions, hormones, and many other factors may cause a temporary rise in pressure. See the article, "High Blood Pressure Control,"[9] for additional information.

Materials

1. Worksheets: "Profile of a Chronic Illness or Disorder"; "Sources of Information".

2. Library reference materials.

3. Optional: American Cancer Society films (deleting the section on coping with mastectomy surgery); "Betsy" breast model; sphygmomanometer; stethoscope; and speculum.

Evaluation

1. Objective one may be met by asking students to investigate one of the following 30 illnesses and carefully complete the worksheet: "Profile of a Chronic Illness or Disorder" (sample copy included): arteriosclerosis, asthma, breast cancer, cancer of the colon-rectum, cerebral palsy, cirrhosis, chronic bronchitis, cystic fibrosis, diabetes, Down's syndrome, emphysema, epilepsy, glaucoma, gout, heart disease, hemophilia, herpes, hepatitis, hypertension, juvenile rheumatoid arthritis, leukemia, lung cancer, multiple sclerosis, muscular dystrophy, myasthenia gravis, Reye's syndrome, skin cancer, Tay-Sachs disease, tuberculosis, uterine cancer, etc.

2. Objective two can be met by requiring students to complete the "Sources of Information" worksheets included in this book.

3. The following "Who Am I?" questions may be used as additional Chronic Illness game cards when evaluating student recognition of chronic illnesses and their symptoms:
   —I am caused by an accumulation of materials on the inside of the arteries, thereby blocking the flow of some blood to the heart and other body tissues. Who am I? (Atherosclerosis)
   —I cause cells to go out of control! Some of my cells grow and spread to other parts of the body replacing normal tissue. I am not one disease but many. Who am I? (Cancer)
   —I cause inflammation of the joints—this means pain, swelling, warmth, redness, and stiffness. There is no known way to prevent any of my various forms. Who am I? (Arthritis)
   —I am caused by abnormally high pressure in the eyeball due to fluid produced by the ciliary cells that cannot get through some small openings in the eye. This pressure can damage the optic nerve and result in blindness. Who am I? (Glaucoma)

4. Answers to Environmental Health Hazards Quiz: (1) C,F; (2) A; (3) H; (4) C; (5) I; (6) A,C; (7) D; (8) C; (9) J,D; (10) F; (11) E; (12) G.

5. Extra credit may be given to students who can properly measure and record another student's blood pressure or who are able to properly demonstrate the technique of BSE using a Betsy Breast model and explain what kinds of changes they are looking for (lump, hard knot or thickening, dimpling of skin or discharge from nipple).

Worksheet: *Profile of a Chronic Illness or Disorder*

Name of illness or disorder: _____

Part/s of body affected: _____

Signs and Symptoms: _____

_____

_____

Prevalence/Incidence: (How common is it? Who is most likely to get it? Where does it usually occur?)

_____

_____

_____

Possible Causes: _____

_____

Treatment (Is it curable?): _____

_____

_____

Disabilities and far-reaching effects: _____

_____

_____

_____

Prevention: _____

_____

_____

_____

Additional comments: _____

_____

_____

Worksheet: *"Sources of Information"*

Topic to be investigated: _____

  I. *Textbook* or other type of book

    A. Title of book: _____

    B. Author or Editor: _____

    C. Publisher: _____

    D. Copyright date: _____

    E. Content value to you: (Circle one) Excellent Good Fair Poor

    F. Comments: _____

  II. *Professional Journal*

    A. Title of journal: _____

    B. Month and year: _____

    C. Title of a current article: _____

    D. Author: _____

    E. Content value to you: (Circle one) Excellent Good Fair Poor

    F. Comments: _____

  III. *"Popular" Magazine*

    A. Title of magazine: _____

    B. Month and year: _____

C. Title of article: _____

D. Author: _____

E. Content value to you: (Circle one) Excellent Good Fair Poor

F. Comments: _____

IV. *Pamphlet* (Attach a copy to this report)

A. Title of pamphlet: _____

B. Author: _____

C. Source address: _____

D. Copyright date: _____

E. Content value to you: (Circle one) Excellent Good Fair Poor

F. Comments: _____

V. *Filmstrip*

A. Title of filmstrip: _____

B. Black and White or Color (Circle one)

C. Running time: _____

D. Does filmstrip include a record or cassette tape? _____

E. Source address: _____

F. Is this filmstrip available locally? (Where?) _____

G. Content value to you: (Circle one) Excellent Good Fair Poor

H. Comments: _____

VI: *Film* (16mm)

A. Title of film: _____

B. Black and White or Color   (Circle one)

C. Running time: _____

D. Source address: _____

E. Is this film available locally? (Where?) _____

F. Content value to you: (Circle one) Excellent Good Fair Poor

G. Comments: _____

VII: *Organization* concerned with this problem

A. Name of organization: _____

B. Address of national headquarters: _____

C. Address of branch closest to you: _____

D. Available services: _____

_____

_____

E. Content value to you: (Circle one) Excellent Good Fair Poor

F. Comments: _____

VIII: *Official* agencies; (State Health Department)

    A. Does your State Health Department offer any type of assistance regarding this topic? (Pamphlets, films, etc.) _____

    _____

    B. Address: _____

    C. Contact person (or department): _____

    D. Telephone number: _____

    E. Content value to you: (Circle one) Excellent Good Fair Poor

    F. Comments: _____

IX: *Country or Local Health Department*

    A. Does your County or Local Health Department offer any type of assistance regarding this topic? (Pamphlets, films, etc.)

    _____

    B. Address: _____

    C. Contact person or division: _____

    D. Telephone number: _____

    E. Content value to you: (Circle one) Excellent Good Fair Poor

    F. Comments: _____

X: *Resource Person*

    A. Name of health professional willing to speak to your class concerning this topic: _____

    B. Name of individual with a chronic condition you are investigating and were able to interview: _____

    Telephone # of "A" _____; of "B" _____

Diseases and Disorders
Planning for Your Well-being
(Early Detection and Prevention)

Objectives

1. In an effort to assume more responsibility for their well-being, the students will:
   a. assess their exercise, diet, smoking, drinking, and safety habits;
   b. assess their susceptibility to stress-induced illness and ability to cope with the stresses of living; and
   c. assess their susceptibility to major diseases, including heart disease and stroke; diabetes; tuberculosis; glaucoma; gout; and sexually-transmitted diseases.

2. Each student will develop personal "Life Plan Goals" in an effort to improve his/her chances for a long, healthy life.

3. The student will be able to describe a lifestyle that incorporates at least fifteen factors that contribute to longevity.

Sources

1. Donald M. Vickery, M.D. *Life Plan For Your Health;* Reading, Massachusetts: Addison-Wesley Publishing Company, 1978.

2. Walter D. Sorochan. *Personal Health Appraisal.* New York: John Wiley and Sons, Inc., 1976.

3. John W. Travis, M.D. "Wellness Inventory," Wellness Resource Center, 42 Miller Avenue, Mill Valley, California 94941, 1977.

4. Thomas H. Holmes, M.D. and R.H. Rahe. "The Social Readjustment Rating Scale," *Journal of Psychosomatic Research II,* 1967, p. 213.

Content and Procedures

A Life Plan

Have you ever tried to figure out your estimated life expectancy by using tables developed by life insurance companies? Most people are interested in trying to determine how many years they have left on earth, but often they do not consider the quality of those years. Is life worth living if you get short of breath with only the slightest exertion, or if pain is a constant companion?

By appraising your susceptibility to major diseases and disorders, and then developing a "Life Plan" that works to change some of your present habits and personal behaviors, you can significantly improve your chances for living a long and healthy life.

Activity

Purchase and use the book, *Life Plan for Your Health,* by Dr. Vickery.[1] Not only are Life Score Worksheets provided for recording your present scores related to habits (exercise, weight, diet, smoking, alcohol, accidents, contraception), mental health (stress), immunizations, personal history, family history, and medical care, but abundant information is included that will help motivate you to change some of your health behaviors and improve your Life Score.

Personal Health Appraisal, by Walter Sorochan,[2] is another excellent source of information. It includes a "Susceptibility to Cardiovascular Disorders Inventory" that asks students to circle the lifestyle factors (age, heredity, medical checkups, coffee drinking, cigarette smoking, occupation, emotional stress, quality of exercise, body weights, eating habits, and symptoms) that most closely apply to them and contribute to cardiovascular disease. Similar inventories, procedures and interpretations for cancer, stress, etc. may also be found in this book.

The *Wellness Inventory*[3] is a short pamphlet by Dr. John Travis that may be purchased for 50¢. The student is asked to place a mark before each statement which is true for them. The questionnaire contains short descriptions related to: (a) productivity, relaxation, sleep; (b) personal care and home safety; (c) nutritional awareness; (d) environmental awareness; (e) physical activity; (f) expression of emotions and feelings; (g) community involvement; (h) creativity, self-expression; (i) automobile safety; and (j) parenting.

After the students have determined their present health status, ask them if they are content with the results or if they are interested in learning how to improve their chances for a long, healthy life. Self-improvement means setting realistic goals that can be followed for life—this may be a long time if one is sincere about assuming responsibility for his/her well-being. Duplicate one copy of "Setting Your Life Plan Goals," for each student, and fill out one for yourself too.

Some students may be interested to know that several commercial companies offer health appraisal screening and risk analysis for the ten leading causes of death, based on a person's age, sex, and present lifestyle. Write to the following companies for more information:

1. Database Acquisition for Student Health (DASH) Medical Datanation, Inc., Southwest and Harrison, Bellevue, Ohio 44811.
2. Interhealth, 2970 5th Avenue, San Diego, California 92103.
3. Pacific Research Systems, 2222 Cornith Avenue, Los Angeles, California 90064.

Many factors seem to contribute to longevity. List as many as the class can think of on the chalkboard and discuss why these factors are important. (Heredity, optimum weight, nonsmoker, nonabuse of alcohol and drugs, good health (few illnesses and diseases), a challenging job, a purpose in life, time for recreation and leisure, minimum stress, satisfying sex life, close family unit, diet low in saturated fats, involvement in community activities, regular, vigorous exercise, optimistic attitude, good sanitation, freedom from environmental hazards (such as asbestos, lead, vinyl chloride), ability to adjust, above average intelligence, satisfaction with one's lifestyle and life in general.)

Setting Your Lifeplan Goals[*]

I. Habits

Exercise: My goal is _____

_____

_____

(Ideal: Within reason, the more the better, but raising your heart beat to 120 beats per minute or more, for 15 minutes three times per week is known to benefit the heart. (Minimum); An optimal program would be approximately 45 minutes per day, but 45 minutes three times per week is probably adequate.[1]
(p. 111)

Healthful hints: Climb stairs rather than ride elevators; and participate in both strenuous sports and stretching-limbering exercises.

Weight: My goal is _____
(Ideal: Stay within five pounds of your ideal weight according to weight tables available from the National Dairy Council or Metropolitan Life Insurance Company)

Diet: My goal is _____

_____

_____

(Ideal: Eat a variety of foods from the Four Food Groups every day; Avoid saturated fats and cholesterol)

Healthful hints: Try to eat at least one uncooked fruit or vegetable each day; avoid adding extra sugar or salt to your foods; read food labels; reduce consumption of coffee or tea to less than three cups a day.

*Adapted from "Setting Your LifePlan goals," *LifePlan-For Your Health,* by Donald M. Vickery (pp. 75–77) copyright © 1978, by permission of Addison-Wesley Publishing Company, Reading, Mass.

Smoking: My goal is _____
(Ideal: No smoking; Second best is to reduce amount or switch to pipe or cigar)

Drinking: My goal is _____
(Ideal: Zero to five alcoholic beverages—including beer—per week)

Seat Belts: My goal is _____
(Ideal: Worn 100% of time while driving or riding in a car)

Contraception: My goal is _____

_____
(Ideal: The safest method acceptable to you)

II. Mental Health
Stress: My goal is _____

_____

_____

Holmes score[4] _____
(Ideal: Holmes score less than 150 in a year)

Healthful hints: Complete Dr. Vickery's informal "Looking For Satisfaction" questionnaire[1] (pp. 180–183);

Consider the subject of stress in your life by completing the Holmes Scale[4]—this scale also appears in Dr. Vickery's book[1] (pp. 184–185);

Walter Sorochan also includes a "Life-change-illness" scale[2] in his book, and asks students to check the events that happened to them during the past year. Discuss ways of reducing high risk to major illness and depression.

III. Immunizations (See next chapter)

My immunization goal is _____
(Ideal: All immunizations up-to-date)

Healthful hints: Adults need a Tetanus shot every 10 years unless they receive a "very dirty" wound. Diphtheria shots are usually only given to adults who have a high risk of exposure.

IV. Major Diseases

Heart Disease and Stroke: My goal is to reduce my risk of dying from heart disease or stroke by _____

_____

(Ideal: Blood pressure checked once a year; regular exercise; weight within five pounds of ideal; no smoking; reduce stress; reduce intake of saturated fats, cholesterol, and caffeine.)

Cancer of the Lung: My goal is to reduce my risk of dying from lung cancer by _____

_____

(Ideal: No smoking; avoid air pollution; avoid exposure to asbestos)

Cancer of the Breast: My goal is to reduce my risk of dying from breast cancer by _____

_____

(Ideal: Monthly self-examination; annual examination by a physician; Xeromammography after age 40 if mother or sister had breast cancer)

Cancer of the Uterus: My goal is to reduce my risk of dying from cancer of the uterus by _____

_____

(Ideal: Pap smear every year or two and pelvic exam if sexually active or over age 20. A person who has Herpes Simplex-2 should have a Pap test every six months)

Cancer of the Colon and Rectum: My goal is to reduce my risk of cancer by _____

_____

(Ideal: Proctosigmoidoscopy examination after age 50; Test stool for hidden blood every two years after age 40, yearly after age 50)

Cancer of the Thyroid: My goal is to reduce my risk of cancer by _____
(Ideal: Yearly examination by a physician if you have had radiation treatment of tonsils, adenoids, acne or ringworm of the scalp)

Cancer of the Liver: My goal is to reduce my risk of liver damage by _____

_____

(Ideal: Less than three alcoholic beverages a day; avoid exposure to vinyl chloride)

Cancer of the Skin: My goal is to reduce my risk of skin cancer by

_____

_____

(Ideal: Avoid prolonged, excessive exposure to the sun; consider monthly self-examination)

Diabetes: My goal is to reduce my risk of diabetes by _____

_____

(Ideal: Stay within five pounds of ideal weight)

Tuberculosis: My goal is to reduce my risk of tuberculosis by

_____

_____

(Ideal: Skin test (PPD or Tine) every five to 10 years if no history of exposure; good living conditions; limit exposure to known cases as far as possible)

Glaucoma: My goal is to reduce my risk of blindness from glaucoma by _____
(Ideal: Tonometry every four to five years after age 40—after age 30 if there is a family history of glaucoma)

Gout: My goal is to reduce my risk of gout by _____

_____

(Ideal: Middle-aged men with a history of gout in their family should be careful to stay within five pounds of their ideal weight and may want to avoid consumption of alcohol)

Sexually-Transmitted diseases: My goal is to avoid contracting VD by

_____

(Ideal: Avoid frequent sexual activity with many different partners; men should wear a condom; blood test (VDRL) every five to six years while sexually active)

Materials

1. Suggested health inventories and appraisals.

2. Copies of "Setting Your Life Plan Goals" (sample included under content).

Evaluation

1. The teacher observes active student participation in the completion of at least one health assessment tool.

2. The student shows interest in developing personal "Life Plan Goals" that are realistic and health-promoting.

3. The teacher observes that the student is eager to share his "Life Plan Goals" with friends, family, and others.

4. The student demonstrates an awareness of the importance of heredity, environment, and lifestyle factors by including them in a one-page essay where he/she is asked to describe a lifestyle that incorporates at least fifteen factors that contribute to longevity.

Selected Learning Activities

Diseases and Disorders

_____ Prepare several graphs that illustrate the incidence of various types of diseases by race, age, and sex. Graphs may also be developed that compare death rates for a given disease over a ten or twenty year period.

_____ Select a chronic disease to investigate. Write a paper that focuses on the psycho-social impact it may have on an individual.

_____ Invite a nutritionist to speak on the subject of preventing birth defects through proper nutrition.

_____ Develop a slide or puppet show depicting current methods for treating diseases such as chemotherapy, dietary therapy, physical therapy, psychotherapy, or surgery.

_____ Tape record your interview with an individual who has a chronic health condition.

_____ Using a world map, identify areas that have high concentrations of nutritionally related diseases such as anemia, ariboflavirosis, beriberi, goiter, heart diseases, pellagra, rickets, and scurvy.

_____ Seek permission to distribute March of Dimes educational materials to hospitals, public health and welfare office waiting rooms, YWCA, etc.

_____ Select a disease or a disorder and make a word search using at least six words related to the disease or disorder.

_____ Design a pamphlet that describes either a disease or a disorder.

_____ Make a disease and disorder bingo game. Use cardboard paper for the board itself and construction paper to make the markers.

_____ Make a poster that has to do with screening for a particular disease or disorder. The poster should clarify at least one health fact.

_____ Have a disease-disorder spelling bee. The words or terms should get harder as the spelling bee progresses.

_____ Develop a list of contributing causes of cancer.

_____ Describe how risk factors of heart disease can be minimized.

_____ Have a panel discussion on the following topic: All drinking water should have fluoride.

_____ In groups of three present a skit about bronchitis, emphysema and asthma. Make sure the signs and symptoms, care and treatment are emphasized.

_____ Conduct a survey to determine the extent of concern among peers about acne.

_____ Invite a speaker from The American Cancer Society to talk about cancer in adolescence.

_____ Ask students to develop a list of what they feel are the most significant diseases and disorders. Ask their parents to do the same. Tally the frequencies in class and discuss the similarities and dissimiliarities.

_____ For each of the body systems, develop a chart which identifies at least five diseases or disorders.

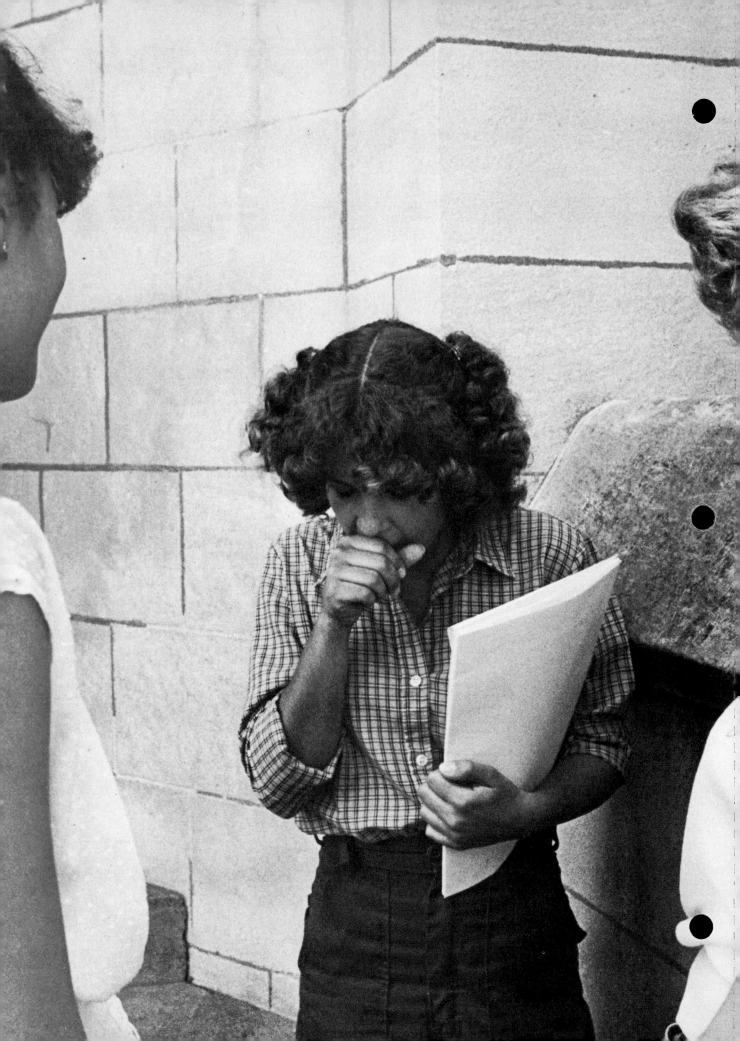

Teaching about Communicable Disease

Every day of our lives each of us is exposed to the potentially dangerous pathogens which cause communicable diseases. Whether or not we become infected with one of the many diseases of this type depends largely upon the type of health behavior we select. We can be careful to observe health practices which minimize disease, and we can also heed the body's early warning signals. In addition, when we are afflicted with disease the recovery period can also be shortened by our behavior choices. This chapter contains an outline of Suggested Topics for Teaching About Communicable Diseases, Three Detailed Sample Lessons which provide the student with the accurate information needed to make wise choices, and additional Selected Learning Activities.

The first lesson, **Signs of Disease,** provides a review of the major childhood diseases for the middle and secondary school student. Because of the previous bouts of illness in the elementary school, the adolescent years are generally free of communicable diseases. The student learns about the Big Seven and about the importance of immunization.

In the second lesson, **In Self-defense,** the student learns about the body's early warning signs of possible danger in either the internal or external environment. The student learns the six principal types of disease-producing organisms and how diseases are transmitted. As examination of the ways in which an individual can assist in the control and prevention of communicable disease adds to the emphasis on responsible decision-making.

Sexually Transmissible Diseases are discussed in the third lesson. Such diseases are especially prevalent in the teenage population, and the student needs to possess important information about each of these diseases, in addition to examining his feelings and looking at the responsibility for personal behavior.

Suggested Topics

Communicable Diseases

I. Disease-causing Microorganisms
   A. Bacteria
   B. Viruses
   C. Rickettsiae

Photo by Bob Coyle

         D. Fungi
         E. Parasitic Protozoa
         F. Parasitic Worms
    II. Methods of Transmission
         A. Direct Contact
              1. Intimate, Direct Personal Contact
              2. Droplet Spray From An Infected Human
              3. Contact With An Infected Animal
              4. Direct Exposure to Microorganisms in Soil, Animal Feces, or Decaying
                 Vegetable Matter
         B. Indirect Contact
              1. Contaminated Materials or Objects
              2. Contaminated Food, Water, or Milk
              3. Contaminated Biological Products, e.g. blood serum
              4. By Insects
              5. Airborne—Microbial Aerosols
   III. Natural Body Defenses
   IV. Characteristics of Immunity
         A. Active
              1. Natural
              2. Artificial
         B. Passive
              1. Natural
              2. Artificial
    V. Common Communicable Diseases: Causes; Symptoms; Treatment; and Pre-
       vention
         A. The Common Cold
         B. Influenza
         C. Mononucleosis
         D. Infectious Hepatitis
         E. Tuberculosis
         F. Measles
         G. Rubella
         H. Chicken Pox
         I. Mumps
         J. Whooping Cough
         K. Pneumonia
         L. Rabies
         M. Rheumatic Fever
         N. Gonorrhea
         O. Syphilis
         P. Herpes Simplex
         Q. Trichomoniasis

Lesson Plans

Communicable Disease
Signs of Disease

Objectives

1. Given a list of symptoms, the student will identify those symptoms he/
   she believes justifies keeping a child home from school.

2. The student will be able to recognize common symptoms of at least ten
   childhood diseases.

3. The student will correctly name all seven of the childhood diseases that
   can be prevented through proper immunizations.

4. The student will demonstrate his/her knowledge of communicable disease by accurately completing "The Big 7" Childhood Communicable Disease crossword puzzle.

5. The student will further demonstrate his/her knowledge of communicable diseases by locating at least 30 (out of 33) words related to immunization and disease in the "Immunization" word search puzzle and correctly use at least twenty of those words in no more than fifteen sentences.

Sources

1. Cecil Slome, M.D., W. Lednar, D. Roberts, D. Basco. "Should James Go To School? Mothers' Responses to Symptoms," *The Journal of School Health,* pp. 106–110, February, 1977.

2. Eileen McCurdy, T. Halpin, M.D., P. Grover. "Why Should You and Your Family Be Immunized Against "The Big Seven"?" The Ohio Department of Health, Columbus, Ohio.

3. Abram S. Benenson, Editor. *Control of Communicable Diseases in Man.* Washington, D.C.: The American Public Health Association, 1975.

4. Donald M. Vickery, M.D., J. Fries, M.D. *Take Care of Yourself: A Consumer's Guide to Medical Care.* Reading, Massachusetts: Addison-Wesley Publishing Company, 1976.

5. John J. Burt, L. Meeks, S. Pottebaum. *Toward A Healthy Lifestyle Through Elementary Health Education.* Belmont, California: Wadsworth Publishing Company, 1980.

Content and Procedures

Why Learn about Disease?

"Reports indicate threats of epidemic polio and measles, especially in central-city poverty areas and some rural areas. . ." "Childhood Diseases Threaten Lives. . ." "Health Officials Trying To Keep Smallpox Out. . ." Are these the headlines of another era? Unfortunately, they are items that appear in newspapers during the 1970's. But why should communicable diseases be of concern to teenagers? After all, "childhood diseases" are much more prevalent among the very young.

This does not mean, however, that a 16-year-old high school student cannot suddenly contract mumps. Do you think he or she will get as ill as the unimmunized six-year-old? Fact: The teenage or adult form of mumps is usually much more severe than the childhood form. While both age groups suffer with swelling and tenderness of the salivary (parotid) glands near the jaw, and a fever of up to 103 degrees, the virus may also settle in a man's testes or a woman's ovaries and result in sterility. Since more than one in five individuals who get mumps after childhood also develop an inflammation of the reproductive organs, this is no minor matter.

Many teenagers also have the opportunity to work with young children, either as baby-sitters or in day care centers. By learning how to identify common symptoms of communicable diseases and by practicing common sense prevention and control measures, the teenager can help to prevent the spread of many diseases, as well as reduce their severity by encouraging early medical care.

Teens thinking of becoming parents one day should understand that their knowledge and beliefs regarding illness, as well as their subjective response to overt symptoms, will contribute to the decision as to whether they will keep their children home from school some day. A means of stimulating thought in this area is to ask each student to complete the questionnaire, "Should James Go To School?"[1] Directions: Place a checkmark next to the symptoms that would cause you to keep your child home from school. After the questionnaires have been completed, have the students tabulate the percentage of students who would keep their child home for each symptom, and rank order the symptoms, beginning with the most important. The students may also wish to examine their data with regard to sex and race, or to compare their results with a group of Delaware mothers who were asked to complete a similar survey.[1] Do the students think they would have rated each symptom the same way if they would have had to take off from work to stay home with their child?

Common Symptoms of Communicable Disease

Knowledge of some common symptoms of communicable diseases can be more meaningful to students if they share the information with other people. Students may wish to develop the following script and present the skit to day care workers, other students, etc.

Ten Little Children

Scene opens with ten little children playing together and singing or saying:

> We are 10 Little Children,
> Life seems so fine,
> But Tom developed Polio,
> And now we are nine.

Polio character takes Tom away.

Narrator I: Polio was a dreaded killer until a polio vaccine was developed in the 1950's and children started receiving four doses of vaccine, which offered complete protection. Polio attacks the nervous system and may cause permanent paralysis, deformity, or even death; however, fever, sore throat, stomach aches, headaches, and stiffness are the first symptoms of this killer disease.

Nine children singing:

> We are 9 Little Children,
> Who will keep on tempting fate,
> But Sue just caught Diphtheria,
> And now we are eight.

Diphtheria character takes Sue away.

Narrator 2: Diphtheria usually develops in the throat, as a patch or patches of greyish membranes. Early symptoms are a sore throat, fever, and chills. If the membrane continues to grow, it can interfere with swallowing or block the breathing passage. Although very contagious, can be prevented with five special "3-in-one" doses of vaccine.[2,3]

Eight children singing:

> We are 8 Little Children,
> Watching TV until eleven,
> But Measles waylaid Bill,
> And now we are seven.

Measles character takes Bill away.

Narrator 3: Measles is also called red measles and 10-day measles. It is the most serious of the common childhood diseases and may lead to bacterial complications, such as ear infections and pneumonia. It begins with cold-like symptoms, along with a very high temperature. After a few days, a blotchy red rash appears, first on the face and spreads from head to chest to abdomen, and finally to the arms and legs. Measles can be prevented with one dose of vaccine.[2,3]

Seven children singing:

> We are 7 Little Children,
> Talking just for kicks,
> But Mary began to cough,
> And now we are six.

Whooping cough character takes Mary away.

Narrator 4: Whooping cough or pertussis is very contagious and acts like a common cold with a bad cough. In severe cases pertussis can cause lungs to collapse, convulsions, and brain damage; however it can also be prevented with five special "3-in-one" doses of vaccine.[2,3,4]

Six children singing:

> We are 6 Little Children,
> Still full of pep and drive,
> Until Impetigo slowed down Bob,
> And left us as five.

Impetigo character takes Bob away.

Narrator 5: Impetigo is most common between ages one and ten and is characterized by sores covered with thick, soft, golden yellow "stuck-on" crusts of dried pus. If the lesions do not show prompt improvement or seem to spread, a physician should be consulted so that an antibiotic may be prescribed.[4]

Five children singing:

> We are 5 Little Children,
> Sifting sand by the shore,
> But Mumps bumped Paula,
> And now we are four.

Mumps character takes away Paula.

Narrator 6: Mumps is a common disease of children that results in swollen glands in the face and neck, fever, headache, and earache. Usually mumps is a mild infection, however adult men are more likely to develop complications. Mumps can be prevented with one dose of vaccine.[2,3,4]

Four children singing:

> We are 4 Little Children,
> Jumping from a tree,
> But Rusty fell on a dirty nail,
> And now we are three.

Tetanus character takes Rusty away.

Narrator 7: Tetanus, or lockjaw, is caused by a bacterium that is present just about everywhere, but mostly in soil and dust. Tetanus germs enter the body through a small cut or wound and cause stiffness of the neck and jaw muscles. Lung and windpipe paralysis may also result. Since this disease kills about half of its victims, it is very important that its occurence be prevented with five special "3-in-one" doses of vaccine.[2,3]

Three children singing:

> We are 3 Little Children,
> With bedtime overdue,
> But Beth developed Rubella,
> And that left only two.

Rubella character takes Beth away.

Narrator 8: Rubella is also called German Measles and 3-day measles. Although it is a common and usually mild disease of childhood, it is extremely dangerous to the unborn child of a woman who contracts the disease early in her pregnancy. The baby may be born with defects of the eyes, ears, heart, and other physical deformities or mental problems. The usual symptoms are a slight fever and a rash on the face and neck, which spreads to the trunk and extremities. It can be prevented with one dose of a vaccine.[2,3,4]

Two children singing:

> We are 2 Little Children,
> Always on the run,
> But Chickenpox caught Peter,
> And ruined all our fun.

Chickenpox character takes Peter away.

Narrator 9: Chicken Pox is a communicable disease that first appears as flat red splotches. The rash then becomes raised and may resemble small pimples before developing into small, fragile blisters. As the blisters break, the sores form a crust and itching is often intense. It is important to gently wash all of the skin in order to prevent a complicating bacterial infection.[3,4]

One child singing:

> Only one young child is left,
> Who's still alert and brisk,
> That's because I know the figures show,
> That immunizations cut my risk!

Immunization

Have you been fully immunized? See if you can check off all the boxes in the following chart.

Immunization Schedule for Normal Infants and Children[2]

Age	Vaccines	
2 months	Polio I	_____
	DTP I (Diphtheria, Tetanus, Pertussis)	_____
4 months	Polio II	_____
	DTP II	_____
6 months	DTP III	_____
15 months	Measles	_____
	Rubella	_____
	Mumps	_____
18 months	Polio III	_____
	DTP IV	_____
Before school	Polio IV	_____
	DTP V	_____

If you cannot check each box, you're not fully immunized. It is not too late however to call your local Health Department for free shots, or to visit your family doctor.

Disease Detective Games

In groups of four or five students, develop an original game that tests a player's knowledge of at least eight common communicable diseases, including symptoms. The construction of game boards, word games, relays, etc. are all permissible, however, the game must incorporate proven facts. The study sheets, "Communicable Disease Symptoms and Control Measures,"[5] as well as other sources of information may be used.

Materials

1. Questionnaire: "Should James Go To School?"

2. Materials for the development of Disease Detective games.

3. Study sheets: "Communicable Disease Symptoms and Control Measures."

4. "The Big 7" Childhood Communicable Disease Crossword Puzzle.

5. "Immunization" Word Search Puzzle.

Evaluation

1. Objective one is satisfied with the "Should James Go To School?" questionnaire/activity.

2. The following matching activity may be used to test recognition of common symptoms that accompany communicable diseases of childhood:

Directions: Match the letter of the symptoms in the right column with the disease in the left column that it most accurately describes.

Diseases

D	1. Chicken Pox
J	2. Common Cold
H	3. Diphtheria
B	4. Headlice
K	5. Impetigo
A	6. Measles
C	7. Mumps
F	8. Polio
I	9. Rubella
E	10. Tetanus
G	11. Whooping Cough

Symptoms

A. Cold-like symptoms and a high fever, followed by a blotchy red rash.

B. Irritation and itching of the scalp; presence of small, light gray insects or eggs.

C. Swollen glands in the face and neck, fever, and headache.

D. Red skin rash turns into blisters that form crusty scabs and cause lots of itching.

E. An often fatal illness, causing stiffness of the neck and jaw muscles following a cut or wound.

F. Fever, stiff neck, headache, paralysis of the legs or lungs.

G. Cold-like symptoms with a bad cough.

H. Sore throat, fever, and chills, followed by a patch of greyish membrane that can block air pipe.

I. Skin rash and slight fever in most cases, but extremely dangerous to unborn babies.

J. Irritated throat, watery discharge from eyes and nose; sneezing, and chilliness.

K. Blister-like sores which develop crusts of dried pus.

3. Answers to objective three: Polio, Diphtheria, Tetanus (or lockjaw), Pertussis (or Whooping cough), Measles, Rubella, and Mumps.

4. Answers to "The Big 7" Childhood Communicable Disease Crossword Puzzle are given below:

Across: 1. Diphtheria; 2. Immunization; 4. Polio; 6. Measles; 8. German; 10. Rubella; 12. Tetanus.
Down: 1. DTP; 3. Pertussis; 5. Rash; 7. Two; 9. Record; 11. Health; 13. Mumps.

5. The following words may be found in the "Immunization" word search puzzle:

rash	deformities	doctor
oral	cough	death
record	blindness	swell
lockjaw	immunization	German
polio	tetanus	pertussis
fever	sneeze	measles
whooping	vaccine	DTP
diphtheria	rubella	deafness
glands	hoarseness	pregnant
booster	pain	contagious
paralysis	throat	mumps

"Should James Go To School?"[1]

(optional) Sex _____

(optional) Race _____
Place a checkmark next to the symptoms that would cause you to keep your child home from school.

_____ Constipation	_____ Fever, Stomachache,
_____ Cough	Diarrhea
_____ Diarrhea	_____ Headache
_____ Dizziness	_____ Loss of Appetite
_____ Earache	_____ Nervousness
_____ Fever	_____ Overtired
_____ Fever, Cough	_____ Pain in Chest
_____ Fever, Cough, Running Nose	_____ Rash
_____ Fever, Cough, Sore Throat	_____ Running Nose
_____ Fever, Earache	_____ Sneezing
_____ Fever, Headache,	_____ Sore Throat
Stomachache	_____ Stiff Neck or Back
_____ Fever, Hurts All Over	_____ Stomachache
_____ Fever, Running Nose	_____ Stomachache, Diarrhea
_____ Fever, Sore Throat	

Adapted from Table 1: p. 107

Study sheets: "Communicable Disease Symptoms and Control Measures" [5]

Communicable Disease	Incubation Period	Common Symptoms	Control Measures
Measles (Rubeola)	Usually 10 days; about 14 days before rash appears	Cough, watery eyes, runny nose, fever, followed by red blotchy rash. Possible red spots on cheeks inside mouth.	Exclude from school for at least 7 days following appearance of rash. Encourage immunization.
Rubella (3-day Measles)	14–21 days; usually 18 days.	Skin rash and mild fever. Glands at back of head, behind ears may be swollen.	Exclude from school at least four days from onset of symptoms or appearance of rash. Encourage immunization.
Chicken Pox	2–3 weeks, usually 13–17 days.	Skin rash with small blisters which leave a scab. Erupts in crops.	Exclude from school for at least 7 days from appearance of first crop of blisters. May return if only dry scales remain.
Common Cold	12–72 hours; usually 24 hours.	Irritated throat, watery discharge from eyes and nose; sneezing; chilliness, general body discomfort.	Exclude from school. Symptoms may precede other communicable diseases.
Impetigo	4–10 days, occasionally longer.	Blister-like lesions which later develop into crusted pus-like sores.	Exclude from school until adequately treated and sores no longer drain. Infected persons should use separate towels and washcloths.
Conjunctivitis (Pinkeye)	24–72 hours.	Redness and swelling of membranes of the eye with burning or itching; thick, yellow discharge; light sensitivity.	Exclude from school until discharge from eyes has ceased. Use separate towels.
Infectious Hepatitis	10–50 days; commonly 30–35 days.	Loss of appetite, fever, nausea, fatigue, jaundice may appear.	Exclude from school during first 14 days of illness and at least 7 days after onset of jaundice, or longer if physician recommends.
Mumps	12–26 days; usually 18 days.	Fever, painful swelling under jaw or in front of ear.	Exclude from school at least 9 days from onset of swelling or until swelling is gone. Immunize.

Communicable Disease	Incubation Period	Common Symptoms	Control Measures
Scabies (Itch)	Several days to weeks before itching is noticed.	Small raised areas of skin containing fluid. Tiny burrow lines frequently in finger webs. Intense itching.	Exclude from school until adequately treated. Use individual towels. Observe for signs in other family members.
Headlice (Pediculosis)	Eggs (nits) of lice hatch in one week, reach sexual maturity in two weeks.	Irritation and itching of the scalp; presence of small, light gray insects or eggs attached to hairs, especially behind ears and at nape of neck.	Exclude from school until disinfestation is completed; All family members should be inspected. Treat all head gear of infected persons.
Ringworm of the Skin	10–14 days.	Ring-like lesions with slightly raised edges, gradually enlarging in size. Itching and burning possible.	Exclude from school until under medical treatment. Exclude from gym and swimming pools. Avoid common use of towels. Examine family members and pets.
Ringworm of the Foot (Athlete's Foot)	Unknown	Scaling, cracking of skin, especially between toes. Blisters containing thin fluid.	Exclusion not feasible since organism is widely distributed, however, severe cases should not be permitted in school showers. Wear socks with shoes.
Streptococcal Sore Throat/Scarlet Fever	2–5 days	Scarlet Fever—sudden onset, fever, headache, sore throat, vomiting and rash, followed by peeling of the skin. "Strep" sore throat same as above without rash or peeling.	Exclude from school for duration of illness and until discharged from isolation requirements by physician; early diagnosis and treatment are essential to prevent serious complications.
Sore Throats and Fevers	Sudden Onset	Headache, eyes may burn, general body discomfort.	Exclude from school until recovery is complete. It is suggested that students should be fever free for 24 hours before returning to school.
Whooping Cough	7–21 days	Cold-like symptoms, cough, whoop develops in about two weeks and cough may end in vomiting.	Exclude from school for at least 10 days from onset or until recovery is complete. Immunize.

"The Big 7" Childhood Communicable Disease Crossword Puzzle[2]

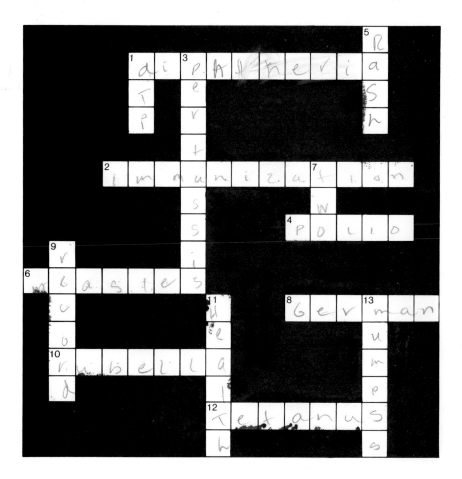

Across:

1. Contagious disease that can result in blocked breathing passages:
2. The safe and effective way to prevent diseases:
4. Before the vaccine was developed in the 1950's, _____ was a killer disease.
6. Also called red measles, and is the most serious of the common childhood diseases.
8. Rubella is also called _____ measles and 3 day measles.
10. _____ causes the greatest danger to an unborn child of a pregnant woman.
12. _____, or lockjaw, is a noncontagious disease, and picked up from dirt and dust.

Down:

1. "Short name" for a combined immunization for diphtheria, tetanus, and pertussis:
3. Also called whooping cough and may result in collapsed lung:
5. A common symptom of both rubella and rubeola is _____.
7. By the age of _____ months, 1 polio and 1 DTP immunizations should be given.
9. You and your doctor should keep a _____ of your immunizations.
11. For information about immunizations, call your local _____ department.
13. Painful, swollen glands in the face and neck and fever are symptoms of this common childhood disease:

"Immunization" Word Search Puzzle

Directions: Can you find all 33 words (including rash) related to immunization and disease in the puzzle below?

```
C A R C O N T A G I O U S X T I Z R M P
A L L E B U R R E E D R Z F R Q S I N A
B J O L J H G B C D I A O F R A S M X R
L P D E A F N E S S P S N E E Z E M D A
I O D M S S I E R X H H Y V R S N U O L
N E C R N N P A I N T O O E A E E N C Y
D R T K X D O C S T H R G R R I S I T S
N H R O J A O R A L E C L D R H R Z O I
E N T S R A H T Z R R B A I E G A A R S
S N E L X U W S C S I A N N V F O T M K
S M T U A I O R O R A T D E A T H I T L
R T A O P E R T U S S I S O C M J O N S
R C N B A A T U G P W A O R C P R N A W
E D U E P A T V H M V R U E I X I E N E
C I S E O W Y L N U T S T R N R A T G L
O U K R L P G H M M E A S L E S T S E L
R O H J I T S O B O O S T E R R O A R C
D T I F O D E F O R M I T I E S A P P L
```

Correctly use at least twenty of those words in no more than fifteen sentences.

Communicable Disease

Objectives

In Self-defense

After completing the activities suggested in this unit,

1. The student will be able to identify ten of the body's early-warning signs of possible danger in either their internal or external environment.

2. The student will be able to name the six main types of disease-producing organisms and a disease that is caused by each type of pathogen.

3. The student will be able to name five common ways in which infectious diseases may be transmitted to humans and an example of the diseases spread.

4. The student will be able to list at least five ways individuals can assist in the control and prevention of infectious diseases.

5. The student will be able to name four ways that disease germs may enter the body.

6. The student will be able to discuss how the body uses structural barriers, chemical barriers, cellular barriers, and antibodies, as defenses against infectious organisms.

7. The student will be able to discuss three major differences between active immunity and passive immunity.

8. The student will be able to differentiate between a vaccine, toxoid, antiserum, and antitoxin.

9. The student will be able to name the two most well known groups of chemotherapeutic agents used for the treatment of infectious diseases.

10. By playing "Health Detective—An Epidemiologic Instructional Simulation Game," the student will learn the basic strategy utilized by epidemiologists in their determination of the source or sources of an outbreak of a disease, condition, or disorder.

Sources

1. "What's A Germ?" *Current Health 2*, May, 1978, pp. 20-21.

2. Abram S. Benenson, Editor. *Control of Communicable Diseases in Man.* Washington, D.C.: The American Public Health Association, Twelfth Edition, 1975.

3. "The Self-Defense System," *Current Health 2*, November, 1977, pp. 3-11.

4. "Out On A Lymph With Burt Bacteria," *Go To Health*. New York: Dell Publishing Company, Inc., 1972, (Communications Research Machines, Inc.) pp. 129-136.

5. "Antibiotics: Miracle or Menace?" *Current Health 2*, September, 1977, pp. 20-21.

6. Niles L. Kaplan. "Health Detective— An Epidemiologic Instructional Simulation Game," *The Journal of School Health*, June, 1977, pp. 367-369.

Content and Procedures

Although our health and well-being is influenced by the presence or absence of various microorganisms in the environment, we usually do not give much thought to this constant interaction. Take a few minutes to see whether you can answer the following questions:

Pre and Post Test

1. Identify ten signals or signs that our bodies may use to warn us that something is wrong either within us or in our environment.

2. Name the six main types of disease-producing organisms (pathogens), and a disease that is caused by each pathogen.

3. Name five common ways in which infectious diseases may be transmitted to humans, and an example of the diseases' spread.

4. Name four ways that disease germs may enter the body.

5. Discuss how the body uses structural barriers, chemical barriers, cellular barriers, and antibodies, as defenses against infectious organisms.

6. Discuss three major differences between active immunity and passive immunity.

7. Explain the differences between a vaccine, toxoid, antiserum, and antitoxin.

8. What are the two most well-known groups of chemotherapeutic agents used for the treatment of infectious diseases?

9. Briefly describe the function of an Epidemiologist.

Warning Signs

How might the following senses detect conditions or substances in the environment that could be dangerous to us?

A. Our eyes _____ .

B. Our ears _____ .

C. Our nose _____ .

D. Our mouth _____ .

E. Our skin _____ .

(Discuss changes in light intensity, irritating noise and air pressure changes, toxic odors and noxious fumes, allergic substances, irritating chemicals and dusts, etc.)

When we are exposed to an irritating or harmful substance or organism, our body may react with some of the following symptoms: cough or throat irritation, watery eyes, runny nose, fever, sneezing, difficulty in breathing, ear ache or ringing in ears, skin that itches or is irritated, pain, headache, dizziness, loss of appetite, stomach ache, nausea, fatigue, swollen glands, chilliness, and general body discomfort.

Disease-producing Organisms

Many of the microorganisms living in, on, and around us, are beneficial. They destroy harmful microorganisms, help us digest our food and use vitamins, and turn waste matter into rich soil. Some of these microorganisms, however, are *pathogenic* (disease-producing). Each variety of pathogen causes its own disease and enters the body in its own special way. Once inside the body, these microscopic organisms head for their favorite areas in which to reproduce. For instance, the poliomyelitis virus likes nerve cells, and the typhoid bacillus chooses the cells of the lymphoid tissue of the intestinal wall.

Six Types of Disease-Producing Organisms

There are six main types of disease-producing organisms: (a) *Bacteria:* "Bacteria are single-celled, plant-like organisms which lack chlorophyll (the green coloring matter of plants)."[1] Microscopic in size, they sometimes form spores and exist for years in a dormant state until they find a suitable environment. Other bacteria, like the gonococcus which causes gonorrhea, need moisture to survive. Most diseases caused by bacteria respond to antibiotic drugs.

(Use the transparency: "Pathogenic Microorganisms" to illustrate the following organisms)

1. *Cocci* bacteria are round in shape and may appear singly (micrococci); in pairs (diplococci); in chains (streptococci); or in groups (staphylococci). They can cause diseases such as scarlet fever, boils, pneumonia, or meningitis.[1]
2. *Bacilli* bacteria are rod-shaped and may cause diseases such as tuberculosis, diphtheria, typhoid fever, tetanus, and leprosy. How would you draw streptobacilli?
3. *Spirilla* bacteria are spiral or corkscrew-shaped. They can cause diseases such as syphilis, cholera, and yaws.

(b) *Viruses:* Viruses are smaller than bacteria and different in basic structure. They are composed of a protein coat surrounding a core of nucleic acid. The core is composed of RNA or DNA. Viruses resemble nonliving crystals when they are not infecting a living cell. However, once inside a cell, they multiply, disorganize cells, and convert the cell proteins into more viruses. Scientists have identified more than 200 viruses that are capable of causing disease in humans. "Like bacteria, viruses are grouped into strains or types. For example: Adenoviruses cause respiratory disorders; Coxsackie viruses invade the digestive tract; Enteroviruses cause meningitis, and Herpes viruses cause fever blisters and a sexually-transmitted disease."[1] Influenza, the common cold, infectious mononucleosis, measles, chickenpox, mumps, rabies, infantile paralysis, smallpox, and yellow fever, are other examples of viral diseases. Unlike bacteria, viruses do not respond to antibiotics; however, vaccines have been produced that are effective in preventing some of these diseases.

(c)*Rickettsiae:* Rickettsiae are smaller than bacteria but larger than viruses. Although they resemble rod-shaped bacteria, they are like viruses in that they can grow only inside a living cell. Rickettsial diseases are usually carried by some sort of insect. For example, typhus fever is carried by body lice; Rocky Mountain Spotted fever results from a tick bite; and Encephalitis is spread by mosquitoes. Antibiotics are used to treat victims, and insecticides can be used to help eliminate the insects that spread the diseases.

(d) *Fungi:* Fungi are responsible for such infections as ringworm of the scalp or skin, athlete's foot, certain lung and ear diseases, and thrush, an infection of the lining of the mouth. Fungus plants occur in a variety of forms and sizes, ranging from large mushrooms to microscopic yeast. Griseofulvin, an oral drug, and topical fungicides are used for treatment.[2]

(e) *Parasitic Protozoa:* These are single-celled, microscopic animals that can cause amebic dysentery, African Sleeping Sickness, (through the bite of a Tsetse fly), and malaria (through the bite of a female Anopheles mosquito).

(f) *Parasitic Worms:* Parasitic worms spend part of their life cycle inside other animals. They can be seen with the unaided eye and range from small worms the size of a pinhead, to Tapeworms of 30 feet. Tapeworms may result from eating uncooked, infected fish, beef, or pork. A small roundworm can be transmitted to humans by eating insufficiently cooked pork products, with Trichinosis as the result. Pinworm disease, often found in school-age children, is also caused by an intestinal round worm.[2]

The Spread and Control of Microorganisms

The way a pathogen travels from one person to another is fascinating. How could you catch a cold from someone you did not come within a mile of? Ask the class to name typical ways various diseases are transmitted.

Activity: Using the study sheets: Transmission of Infectious Agents, as a resource, write the names of different diseases on a set of notecards. Be sure to select enough diseases so each student will be able to draw a card from a box. After each student has randomly selected his or her disease, ask them to complete the worksheet: The Transmission and Prevention of an Infectious Disease. The completed sheets may be combined in a three-ring notebook for use as a resource book throughout the year.

Activity: Another classroom activity involves shuffling the previously made disease notecards and asking each student to draw one at random from a box. Instruct the students to pin or tape the card to their clothes, and without talking, gather together in groups, depending on their disease's mode of transmission. After the groups have formed, have the students write the mode of transmission they think they have in common on a piece of paper. Distribute the study sheets, Transmission of Infectious Agents, so students can verify or correct their placement. Ask each group to think for a few minutes, then list at least five ways individuals can assist in the control and prevention of their type of infectious diseases. Share the findings.

Portals of Entry

Show the class an illustration of the human body and discuss various "portals of entry" or ways that "germs" may enter the body, e.g. broken skin; eyes; ears; nose—leading to other respiratory organs; mouth—leading to other organs of digestion; and mucous membranes of the urogenital tract.

Natural Body Defenses

Introduce the importance of natural defenses against disease organisms by describing individuals (such as infants and old people) who have weakened immunity systems. Diseases, treatment with certain drugs, and radiation, can also impair the immunity system. What do you think it would be like to spend your entire life in germ-free isolation rooms because you had been born with a rare *immunodeficiency* disease? Since your bone marrow would not produce lymphocytes and other disease fighting cells, a common cold virus could be a deadly enemy!

What type of *structural* defenses comprise the body's first line of defense? (Unbroken skin, eyelashes and tears, cilia, and sticky mucous membranes that trap microorganisms and produce chemicals that kill germs.) Special reports may be written about the following parts of the immune system: lymph nodes, spleen, bone marrow, thymus gland, and Peyer's patches.

Students may use a medical dictionary to define the following terms: Reticuloendothelial system; phagocytes; B-lymphocytes (also called B-cells); T-lymphocytes (also called T-cells); antigens; macrophage; antibodies; interferon; immunoglobulins; and inflammation.

A further understanding of natural body defenses may be obtained by reading "The Self-Defense System,"[3] and the cartoon story, "Out On A Lymph With Burt Bacteria."[4]

Immunity

Immunity is a state of high resistance to a particular disease. It is achieved by increasing the number of antibodies in a person.

	Active Immunity	Passive Immunity
Natural	1. Results from having had the disease. (The pathogenic microorganisms stimulate the body to produce antibodies which fight the disease-causing organisms) 2. Usually life-time immunity for a specific disease.	1. Results from the placental transfer of antibodies from the mother to the unborn fetus. 2. The newborn infant may acquire additional antibody protection from the first milk (colostrum) of the mother. 3. Temporary immunity against certain diseases.
Artificial (Acquired)	1. Results from being given a substance which contains either the dead or attenuated disease-causing organisms (a vaccine) or the product of the organisms (a toxoid). This stimulates the production of protective antibodies.	1. Results from being given a substance which contains the specific antibodies to fight a disease. (Antiserum) 2. This is given for protection after you have been exposed to a specific disease.

	Characteristics of Active Immunity	Characteristics of Passive Immunity
	1. The individual *produces* the antibodies within his/her own body. 2. Immunity is long-lasting. 3. There is a lapse of time before the body starts producing protective antibodies.	1. The individual *receives* the antibodies directly and does not produce them. 2. Immunity lasts only a short time. 3. Protection is acquired immediately.

Help for Body Defenses

Vaccines are given to stimulate the development of specific defense mechanisms in the body, which result in more or less permanent protection against the disease, without the risk of illness.

Nature of Vaccine	Example of Diseases Prevented
1. Vaccine contains *live, but weakened,* infectious organisms.	Smallpox, Polio (Sabin vaccine), Measles, Tuberculosis, and Yellow Fever.
2. Vaccine contains infectious organisms that have been *killed* by physical or chemical means.	Typhoid fever, Whooping cough, Polio (Salk vaccine), Rabies. Less reliable against Cholera, Dysentery, Undulant Fever.
3. *Toxoid*-vaccine contains a toxin (poison) that has been chemically treated to make it harmless.	Diphtheria, Tetanus.

Use the transparency, "Help For Body Defenses," to explain the differences between a vaccine, toxoid, antiserum, and antitoxin.

Treatment of Infectious Diseases

It was not until the early 1900's that a specific drug capable of curing disease, without causing great danger to the patient, was synthesized. Antibiotics and Sulfonamides are perhaps the two most well-known groups of chemical substances that are used for the treatment of infectious diseases.

Antibiotics

Antibiotics differ from most other chemotherapeutic agents in that they are usually obtained from living organisms (bacteria or fungi), but newer antibiotics have been produced in a chemical laboratory. They are most effective against bacterial infections and can sometimes be combined to eliminate organisms that are not completely susceptible to the action of a single antibiotic. Short descriptions of the Penicillins, "Mycins"—including Streptomycin, Cephalosporins, and Tetracyclines, can be found in the article "Antibiotics: Miracle or Menace?"[5] as well as precautions against their abuse.

Sulfonamides

Sulfonamides are a group of compounds that are effective against a wide variety of diseases ranging from urinary infections caused by gram-negative organisms to respiratory infections caused by streptococci and staphylococci. Invite a pharmacist to class to discuss the treatment of infectious diseases by chemotherapy, possible adverse reactions, and ways a consumer can be more cautious and selective in their use of drugs.

Epidemiology

Epidemiology is the division of medical science concerned with defining and explaining the inter-relationships of the host, agent, and environment in causing disease. It is sometimes thought of as medical ecology. People who study the causes of disease and work to stop epidemics, are known as *Epidemiologists.*

Do you know what agency is considered the brain center of disease detective work in the United States? It is the Center for Disease Control (CDC) in Atlanta, Georgia, one of six major agencies of the U.S. Public Health Service. Students interested in learning more about CDC should read the article, "CDC—The U.S.'s Disease Detectives," *Current Health 2,* April, 1977.

Activity: "Health Detective—An Epidemiologic Instructional Simulation Game,"[6] is an excellent class activity for depicting the basic strategy utilized by epidemiologists in their determination of the source or sources of an outbreak of a disease, condition, or disorder. After students try their luck at tracking down the contaminated food or foods that caused nine picnikers at Goodgrove Park to suffer the effects of Salmonella poisoning, they may want to devise their own "epidemic" using the same basic strategy.

Materials

1. Transparencies: "Pathogenic Microorganisms" (Included) and "Help For Body Defenses." (Included)

2. Notecards and straight pins.

3. Worksheets for each student—"The Transmission and Prevention of an Infectious Disease" (Sample included)

4. Study sheets— "Transmission of Infectious Agents" (Sample included)

5. Medical dictionary

6. Recommended Articles: "The Self-Defense System,"[3] "Out On A Lymph With Burt Bacteria,"[4] and "Health Detective—An Epidemiologic Instructional Simulation Game."[6]

7. Sample Matching Questions (Evaluation Tool) Included

Evaluation

1. Administer the Pre and Post Test again to verify an improved understanding of objectives # 1–9.

2. Students who read the cartoon story, "Out On A Lymph With Burt Bacteria,"[4] can test their understanding of the story by answering the twelve multiple choice questions that follow the article.

3. Answers to sample Matching Questions: 1. G; 2. I; 3. K; 4. J; 5. L; 6. N; 7. R; 8. S; 9. Q; 10. U; 11. Z; 12. X; 13. A; 14. B; 15. C.

_____ 1. Microorganisms that cause disease. (general term)

_____ 2. When germs cause an increase in the number of white blood cells.

_____ 3. Protection resulting from having had the disease.

_____ 4. A vaccine provides this type of immunity.

_____ 5. A newborn infant has this type of immunity.

_____ 6. The type of microorganism responsible for the common cold, mumps, and chickenpox.

_____ 7. The type of microorganism responsible for pneumonia, diphtheria, and tetanus.

_____ 8. The type of microorganism responsible for diseases that are usually carried by an insect, e. g. malaria.

_____ 9. The type of microorganism responsible for ringworm of the scalp or skin.

_____ 10. A substance used after exposure to a poison, e. g. botulism.

_____ 11. A substance used to produce immunity before exposure to germs that make a poison.

_____ 12. A substance used to produce immunity to germs before exposure.

_____ 13. Cells said to have "immunological memory" because they have the ability to remember a particular antigen.

_____ 14. Cells which are precursors of plasma cells.

_____ 15. Cells that secrete antibody

A. T-cells

B. B-cells

C. Plasma cells

D. PMNs

E. Lysozomes

F. Phagocytes

G. Pathogens

H. Immunoglobulins

I. Infection

J. Active, Artificial Immunity

K. Active, Natural Immunity

L. Passive, Natural Immunity

M. Passive, Artificial Immunity

N. Viruses

O. Parasitic Worms

P. Parasitic Protozoa

Q. Fungi

R. Bacteria

S. Rickettsiae

T. Toxin

U. Antitoxin

V. Antiserum

W. Interferon

X. Vaccine

Y. Allergoids

Z. Toxoid

Pathogenic Microorganisms

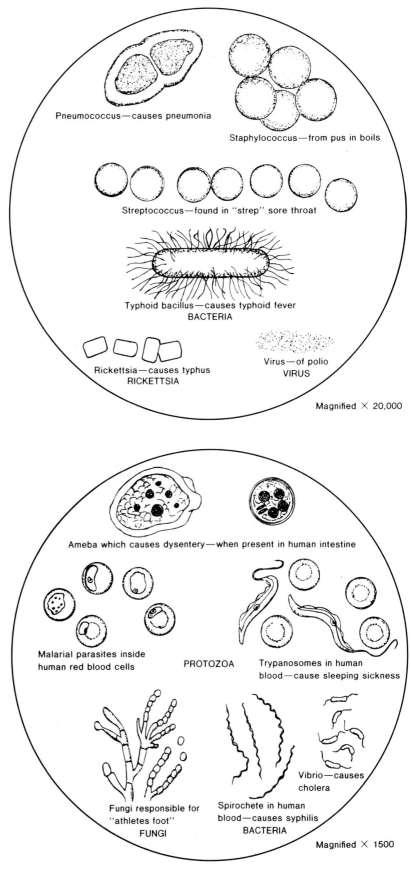

Pneumococcus—causes pneumonia

Staphylococcus—from pus in boils

Streptococcus—found in "strep" sore throat

Typhoid bacillus—causes typhoid fever
BACTERIA

Rickettsia—causes typhus
RICKETTSIA

Virus—of polio
VIRUS

Magnified × 20,000

Ameba which causes dysentery—when present in human intestine

Malarial parasites inside
human red blood cells

PROTOZOA

Trypanosomes in human
blood—cause sleeping sickness

Fungi responsible for
"athletes foot"
FUNGI

Spirochete in human
blood—causes syphilis
BACTERIA

Vibrio—causes
cholera

Magnified × 1500

Current Health 2, May, 1978, Vol. 4 #9 Curriculum Innovations, Inc.

Worksheet: *The Transmission and Prevention of an Infectious Disease*

Name of Disease: _____

How the disease can be identified: _____

_____

_____

_____

Occurrence: (How common is it? Who is most likely to get it? Where does it usually occur?)

_____

_____

_____

Infectious Agent: (The organism capable of producing the infection)

_____

Reservoir: (Where the infectious agent normally lives and multiplies, and on which it depends primarily for survival.)

_____

Mode of Transmission: _____

Incubation Period: (The time interval between exposure to an infectious agent and appearance of the first sign or symptom of the disease)

_____

Period of Communicability: _____

Preventive Measures: _____

_____

_____

_____

Specific Treatment: _____

_____

Study Sheet: Transmission of Infectious Agents[2] (pp 386–388)

(Any mechanism by which a susceptible human host is exposed to an infectious agent)

Mode of Transmission	Examples of Diseases Spread

Direct Transmission: Direct and essentially immediate transfer of infectious agents to a receptive portal of entry in man.

1. *Intimate, direct contact* with an infected human through:
  a. touching moist lesions of skin and mucous membrane;
  b. kissing (Infected saliva);
  c. sexual intercourse.
Organisms may enter through a break in the skin, mucous membranes, or urogenital tract.
	Sexually transmitted diseases including Syphilis, Gonorrhea, and Chancroid; Urethritis; Yaws; Impetigo; Boils; Athlete's Foot; Ringworm of the body; Conjunctivitis; Scabies; Scarlet Fever; Mumps; Mononucleosis.

2. Direct projection of *droplet spray* from an infected human through:
  a. sneezing
  b. coughing
  c. spitting
  d. singing, talking, etc.
Organisms may enter the conjunctiva (membrane lining eyelids), or through mucous membranes of the nose or mouth.
	Colds; Diphtheria; Scarlet Fever; Poliomyelitis; Pneumonia; Smallpox; Whooping Cough; Chickenpox; Measles; Rubella; Mumps; Influenza;

3. *Direct exposure* of susceptible tissue to:
  a. microorganisms in the soil;
  b. microorganisms in compost or decaying vegetable matter;
  c. microorganisms in animal feces.
Organisms enter through broken skin, often on the feet.
	Tetanus; Hookworm; Anthrax; Leptospirosis.

4. Direct contact with an infected *animal:*
  a. biting
  b. scratching
  c. licking
Organisms enter through a break in the skin.
	Anthrax; Rabies; Cat-Scratch Fever; Brucellosis (Undulant fever); Tularemia; Rat-Bite Fever.

Indirect Transmission

5. *Vehicle-Borne:* Infectious agent is transported into the mouth or other portal of entry through:

   a. contaminated materials or objects such as toys, handkerchiefs, soiled clothes, bedding, cooking or eating utensils, surgical instruments, or dressings.

   b. contaminated *food;*

   c. contaminated *water;*

   d. contaminated *milk;*

   e. contaminated *biological products,* including serum and plasma.

(The agent may or may not have multiplied or developed in or on the vehicle before being introduced into man.)

Athlete's Foot; Ringworm of the scalp; Ringworm of the body; Chickenpox; Measles; Rubella; Influenza; Pinworm; Typhoid Fever; Paratyphoid Fever; Shigellosis; Septic Sore Throat; Diphtheria; Brucellosis; Infectious Hepatitis; Amebic Dysentery; Cholera; Trichinosis; Salmonellosis; Botulism; other types of food poisoning and various eye-ear-nose-and throat infections.

6. *Vector-Borne:*

   a. *Mechanical:* Organism is carried by an insect that has soiled its feet or proboscis, or by passage of organisms through its gastrointestinal tract. (This does not require multiplication or development of the organism.)

   b. *Biological:* Organisms infect an insect, multiply and develop, and are then transmitted to man in saliva during biting, or by regurgitation or deposition on the skin of feces or other material that may enter a bite wound or irritated area.

Bubonic Plague (rat fleas); Rocky Mountain Spotted Fever (ticks); Typhus Fever (Body louse); Malaria (Anopheles mosquito); Typhoid Fever (House Fly); Encephalitis (mosquito); Yellow Fever (mosquito); Colorado Tick Fever (Tick);

7. *Airborne:* The dissemination of microbial aerosols to a suitable portal of entry, usually the respiratory tract. Microbial aerosols are suspensions in the air of tiny particles consisting partially or wholly of microorganisms (e. g. fungus spores). Unlike droplets and other large particles, identified under Direct Transmission, aerosols may remain suspended in the air for long periods of time.

Tuberculosis; Rubella; Influenza; Chickenpox; Histoplasmosis; Q Fever; Smallpox;

Help for Body Defenses

Vaccine—used to produce immunity to germs before exposure
  A. Germs (polio) are grown and then weakened
  B. Weakened germs are given to man as a vaccine
  C. Man then forms antibodies to polio
    germs without becoming ill
    He is now protected against the disease

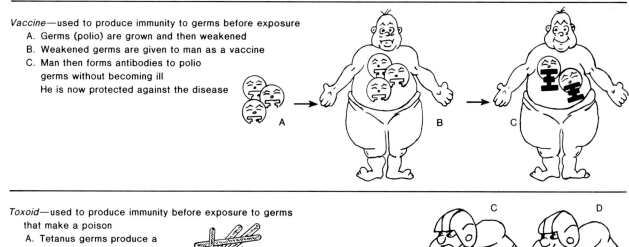

Toxoid—used to produce immunity before exposure to germs
    that make a poison
  A. Tetanus germs produce a
    poison
  B. Poison is diluted
  C. Diluted poison is given to man
  D. Man forms antibodies to weakened
    poison and is now protected against
    tetanus

Antiserum—used after exposure to a germ when there is no
time for the body to form its own antibodies
  A. Antibodies to tetanus are taken from human blood
  B. Man has been exposed to tetanus and has no antibodies
  C. Antibodies from human blood given to man to cause
    instant short-term immunity, so man survives

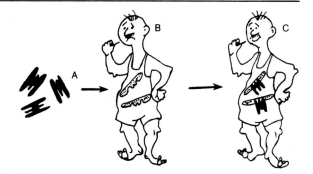

Antitoxin—used after exposure to poison
  A. Botulism germs which cause food poisoning
  B. Germs make a poison which
    is diluted
  C. Diluted poison is injected
    into horse
  D. Horse forms antibodies to poison
  E. These antibodies are given to man
    exposed to botulism
  F. Horse's antitoxin neutralizes poison,
    and man survives

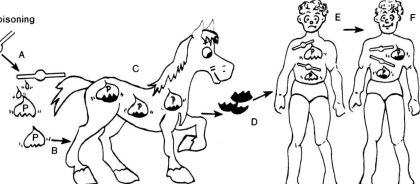

Current Health 2, Vol. 4 # 3 November, 1977 Curriculum Innovations Inc.

Objectives

1. The student will be able to recognize the signs and symptoms of Gonorrhea, Syphilis, Trichomoniasis, Herpes Simplex-2, and Candidiasis, as well as describe how these diseases are diagnosed and treated.

2. The student will be able to describe four simple measures that help to reduce one's chances of contracting a sexually transmissible disease.

3. The students will clarify their values regarding sexually-transmissible diseases by:
   a. analyzing their feelings toward people that have or had VD;
   b. placing themselves on a continuum between two extreme and polar positions; and
   c. responding to "What Would You Do If?" situations, either individually or in small groups.

4. Given a hypothetical situation in which one person of a young couple believes he or she has VD, the students (acting as the couple) will:
   a. tentatively identify the disease, based on the symptoms given to them;
   b. discuss what they will do and whom they will tell;
   c. discuss where they can go to find out if it is VD;
   d. discuss how they can prevent it from spreading and what they consider to be their responsibilities.

Sources

1. Donna Cherniak and Allan Feingold. *VD Handbook* third edition Montreal Health Press, Inc. P. O. Box 1000, Station G, Montreal, Quebec, H2W2N1, 1977.

2. Sol Gordon, Roger Conant. "VD Claptrap," Syracuse, New York: Ed-U Press, 1971. New, completely revised, 1975.

3. Warren L. McNab. "The Other" Venereal Diseases: Herpes Simplex, Trichomoniasis and Candidiasis," *The Journal of School Health,* February, 1979, pp. 79–83.

4. Theodor Rosebury. *Microbes and Morals.* New York: Ballantine Books, A division of Random House, Inc., 1971.

5. Don Breckon, Don Sweeney. "Use of Value Clarification Methods in Venereal Disease Education," *The Journal of School Health,* March, 1978, pp. 181–183.

6. Stephen J. Jerrick. "Federal Efforts To Control Sexually Transmitted Diseases," *The Journal of School Health,* September, 1978, pp. 428–432.

7. Yarber, William L. "New Directions in Venereal Disease Education," *The Family Coordinator,* April, 1978.

8. Yarber, William L. "Waging War on V. D.," *The Science Teacher,* 45:5, May, 1978.

Content and Procedures

Why Learn about STDS?

"In 1974 there were approximately three million cases of gonorrhea and one hundred thousand cases of infectious syphilis in North America. In some communities, 10–20% of young people have gonorrhea, and it is the fortunate individual who has several lovers without catching gonorrhea from one of them. The situation has reached a critical point and requires immediate action, for VD is not only an unpleasant hindrance to the free expression of human sexuality, it is also a significant drain on the health of North Americans."[1]

Critical! Various sources may not agree on the number of new cases of Gonorrhea, Syphilis, Genital Herpes, etc. in a given year, but they are of one voice in crying for immediate action. Nevertheless, only seven states (Arkansas, Florida, Hawaii, Iowa, New Hampshire, Ohio, Tennessee) and the District of Columbia, mandate instruction on venereal diseases in their schools.[6] Even in these states the quality of VD education activities is often far from optimal.

Do you think it is important for all students to go through a VD education program at least once in junior high school and once in senior high school? A higher rate of increase in new cases of gonorrhea in the U.S. is in the 0–14 age group.[5] Do you think VD education should also occur in upper elementary school?

Many experts believe that a VD unit should be taught as part of a communicable disease unit, with the sexual aspects coming out naturally as the discussion progresses, rather than as a spin-off of a basic sex education class. What do you think?

What kind of teaching methods should be used? Facts are important, and some will be included in this unit. However, it may be more beneficial to engage students in gathering pertinent information and analyzing it while formulating possible solutions, rather than presenting the material to them in lecture form. As in other areas, facts alone are not sufficient in motivating the individual to seek treatment and cooperate in the epidemiologic process, therefore, techni-ques that help students clarify their feelings, attitudes, and prejudices, have also been included.

"Venereal" (pertaining to Venus, goddess of love) Disease has traditionally referred to gonorrhea and syphilis, although some experts have always thought of it in the broader sense, i. e. "any disease that *can be* transmitted by sexual contact, which means contact between the genital organs, either of one sex with the other, as in heterosexual intercourse, or between two members of the same sex, or of the genitals of one person with any moist surface of another."[4] Some diseases, such as "crabs" (crab lice) and scabies, are not necessarily transmitted by sexual contact; and the term has brought forth unnecessary anguish in some cases.

Since other venereal diseases such as Herpes Simplex, Trichomoniasis and Candidiasis are becoming so prevalent,[3] there has been a recent movement to broaden teaching efforts to include these diseases, along with syphilis and gonorrhea, under the heading of Sexually Transmissible Diseases (STDs). These diseases not only threaten the health of millions of Americans—particularly those between the ages of 15 and 30 years, but they affect adversely the offspring of infected females.

A brief description of specific disease characteristics of some of the more common STDs (listed in order of their estimated 1976 incidence) are described below:[1,3,6]

Trichomoniasis

The most widespread sexually transmissible disease in America.

Caused by Trichomonas vaginalis, a protozoan that lives in the vagina. (As many as 50% of all women may harbor this organism; rarely produces symptoms in men)

Symptoms include intense itching and burning of the vagina and a thin foamy, yellowish discharge that may have a foul odor and cause unsightly staining.

Diagnosis can be made by microscopic examination of discharges, or by culture.

Treated with Flagyl, an oral medication.

Gonorrhea

Until recently, the incidence of gonorrhea in the U.S. had been steadily increasing for 25 years. It is still at epidemic proportions, with an estimated 2–3 million cases a year.

Caused by Gonococcus bacteria. (Outside the human body the Gonococcus dies within a few seconds)

Symptoms include a yellowish pus discharge from the penis or a burning feeling while urinating; females *may* have a discharge from the vagina and a burning sensation while urinating.

Diagnosis can be confirmed with a bacteriologic culture on special media.

Treated with more than 4 million units of penicillin, although a new threat has been posed recently by the emergence of a strain of gonorrhea resistant to penicillin.

Gonorrhea is believed to be responsible for a significant incidence of pelvic inflammatory disease and it is associated infertility and other complications, therefore, early diagnosis is very important.

Non-Gonococcal Urethritis (NGU)

A common clinical syndrome with symptoms resembling those of gonorrhea in males (urethral pain and discharge).

The incidence of NGU has increased rapidly over the past 15 years. NGU is not known to occur in women, (clinical symptoms) although they may carry the disease causing organisms in their vaginas.

Causative organisms have not been clearly established, however research studies indicate that about 40% of all cases are caused by Chlamydia and 20% by Mycoplasma.

Diagnosis of NGU is often missed because many doctors assume that any discharge from the penis is caused by gonorrhea. Urethral discharge should be tested for gonorrhea.

Treatment is often not needed, since many cases of NGU will disappear within 14 days; however, Tetracycline taken orally will eliminate the symptoms and cure the disease more quickly.

Genital Herpes (Herpes simplex virus type-2)

Genital herpes is not a reportable communicable disease, therefore no statistics are available on the exact number of people infected each year. However, it is estimated that it ranks close to gonorrhea as a commonly sexually transmissible disease.

Caused by Herpes simplex virus.

Herpes simplex is a specific name for a virus that often causes many skin problems. Type 1 attacks the upper part of the body above the waist (cold sores, fever blisters); Type 2 (genital herpes) attacks below the waist and causes repeated recurrent localized lesions that may break open and cause intense itching and extreme pain, especially during intercourse. The sores appear on the sex organs and are covered by a yellow-grey secretion.

Diagnosis is confirmed by isolation of the virus from lesions, from oral or genital mucous membranes and from semen. (Diagnosis can also be confirmed by a rise in specific neutralizing antibodies). A cotton swab is passed gently over the sore and its secretions. Cells picked up are smeared on a microscopic slide and are stained by the Pap staining technique.

Treatment can relieve pain and cause the blisters to dry up more quickly, but genital herpes is incurable at the present time.

Women who have herpes genitalis should have a Pap test for cervical cancer every 6 months for the rest of their lives. Pregnant women with this disease are much more likely to spontaneously abort; delivery through an infected canal may expose the child to the virus, irreversible brain damage, and possible death. It is also possible for the virus to spread to the unborn fetus through the placenta during pregnancy resulting in blindness, disfigurement and death.

Venereal Warts

Warts appear on genital organs 1 to 3 months after the infecting sexual intercourse. They tend to grow larger if kept moist by vaginal or urethral discharge caused by diseases such as trichomonal vaginitis and gonorrhea. Pregnancy can stimulate the warts to grow quite large.

Small warts can be easily removed by the surface application of podohyllin. Large genital warts must be removed surgically.

Pubic Lice ("Crabs")

Pubic lice are usually transmitted from person to person by the very close physical contact of sexual intercourse. In some cases, people become infested after sleeping in a bed used by a person who has pubic lice. Some people experience intense itching while other people have no symptoms.

Treatment: Pubic lice and their eggs are not affected by normal soap, but can be killed easily by the local application of a drug sold under the brand name "Kwell." After treatment, the person should have a complete change of clean clothing. (Lice die within 24 hours after separation from their human host)

Gonococcal Pelvic Inflammatory Disease

A serious and often early complication of a gonorrhea infection. Frequently requires hospitalization and may cause permanent sterility (in about one quarter of the women affected).

Syphilis

Syphilis is one of the clearest examples of how all human diseases are affected by people's physical and social environment.[1]

Effective treatment and prevention programs have enormously decreased the serious damage that occurs in late (tertiary) syphilis.

Caused by Treponema pallidum (spirochete bacteria).

Symptoms of primary syphilis occur 10–90 days after sexual intercourse with an infected person. They consist of a sore called a chancre that appears at the spot where the spirochetes entered the body and a swelling of the lymph glands in the groin.

If primary syphilis is not treated, the disease progresses silently for awhile. Two to six months after exposure germs flood through the bloodstream and secondary symptoms appear—a rash, sore throat, fever, and patchy baldness. Like the first stage, this is an extremely contagious time.

These symptoms also go away on their own, leaving the person free of outward clinical signs. (A blood test for Syphilis would be positive)

Permanent damage usually does not result until 15 to 25 years after the infection. (Tertiary Syphilis) This may include heart failure, insanity, paralysis, destruction of bone and cartilage, blindness, nerve deafness, and nonhealing skin ulcers.

Diagnosis is not easy. Syphilis has been called "the great mimic" because it can produce symptoms similar or identical to dozens of other diseases. However, the darkfield microscopic examination is an excellent test for primary syphilis when it is performed by highly trained personnel. Over 200 blood tests for syphilis have been developed, but the VDRL (The letters stand for the Venereal Disease Research Laboratory of the U.S. Public Health Dept., where the test was developed) is considered the basic blood test for syphilis. It cannot give accurate results before the disease has been present for at least 4 to 6 weeks.

Treatment of first choice: Penicillin given by injection.

Candidiasis (Yeast Infection)

Trichomoniasis and candida frequently occur at the same time as infections in the vaginal area.

Caused by the yeast-like organism, candida albicans.

Symptoms include an intense vaginal and vulva itching, vagina becomes red and dry; sexual intercourse is painful; the vaginal discharge is thick, white, curdy and resembles cream cheese.

Diagnosis is made by examining the inner walls of the vagina and through microscopic examination of material taken from a candida patch.

Treatment usually consists of an antibiotic called nystatin (Mycostatin) in the form of vaginal tablets that are inserted high in the vagina each night for at least 4 weeks. Additional nystatin may need to be taken orally.

Students who are interested in reviewing male and female anatomy that concentrates on those structures which are affected by sexually transmissible diseases as well as studying STDs in greater depth, should send for the "VD HANDBOOK, P. O. Box 1000, Station G, Montreal, Quebec, H2W 2N1. Single copies are free, except a small charge for postage and handling. The comic book, *VD Claptrap*,[2] is a short, humorous resource that still manages to be informative.

A sexually active person can help reduce his/her chances of contracting a sexually transmissible disease by "(a) avoiding contact with an infected person; (b) using condoms to reduce the incidence of venereal disease as well as pregnancy; (c) being selective in one's sexual behavior; (d) using soap and water after sexual contact, and (e) urinating by the male after intercourse."[3]

Chiappa and Forish, in their *VD Book* suggest that health educators help their students by informing them of the clinics that diagnose and treat VD in their community (including hours, location, conditions, fees—in any, and whether you would recommend them); distributing the toll free National Operation Venus helpline number (800–523–1885) as well as telephone numbers of their local VD clinics; placing classroom information on VD on school bulletin boards, publishing an article about VDs in the school paper, and making sure their library has an easily interpreted book on VD. (*Microbes and Morals*[4] is a fascinating, thorough study of venereal disease)

Activity: Ask students to plan, write, and produce a play about venereal disease. The characters may include Willy Wise (a knowledgeable student);

Irma Ignorant (a student full of myths and misinformation about venereal diseases); Cathy Clapp (a gonococcus germ); Suzie Syph (a spirochete); and possibly Harry Herpes II. By researching information to be included in the play, the students will become aware of additional facts and materials about sexually-transmitted diseases.

Who's Who in VD

How would you describe a person who contracts venereal diseases? Do you think these people fit into any kind of stereotype?

(Teacher) Select five or six famous people from the following list[4] and ask students to rank order them on the probability that they might have had a venereal disease.

Biblical figures:
    Abraham and Sarah
    the Pharaoh of Genesis
    King Abimelech of Gerar
    Miriam, David, Bath-sheba, Job.

Among Romans:
    Julius Caesar, Cleopatra,
    Herod-King of Judea,
    Tiberius-Emperor.

18th and 19th century
    John Keats, poet
    Franz Schubert, composer
    King Edward VII of England
    Lord Randolph Churchill (father of Sir Winston)
    Van Gogh, artist

(All of these people are believed to have had a venereal disease)

Ask the students to respond to "What Would You Do If?" situations,[5] either individually or in small groups. What would you do if your 14-year old brother tells you he might have VD?

What would you do if you saw your favorite teacher coming out of a VD clinic?[5]

What would you do if your wife told you that she had VD?

Students may want to create other "What If?" situations for the class to answer.

Values Continuum

Ask the student to place him/her self on the following continuums and explain why they chose to be there. Issue: Reward vs Punishment[5]

Specific Strategy: We could significantly reduce the VD epidemic by:

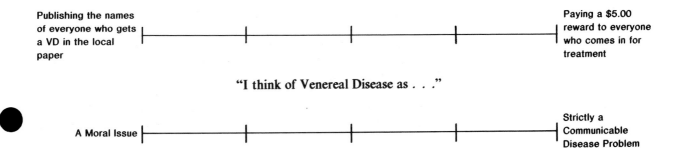

Publishing the names of everyone who gets a VD in the local paper   Paying a $5.00 reward to everyone who comes in for treatment

"I think of Venereal Disease as . . ."

A Moral Issue   Strictly a Communicable Disease Problem

Hypothetical Situation[3]

(Role playing, buzz sessions, or small problem-solving groups)

Prepare some index cards by writing down several symptoms of a sexually transmissible disease on each card. Distribute the cards to your students and instruct them to behave as if they were a young couple who had been dating for a short while, when suddenly one of the individuals develops the symptoms that you have just distributed. Ask the students to:

a. tentatively identify the disease, based on the symptoms given to them;
b. discuss what they will do and whom they will tell;
c. discuss where they can go to find out if it is VD;
d. discuss how they can prevent it from spreading and what they consider to be their responsibilities.

Materials

1. VD Game cards (Included)
2. Index cards, poster board, scissors, drawing materials.
3. Resource materials

Evaluation

1. The recognition of signs and symptoms for Gonorrhea, Syphilis, Trichomoniasis, Herpes Simplex-2, (and perhaps Non-Gonococcal Urethritis, and Candidiasis) can be tested during the hypothetical situation activity, depending upon which symptom cards the teacher chooses to distribute. (See sample cards)

(Gonorrhea)	(Syphilis)
Male partner notices a thick, creamy whitish-yellow discharge from his penis. It also *hurts* to urinate. (He had sex last weekend, 4 days ago)	(Sexually-active) male partner notices a dull red bump about the size of a pea on the fleshy tip of his penis. It changes into an open sore but does not hurt.
(Sexually-active) Female partner becomes very uncomfortable because of a heavy vaginal discharge that is frothy, whitish-yellow, & smells bad.	(Sexually-active) Male partner observes a thin, usually clear discharge coming from his penis. There is a mild pain when he urinates.
(Trichomoniasis)	(Non-Gonococcal Urethritis)

This activity is also useful for evaluating if students understand that these diseases are communicable and usually treatable. It tests a student's knowledge of when and where to seek help.

2. VD Game cards have also been included in this book. (Fifteen statements about Gonorrhea, fifteen statements about Syphilis, and five statements about other sexually-transmitted diseases have been included.) These cards may be cut out and taped to index cards for greater strength. They may be used for individual or small group review purposes. Many other games, such as the one to be described, may also be devised.

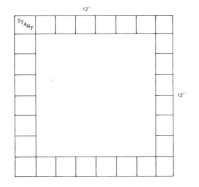

12"

START

12"

A VD Game: (Up to four players in a game) Use a standard checker board (playing area approx. 12" × 12") or make your own—see pattern. Cut out VD Game cards and randomly arrange them around the board; Each outside square may be covered or some squares designated as "Bonus" or "Penalty", may be created. Let each player draw 12 cover cards. (Make cover cards the same size as VD Game cards and write Gonorrhea or Syphilis on them; Since the VD Game cards are not written directly on the board, other Venereal diseases may be added, and cover cards with the names of additional diseases made to match them.)

Roll a die to determine the first player; Move clockwise in turn after that; Throw a die to determine the number of spaces you will move your marker;

Gonorrhea	Only the common cold is more catching than this disease	This disease usually shows up in men two to six days after sexual contact with an infected person	Slang names for this disease include "Clap", "Drip" and "Dose"	A disease caused by Gonococcus bacteria	Germs for this disease require a warm, moist environment, e.g., sexual organs, rectum, mouth, or eye
Gonorrhea	The Gonococcus germ usually has a short incubation period— grows immediately and multiplies continuously	Only 20-40% of infected females will have early warning signs of this disease. Most women are unaware . . .	Some women will have a slight discharge from vagina and a burning sensation. . . . Most of the time there are no signs	90% of all males will have a yellowish pus discharge from penis or a burning feeling while urinating	Later warning signs in the female: pelvic pain, due to infection of the fallopian tubes; Result: Sterility
Gonorrhea	Later warning signs in the male: swollen, painful testicle and heavy discharge from penis; Result: Sterility	Untreated, this disease can cause a form of arthritis, heart trouble, and general bad health	A pregnant female can pass this germ to the baby's eyes during birth process, Result: Blindness	This disease can be cured, but the "germ" is becoming more resistant; No immunity	Described in Book of Leviticus (Old Testament 1500 B.C.)
Syphilis	Commonly called "Syph" or "Pox" or "Bad Blood" "The great imitator"	A disease caused by the bacteria Spirochete	Germs for this disease are delicate and require warm, moist tissue, and rich blood circulation	Some people think Columbus spread this disease throughout Europe	The first sign of this disease is usually a sore called a chancre—does not hurt
Syphilis	A chancre usually appears where the Spirochetes enter the body; Heals within 1-6 weeks, without treatment	First stage of this disease is extremely contagious; occurs from 10 to 90 days after exposure (sore usually appears within 21 days)	90% of females and 40%-60% of males, do not recall chancre because it is painless and often hidden . . . (inside vagina)	A blood test can detect this disease 7-10 days after the sore appears and will continue to be positive	This disease becomes a Total body infection (Systemic)
Syphilis	The second stage of this disease occurs 2-6 months after exposure—extremely contagious (rash, patchy baldness)	After rash disappears, germs become dormant; person is not contagious (Latent stage)	Untreated, this disease can cause damage to heart, brain, bones, eyes, ears, and skin	Disease can be passed via bloodstream from infected mother, thru placenta, to unborn child	Medical treatment of infected pregnant woman prior to 7th month, will cure both mother and child
	A viral disease causing groups of painful sores or blisters on the sex organs—sores break open and ooze yellow-grey pus	Women who have had this disease have higher chance of developing cancer of the cervix; need Pap smear every 6 months	NGU—an infection of the urinary tract, which if left untreated, may spread to a man's prostate gland	"Trich"—a disease that inflames the vagina—redness and itchiness; smelly, foul discharge	An acute, localized, sore, limited infection—painful ulcerations—caused by a bacillus
	Chancroid	Trichomonas Vaginalis	Non-Gonococcal Urethritis	Herpes II	Herpes II

Each square represents a statement about a certain venereal disease. When you land on an uncovered square, determine which venereal disease is being described and cover it with an appropriate cover card. If you land on a square already covered or if you do not have a cover card with the correct answer, better luck next time! Next player moves;

Challenges: If you think another player has laid down an incorrect card, you may challenge. (Turn the VD Game card over to check correct answer) If you're right, you get to lay down the correct card if you have it. (He removes his) If you are wrong, you must keep your card and the original player may put an additional correct cover card on the top of the first;

The winner is the first player to use up all of his cards or have the fewest left after all the squares have been covered.

Selected Learning Activities

Communicable Diseases

_____ Create a bulletin board illustrating various disease sources and ways diseases are spread.

_____ Visit your city health department and learn what is being done to control communicable diseases in your community.

_____ Given a list of common household pets and diseases that can be transmitted from animal to man, match the pet with disease.

_____ Ask various senior citizens to recall outbreaks of cholera, diphtheria, polio, smallpox, etc.

_____ Bring in current news items related to communicable diseases and their prevention.

_____ Ask students to construct a graph which compares the leading communicable diseases in 1900 to those of today.

_____ Select a communicable disease and give a five minute presentation to the class. Among the points to be brought out are causes, signs and symptoms, care, treatment, and prevention.

_____ Write an essay on how to prevent the spread of communicable disease.

_____ Write a position paper on the merits and demerits of vitamin C.

_____ Invite a guest speaker from the local department of health to lecture on the role (s)he plays in halting the spread of disease.

_____ Divide the class in groups of three, play "Stump the Panel." Each of the three panels will present a disease—syphilis, gonorrhea, and herpes simplex II. The remainder of the class must ask questions which the panel must answer. Incorrect answers will score points for the "askers" and correct answers will score points for the "answerers."

_____ Construct a collage about a communicable disease.

_____ Compile a list of possible reasons why communicable diseases are spread.

_____ List five ways diseases can be prevented from spreading in your home.

_____ Write an essay on your most feared communicable disease.

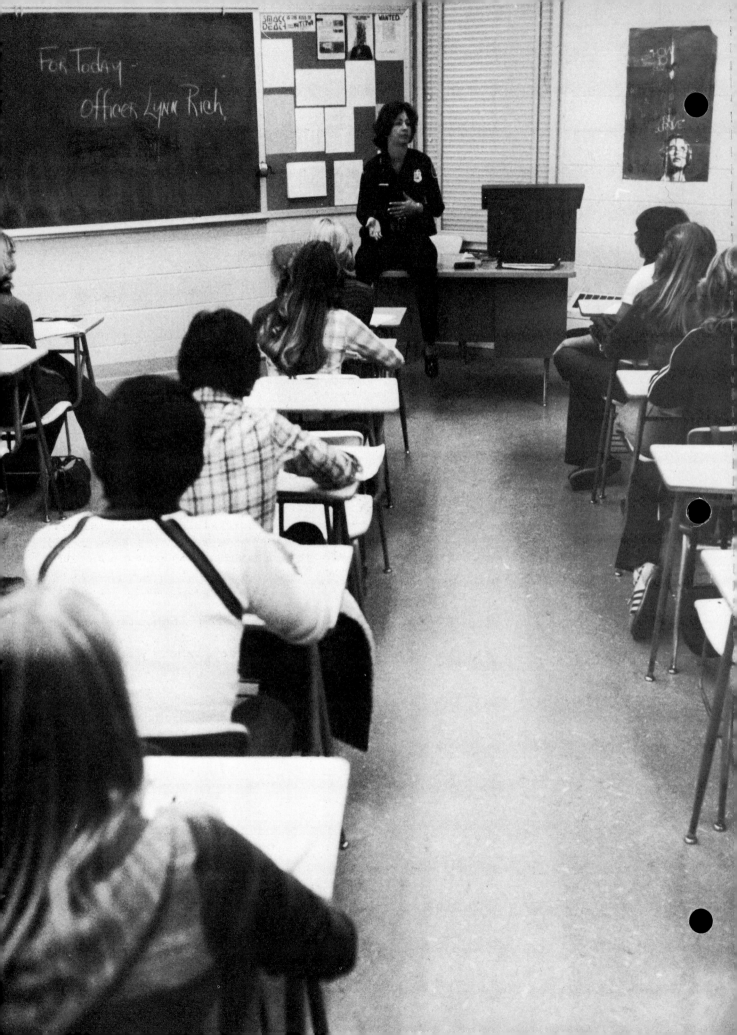

19

Teaching about First Aid and Safety

During the adolescent years the possibility of accidents and the need for first aid are especially prevalent. This chapter includes an outline of Suggested Topics for Teaching About First Aid and Safety, Three Detailed Sample Lessons which deal directly with the most important concerns of adolescence, and additional Suggested Learning Activities.

The first lesson, **First Aid,** identifies the four emergency situations— stoppage of breathing, severe bleeding, poisoning, and shock—which middle and secondary school students might experience. The student learns to demonstrate proper first aid procedures for each of these situations. The lesson also includes information on epilepsy and on dealing with a seizure, as well as information on diabetes and dealing with diabetic coma or with insulin shock. Finally the student is familiarized with the Good Samaritan Laws pertaining to emergency medical services that are applicable to the different States.

The second lesson deals with **Traffic Safety.** With the student beginning to drive or at least thinking about the license in the coming years, traffic safety is an especially important topic. The lesson is particularly directed toward developing sound values and toward enabling the students to identify behaviors that would be helpful in increasing their safety in traffic situations.

In the third lesson, **Accident Prevention,** several types of accidents such as poisoning and fire are discussed. The student examines his or her role in the prevention of accidents.

Suggested Topics

First Aid and Safety

I. Introduction to First Aid
  A. Defining First Aid
  B. Reasons for First Aid
  C. The Value and Purpose of First Aid Training
  D. Good Samaritan Statutes

II. Situations Requiring First Aid
   A. Wounds: Common Causes; Types; Symptoms; Stoppage of Bleeding
   B. Injuries to Specific Body Parts: Appropriate Treatment
   C. Shock: Causes; Symptoms; First Aid
   D. Respiratory Emergencies/CPR
   E. Choking: Causes; Symptoms; First Aid; Prevention
   F. Poisoning and Drug Overdoses: Symptoms; First Aid; Prevention
   G. Burns: Classification; First Aid; Prevention
   H. Frostbite and Exposure to Extreme Cold: Symptoms; First Aid
   I. Stroke, Cramps, or Exhaustion—Due to Heat: Symptoms; First Aid
   J. Sudden Illness
III. Common Athletic Injuries
   A. Causes
   B. Symptoms
   C. Application of Dressings and Bandages
   D. Prevention
IV. Transportation of the Sick and Injured
V. Introduction to Safety
   A. Defining Safety-Related Terms
   B. Understanding Accident Statistics
   C. Accident Causes and Countermeasures
       1. Home Accidents
       2. Yard and Garden Safety
       3. Traffic Safety
       4. Recreational Safety
       5. Water Safety
       6. Safety Around Animals
   D. Accident Proneness
   E. Organizations and Agencies Concerned With Safety
       1. Engineering
       2. Enforcement
       3. Education

Lesson Plans

First Aid and Safety
First Aid

Objectives

1. The student will be able to identify the four emergency situations where aid is urgently needed.

2. The student will be able to demonstrate proper first aid for stoppage of breathing, severe bleeding, poisoning, and shock.

3. The student will be able to distinguish between impending diabetic coma and insulin shock.

4. The student will be able to describe the procedure to be followed when witnessing a *major* epileptic seizure.

5. The student will be able to describe the Good Samaritan laws, pertaining to emergency medical services, that are applicable to his/her state.

Sources

1. "When Will People Help?" *Current Health 2,* November, 1978, p. 24.

2. "The Unconscious Challenge," *Current Health 2,* April, 1979, pp. 20–21.

3. The American National Red Cross. Poster: "When Breathing Stops," (Revised, April, 1978) Garden City, New York: Doubleday and Company, Inc.

4. The Ohio Department of Health. "First Aid For Food Choking," Columbus, Ohio, 1977.

5. The American National Red Cross. *Standard First Aid and Personal Safety.* Garden City, New York: Doubleday and Company, Inc., 1977.

6. John J. Burt, L. Meeks, S. Pottebaum. *Toward a Healthy Lifestyle Through Elementary Health Education.* Belmont, California: Wadsworth Publishing Company, 1980.

7. The American National Red Cross. Poster: "The American Red Cross Attacks Poisons," Garden City, New York: Doubleday and Company, Inc., 1977.

Content and Procedures

What Would You Do?

What would you do if you suddenly came across an apparently unconscious person, lying on his back in an almost dark and nearly empty parking lot?[2]

When "innocent bystanders" fail to aid people in need of help, it is often due to one of four basic reasons:

1. The potential helper may not notice anything is wrong or that help is needed.

2. The potential helper assumes someone else will help.

3. The helper is not willing to take personal responsibility for someone else.

4. The potential helper does not know what to do and "freezes."[1]

What You Could Do?

In the situation given, reasons one and two are probably not applicable; however, when a lot of people are present during an emergency, there is a much greater likelihood that no individual will take the needed action. Reason 4 is perhaps the easiest to avoid. By enrolling in accredited First Aid and CPR courses, an individual can increase his/her ability to react calmly and without error in a life-saving manner. It is desirable to refresh ones memory every few years through instruction offered as a part of on-going safety programs in industries, schools and colleges, and by hospitals, the Red Cross, and fire departments, and to encourage family members to take first aid training as well.

1. As a knowledgeable individual, who has determined that the victim described in our earlier example is indeed unconscious by loudly asking, "Are you awake?", your first concerns are to check for _____ and to look for _____.
Does the chest rise and fall? Can you hear or feel air coming from the victim's nose or mouth? If the person is *not* breathing, follow the procedures described in Table 19.1: "When Breathing Stops."[3] Artificial respiration can be lifesaving when breathing has ceased due to electric shock, drowning, gas poisoning, drugs such as morphine, opium, barbiturates and alcohol, compression of the chest, choking and strangling, and partial obstruction of the breathing passages. Artificial respiration should be continued until the victim begins to breathe for himself, is pronounced

dead by a doctor, or is dead beyond any doubt. *Activity:* Try practicing this technique on a manikin borrowed from your Red Cross or Heart Association.

2. If you seem unable to inflate the lungs, the victim's airway may be obstructed. Skin that appears a dusky *blue* indicates the immediate need for oxygen. By using the "Heimlich Maneuver,"[4] you can exert pressure that forces the diaphragm upward, compressing air into the lungs, and thus expelling the object that is blocking the breathing passage.
   —With the victim lying face up, kneel astride the victim, face to face. With one of your hands on top of the other, place heel of bottom hand on victim's abdomen below the rib cage and slightly above the navel. With a quick upward thrust, press forcefully into the victim's abdomen and repeat several times if necessary.
   —If you reach a choking victim who is still conscious but unable to speak, cough, or breathe, and clutching his throat, stand behind the victim and wrap your arms around the victim's waist. (If the victim is in a sitting position, the rescuer should kneel behind to apply H. M.). Place your fist, thumb-side in, against the victim's abdomen below the rib cage and slightly above the navel. Grasp your fist with the other hand and press the fist forcefully, with a quick upward thrust, into the victim's abdomen. NOTE: The American Red Cross recommends delivering four sharp blows with the heel of your hand over the victim's spine, between the shoulder blades, before administering the abdominal thrusts. *Activity:* Practice the hand positions and general actions of the Heimlich maneuver on each other *without* giving actual back blows or abdominal thrusts.

3. Can you locate evidence of a pulse at the carotid artery, located in the side of the neck? When a person's heart stops, his breathing will also stop within a few seconds. In this case, you must immediately restore both breathing and circulation (CPR—cardiopulmonary resuscitation) or the individual will die. This requires special supplemental instuction and practice with a manikin, but the generel procedure consists of applying a rhythmic pressure over the lower half of the sternum while giving artificial ventilation.

4. If the victim is breathing, but severe bleeding is a problem, what are your four objectives?

_____

_____

Apply *direct pressure* over the wound, using a clean cloth or sterile gauze pad if one is available. It is possible to bleed to death in a matter of minutes if a large artery has been severed, but in most cases the natural clotting process will soon diminish the flow of blood. After the bleeding has been controlled, apply additional layers of cloth without removing the original dressing and disturbing the blood clots; bandage firmly. If there is no evidence of a fracture, it also helps to *elevate* the injured part of the body above the level of the victim's heart in order to reduce blood pressure in the injured area. If bleeding continues, exert pressure with your fingers or hand over the nearest arterial *pressure point* to temporarily compress the artery supplying blood to the affected limb, but do not use a pressure point in conjunction with direct pressure and elevation any longer than is necessary to stop the bleeding. A *tourniquet* (an extremely tight bandage wrapped around an arm or leg to stop hemorrhaging) is a very dangerous device that is rarely justified except in critical emergencies that are life-threatening.[5] *Activity:* Practice treating each other for severe bleeding. NOTE: No attempt should be made to cleanse *serious* wound,

Table 19.1

WHEN BREATHING STOPS[3]

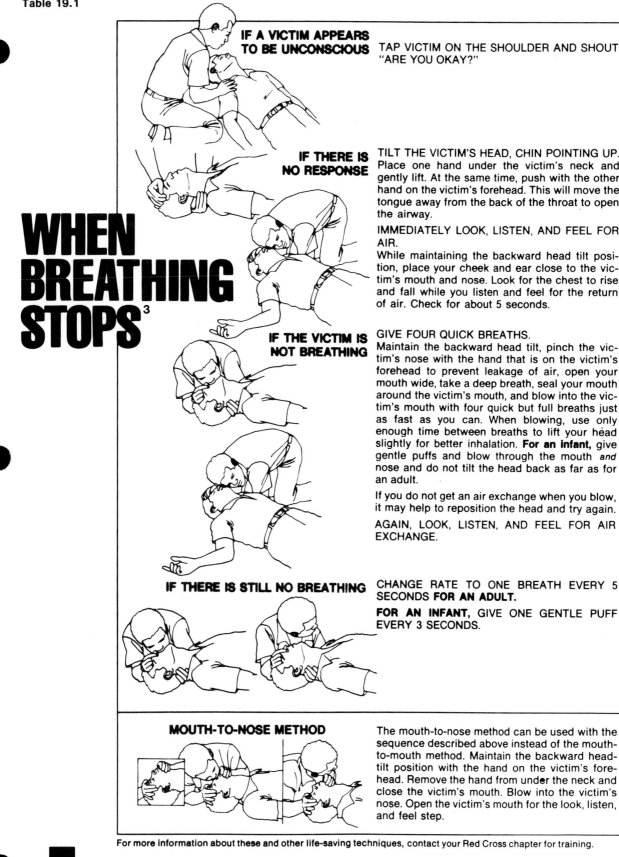

IF A VICTIM APPEARS TO BE UNCONSCIOUS TAP VICTIM ON THE SHOULDER AND SHOUT, "ARE YOU OKAY?"

IF THERE IS NO RESPONSE TILT THE VICTIM'S HEAD, CHIN POINTING UP. Place one hand under the victim's neck and gently lift. At the same time, push with the other hand on the victim's forehead. This will move the tongue away from the back of the throat to open the airway.

IMMEDIATELY LOOK, LISTEN, AND FEEL FOR AIR.

While maintaining the backward head tilt position, place your cheek and ear close to the victim's mouth and nose. Look for the chest to rise and fall while you listen and feel for the return of air. Check for about 5 seconds.

IF THE VICTIM IS NOT BREATHING GIVE FOUR QUICK BREATHS.

Maintain the backward head tilt, pinch the victim's nose with the hand that is on the victim's forehead to prevent leakage of air, open your mouth wide, take a deep breath, seal your mouth around the victim's mouth, and blow into the victim's mouth with four quick but full breaths just as fast as you can. When blowing, use only enough time between breaths to lift your head slightly for better inhalation. **For an infant,** give gentle puffs and blow through the mouth *and* nose and do not tilt the head back as far as for an adult.

If you do not get an air exchange when you blow, it may help to reposition the head and try again.

AGAIN, LOOK, LISTEN, AND FEEL FOR AIR EXCHANGE.

IF THERE IS STILL NO BREATHING CHANGE RATE TO ONE BREATH EVERY 5 SECONDS **FOR AN ADULT.**

FOR AN INFANT, GIVE ONE GENTLE PUFF EVERY 3 SECONDS.

MOUTH-TO-NOSE METHOD The mouth-to-nose method can be used with the sequence described above instead of the mouth-to-mouth method. Maintain the backward head-tilt position with the hand on the victim's forehead. Remove the hand from under the neck and close the victim's mouth. Blow into the victim's nose. Open the victim's mouth for the look, listen, and feel step.

For more information about these and other life-saving techniques, contact your Red Cross chapter for training.

AMERICAN RED CROSS   ARTIFICIAL RESPIRATION

however, when wounds are minor they should be cleansed thoroughly, using soap and water, to lessen the danger of infection. Minor wounds may be blotted dry with a sterile gauze pad and covered with a dry sterile bandage.

5. If the victim's skin color appears *red*, rather than bluish, what might be the trouble? _____

_____

Look for other clues. Smell his breath. If you detect an acetone or peculiar fruity odor, this is another sign of a diabetic coma. See table 19.2 for signs and symptoms of diabetic coma and shock.[6] Check to see if the victim is wearing a *Medic Alert* I.D. for diabetes.

Medic Alert is a foundation that exists to protect the victim of a chronic condition from the risk of wrong treatment or non-recognition of the problem by providing vital data in an emergency situation. A necklace or bracelet may be purchased for a small charge; this bears the Medic Alert emblem, the condition you specify (such as, "Allergic to Penicillin"), an identifying serial number and a telephone number that may be called collect, at any hour of the day or night, by medical personnel, police, etc. The telephone number is that of a central file which contains all relevant information you wish to have available. For further information, write to the Medic Alert Foundation, Turlock, California, 95380.

6. If the victim's tongue has been bitten, he may have just experienced a major epileptic seizure and will probably recover consciousness within a few minutes. A major epileptic seizure does not require expert care or transportation to an emergency room, however, it can be frightening to watch if the bystander does not understand what is happening.

Keep calm. You cannot stop a seizure once it has started. Reassure young observers that the person is not in pain, will be okay very soon, and that they can not "catch it." If you can, ease the person to the floor and try to prevent him from striking his head or body against any hard, sharp, or hot objects, but do not interfere with his movements. *Do not* force a blunt object between the victim's teeth since you may injure the teeth or gums. When the jerking is over, loosen clothing around the neck and turn the person on his side, face pointed downward, so that saliva or vomitus can drain out and not be inhaled. During a seizure there is increased salivation and the saliva may appear frothy and bloody. After the seizure is over the victim may seem groggy, confused or weak and wish to rest before returning to his business. If jerking of the body does not stop within five minutes (time the seizure) or keeps recurring, medical assistance should be obtained.[6]

7. *Look at the victim's eyes.* What do dilated pupils often indicate? Check the skull and the ear canals for blood. What do constricted pupils (pinpoints) indicate? _____
If the pupils are of unequal size, what would you suspect? _____
Elevate the head and shoulders.[2]

8. What would you suspect if you found pill bottles in the victim's pockets, burns around the lips or mouth, or a chemical odor on the breath? ____

_____

See Table 19.3 for more information about this third type of emergency that requires immediate attention.

Table 19.2
Diabetes Emergencies[6]

	Impending Diabetic Coma	Impending Insulin Shock
	(Hyperglycemia, too much sugar in the blood; not enough insulin)	(Too much insulin, or too little food with usual doses of insulin; children are prone to it because of their higher level of activity and lower sugar reserves)
Onset	Unconsciousness is usually fairly slow in developing.	Sudden; fainting may develop without warning.
Hunger and Thirst	Intense thirst; dry mouth. Frequent urination.	Hunger
Skin	Dry, flushed.	Cold sweat, pale.
Breathing	Deep and rapid.	Shallow or normal.
Gastrointestinal	Nausea and vomiting sometimes occur.	Gnawing sensation in stomach.
Other Symptoms	Drowsiness; confusion; breath has a peculiar fruity odor.	Weakness; dizziness; jittery feeling; tremor of the hands; dimness of vision; change in personality.
First Aid	There is no adequate first aid treatment; immediate hospital treatment is necessary, including an injection of insulin.	If conscious, raise blood sugar concentration as quickly as possible—candy, soft drinks, sugar, fruit juice, or anything sweet; hypoglycemia with unconsciousness is an extremely urgent medical emergency—rush person to hospital for an immediate intravenous injection of dextrose or glucagon.

9. Although it is not wise to move a victim unless it is necessary for safety reasons, you should treat for traumatic shock, a condition "resulting from a depressed state of many vital body functions."[5] (p. 60) This is done by positioning the victim so as to improve blood circulation. An unconscious victim should be placed on his side to allow drainage of fluids and to avoid blockage of the airway by vomitus and blood. Be careful to maintain an open airway and to keep the victim from chilling. If the victim is exposed to cold or dampness, place blankets over and under him if possible. *Activity:* Learn how to treat for shock when the victim is conscious.

10. As soon as you attract help, send for medical assistance. Your goal is to keep the victim alive until help comes and to remain in charge until the victim can be turned over to qualified medical personnel. A first-aider does not attempt to diagnose or discuss a victim's condition with bystanders or reporters.

Table 19.3
The American Red Cross Attacks Poisons[7]

IS IT POISON?

Symptoms vary greatly. Base your suspicion that a person has swallowed poison on—
- Information from the victim or an observer
- Presence of a poison container
- Sudden onset of pain or illness
- Burns around the lips or mouth
- Chemical odor on the breath
- Pupils contracted or dilated

FIRST AID FOR POISON BY MOUTH

Conscious victim:
- *Dilute* the poison *with a glass of water or milk* if the victim is not having convulsions.
- *Call the poison control center* or your doctor or dial 0 or 911; call the emergency rescue squad.
- Save the label or container for identification; save vomited material for analysis.
- *Do not* neutralize with counteragents. *Do not* give oils.
- If the victim becomes unconscious, keep his airway open.

Unconscious victim:
- Maintain an open airway.
- Call the emergency rescue squad.
- Give mouth-to-mouth resuscitation or cardiopulmonary resuscitation (CPR) if necessary.
- *Do not* give fluids; *do not* induce vomiting; if the victim is vomiting, position his head so that vomit drains from his mouth.
- Save the label or the container for identification; save vomited material for analysis.

Convulsions:
- Call the emergency squad as soon as possible.
- *Do not* attempt to restrain the victim; try to position him so that he will not injure himself.
- Loosen tight clothing.
- Watch for obstruction of the airway and correct it by tilting the head; give mouth-to-mouth resuscitation or CPR if necessary.
- *Do not* force a hard object or finger between the teeth.
- *Do not* give any fluids.
- *Do not* induce vomiting.

- After a convulsion, turn the victim on his side or in the prone position, with his head turned to allow fluid to drain from his mouth.

Instructions on product labels for specific treatment of poisoning *may* be wrong; contact your doctor or a poison control center for instructions.

Have on hand
These products should be used *only* on the advice of your doctor or the poison control center.
1. *Syrup of ipecac* (to induce vomiting)
2. *Activated charcoal* (to bind, or deactivate, poison)
3. *Epsom salts* (a laxative)

If poisoning occurs where medical help is unavailable (e.g., camping), you may induce vomiting if the victim has taken an overdose of drugs or medication, but *not* if a strong acid, alkali, or petroleum product has been swallowed. Then get the victim to a hospital as quickly as possible.

Emergency telephone numbers

DOCTOR _____

RESCUE SQUAD _____

POISON CONTROL _____
    CENTER

Write in these numbers now! Have the family memorize them. Also place them on your telephone.

The information on this poster is based on a report prepared by the National Academy of Sciences—National Research Council, Committee on Emergency Medical Services.

How did you do? Do you think you could handle a situation involving an unconscious person? It is one of the most challenging emergencies that exists.

You should be aware of the legal implications of your acts and know that, contrary to common belief, you probably will not be held liable for attempting to provide emergency assistance. Check with your state's department of transportation or motor vehicles to learn of the *Good Samaritan laws* that apply within your state. These laws have been enacted in a number of states to counteract the reluctance of many individuals to aid traffic accident victims.

Materials

1. American Red Cross posters: "When Breathing Stops", and "The American Red Cross Attacks Poisons". (Included)

2. Copy of your State Statutes Pertaining to Emergency Medical Services (Good Semaritan Laws).

3. Optional: Samples of Syrup of Ipecac, activated charcoal and Epsom Salts.

Evaluation

1. Using a manikin, ask the student to properly demonstrate how to perform mouth-to-mouth resuscitation on a adult and verbally explain how the procedure is modified when breathing into an infant.

2. Ask the student to demonstrate the proper hand positions and general actions of the Heimlich maneuver on another student *without* giving actual back blows or abdominal thrusts.

3. Ask the student to demonstrate his/her skill at controlling severe bleeding of the lower arm. The student should correctly (a) apply direct pressure over the wound, (b) elevate the injured arm, and (c) exert pressure on the correct pressure point (brachial artery).

4. Ask the student to role-play various emergency situations and demonstate proper first aid techniques. (Include stoppage of breathing, severe bleeding, poisoning, and shock).

5. What should be done for a known diabetic who suddenly becomes pale, sweaty, dizzy and is about to faint? (Treat for impending insulin shock by raising the blood sugar, e.g. give them a candy bar, soft drink, fruit juice, etc.).

6. Ask students to list four actions they would or would not do for a victim of a major epileptic seizure.

7. Ask students to describe the Good Samaritan laws that apply to their state. If no law protects the ordinary citizen in your state, ask the students what they would do if they came across an injured person.

8. Check to see if you filled in the blanks during the lesson with the following answers:

Item 1. Check for *breathing* and look for *severe bleeding*.

Item 4. Objectives when treating severe bleeding: stop the bleeding; protect the wound from contamination and infection; provide treatment for shock; and obtain medical attention.

Item 5. Red skin color may indicate heat stroke, carbon monoxide poisoning, diabetic coma, etc.

Item 7. Dilated pupils may indicate a head injury. Constricted pupils may indicate an overdose of narcotics. Pupils of unequal size are a sign of brain injury.

Item 8. Drug overdose or poisoning.

First Aid and Safety
Traffic Safety

Objectives

1. After reading the pamphlet, "Defensive Driving," the student will be able to identify the correct way to use the "2-second following distance" and will be able to describe the purpose of the "4-second rule" and the "12-second visual lead time."

2. The student who drives on freeways will read the pamphlet "Freeway Driving Demands Special Skills," and be able to identify maintenance steps that should be taken to prepare for freeway driving; describe the importance of and procedures for advance route planning; identify the correct procedures for entering and leaving the freeway, passing, and lane changing; and describe factors that influence lane and speed selection.

3. The student will be able to explore his/her feelings, values, and attitudes regarding drinking and driving and the use of motorcycle helmets, through the use of Value Ranking, Case Situation and Value continuum activities.

4. After reading the articles, "What You Think You Know Can Skill You," and "Safety Restraint Systems," the student will be able to identify myths related to seat belts and explain why these beliefs are not true.

5. After analyzing a series of photographs depicting specific problems concerning lane positioning, the student will be able to ascertain safe ways to react when encountering various traffic situations while cycling.

6. The student will be able to demonstrate how to use a tire gauge, properly examine bicycle tires, adjust a bicycle seat and handlebars for a proper fit, and how to oil and clean the moving parts of a bicycle.

7. The student will be able to identify some behavior or characteristic which they would like to change in order to increase their safety in traffic situations.

Resources

1. Donald LaFond. "10 Traffic Safety Guides", Falls Church, Virginia: American Automobile Association, 1978. (Guides rewritten annually)

2. To ascertain the availability of these or other AAA materials, please contact your local AAA club. If there is no local office listed in your telephone directory, contact the Traffic Engineering and Safety Department, American Automobile Association, Falls Church, Virginia 22047.

3. "Accident Prevention—More Than Hit or Miss," *Current Health 2*, May, 1978, pp. 3-13.

4. Alton L. Thygerson. *Safety Concepts and Instruction*, Second Edition. Englewood Cliffs, New Jersey: Prentice-Hall, Inc., © 1976. pp. 43, 117, 120 reprinted by permission.

5. "Auto Safety Myths—What You Think You Know Can Kill You," *Family Health*, September, 1976, p. 36.

6. "Bicycles—Buy Right, Drive Right." Write to Bicycle Safety, U.S. Consumer Product Safety Commission, Washington, D.C. 20207, or call the toll free consumer Hot Line—800-638-2666 (Maryland residents should call 800-492-2937).

**Content and
Procedures**

As a teacher, you are a key person in guiding the growth and development of your students' traffic habits. The community and your students both benefit when you include instruction about the WHATS, WHYS, and HOWS of traffic safety.

Traffic Accident Prevention Program Checklist

The American Automobile Association has prepared the following "Traffic Accident Prevention Program Checklists" for inclusion in each of their 1979 Teacher's Guides and suggests that you use this list for ongoing evaluation. "Does your school's traffic safety education program:

_____ Analyze school accident records to determine the extent of school traffic problems?

_____ Plan a coordinated traffic accident prevention program?

_____ Conduct an effective traffic safety education program?

_____ Maintain an effective School Safety Patrol?

_____ Stimulate community action to provide safe crossings and play areas?

_____ Evaluate the effectiveness of the program?

In your own classroom traffic safety education program, do you:

_____ Place emphasis on learning what actions to take in traffic?

_____ Prepare students to evaluate high risk traffic situations?

_____ Consider the traffic safety habits of students in after school hours?

_____ Demonstrate proficient pedestrian, driver, and passenger behavior?

_____ Involve parents in the activities?

_____ Evaluate whether students are becoming more self-reliant in traffic situations?"[1]

A classroom traffic safety education program may cover some or all of the following topics:

I. *Safe Use of an Automobile*
   A. Defensive Driving Quiz

_____ 1. Do you know the correct way to use the "2-second following distance"?

_____ 2. Can you describe the purpose of the "4-second rule" and the "12-second visual lead time"?

_____ 3. Can you describe the use of three techniques that are necessary for efficient lateral (side) positioning?

_____ 4. Do you know how to make accurate decisions in traffic and how to efficiently manage time and space?

If you are unsure of the answers to some of these questions, read the American Automobile Association pamphlet, "Defensive Driving—Managing Time and Space."[2] (Stock #3389)

   B. The American Automobile Association will provide drivers with a pamphlet, "How to Go On Ice and Snow," (Stock #3387) which lists steps that should be followed in preparing your car for winter.

C. Ask students who sometimes drive on freeways if they are able to:

_____ 1. identify maintenance steps that should be taken to prepare for freeway driving.

_____ 2. describe the importance of and procedures for advance route planning.

_____ 3. identify the correct procedures for entering and leaving the freeway, passing and lane changing.

_____ 4. describe ways to deal with problems that could occur when entering, exiting and lane changing maneuvers are attempted.

_____ 5. describe factors that influence lane and speed selection.

_____ 6. identify space management techniques that freeway drivers need to employ.

These topics are discussed in the pamphlet, "Freeway Driving Demands Special Skills."[2] (Stock #3396)

D. Discuss the role of alcohol consumption as it relates to the prevalence of traffic injuries and fatalities. According to the Alcohol and Highway Safety Report: "The use of alcohol by drivers and pedestrians leads to some 25,000 deaths and a total of at least 800,000 crashes in the United States each year." Alcohol seems to be a factor in at least half of all fatal auto accidents, with 18 and 19-year olds being the age group most apt to be involved in an accident that involves drinking.[3]

Value Ranking Activities[4] (p. 117)
Rank according to why people drink and drive:
_____ peer pressure
_____ show off
_____ need to drive to and from drinking place
_____ immaturity
Rank according to those you would like legal action taken against:
_____ social drinking driver
_____ problem drinking driver
_____ drug abusing driver
_____ driver convicted of previous manslaughter
_____ underaged driver

Case Situation[4] (pp. 119–120)
Duplicate the following case situation and alternatives for every member of your class. Ask the student to mark his/her choice(s) among the alternatives and then conduct a class discussion centering upon which of the choices is best and why. The teacher may wish to document which of the choices may be the best and give them at the end of the class period.

"You are the parent of Steve who was apprehended for drunken driving. He was fined and had his license revoked. As Steve's parent, which would you do?

_____ 1. Take away his driving privileges for three months after revocation.

_____ 2. Cut off his allowance.

_____ 3. Restrict him to 9:00 p.m. curfew for three months.

_____ 4. Instruct him not to see the friends who were with him.

_____ 5. Make him pay his own fine by working.

_____ 6. Force him to do extra chores around the house as an additional penalty.

_____ 7. Just discuss the situation with him without punishment.

_____ 8. Tell him it is okay if he drinks as long as he doesn't drink and drive.

_____ 9. Let him know you are disappointed in his behavior.

_____10. Emphasize to him that he has shamed the family name.

_____11. Allow him no more driving privileges with the family car(s), even after his license has been reinstated.

E. Safety Restraint Systems: Place a checkmark by the statements that you agree with.

_____ 1. "I am hurting only myself if I don't wear a seat belt."

_____ 2. "It is safer not to wear seat belts and be thrown clear of the car during a collision."

_____ 3. "I don't wear a seat belt because I will be trapped if the car goes off a bridge and lands in water, or if it catches fire."

_____ 4. "It is more important to fasten your safety belt on long trips at high speeds or while driving on freeways or turnpikes."

_____ 5. "A seat belt should be worn loosely in order to prevent severe pelvic and stomach injuries."

_____ 6. "Pregnant women should not wear seat belts."

All of these statements are myths. Read the articles, "What You Think You Know Can Kill You."[5]

II. _Safe Use of Motorcycles and "Mopeds"_ (Motorized Bicycles)

A. Students who ride motorcycles or are considering the purchase of one, should read the booklet, "Guide to Motorcycling."[2] (Stock #3304) This publication includes the proper clothing to wear for added protection; how to check a motorcyle before riding it; how to control a motorcyle and handle dangerous conditions, emergency situations and mechanical problems; how to carry passengers and cargo; and things that often keep cyclists from being in shape to ride. Depending on the interest of your class in motorcycling, you may wish to invite a motorcyle policeman to speak to your class.

Values Continuum: To aid students in seeing issues as having varying degrees of alternative choices, ask them to place a check indicating where they stand on the issue of motorcycle helmets. Students should be asked to defend their positions.

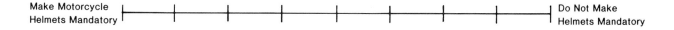

Make Motorcycle Helmets Mandatory   Do Not Make Helmets Mandatory

Reaction Statement—Spark a classroom discussion by writing the statement, "The name of MOTORCYCLES should be changed to MURDERCYCLES,"[4] on the chalkboard. Take a class vote on this issue and ask the students to explain why they voted as they did.

B. A "moped" is a motorized bicycle that is very popular in Europe, but relatively new to the United States. Since they can get anywhere from 120 to 200 miles per gallon, it is predicted that there may be as many as four million mopeds in the United States by the early 1980's. On the other hand, the engine is limited to about two horsepower, with a top speed of only 30 miles per hour and their appearance in the traffic mix may cause some very unique problems.

Class Survey: Survey your class as to possible owners or users of mopeds. If any exist, see if they can bring their vehicle to class and describe its features.[1]

Research: Have a small group of interested students contact your state motor vehicle administration office or license authority and learn the registration requirements, minimum operators age, how the vehicle is defined by law, if the use of a helmet is required, and any other special laws pertaining to their use.

III. Safe Use of a Bicycle

The purchase and use of bicycles for business as well as pleasure have been constantly increasing, but so have the number of serious injuries and fatalities. How can we help reduce these tragedies?

Some concerned private organizations and schools are teaching safe bicycle use. Courses in bike safety are gaining popularity at the college level. Bicycle paths are being developed in some areas, and special lanes are being designed for the use of bicyclists on heavily travelled streets and roads. The U.S. Consumer Product Safety Commission (CPSC) is also launching a nation-wide effort to provide consumers with the information they will need to select, use, and maintain bicycles in a safe way.[6]

As a consumer, you can protect yourself by knowing the rules of the road, by buying a safer bicycle, by maintaining your bicycle on a regular basis, and by being constantly aware of your traffic environment as you drive.

A. Take various photographs that illustrate specific problems concerning lane positioning. Paste the photographs to cardboard and pass the pictures around the class. Ask students to put themselves in the picture as a cyclist and select the lane they would choose to be in if they were continuing straight ahead; making a right turn; making a left turn.

B. Selecting a Bike: The type of bicycle you buy should depend on the kind of riding you do; how much money you have to spend, if you will be able to make repairs and maintain the bike yourself, your size, style preference, and if you have a place to keep your bike. Obtain the pamphlets, "Bike Basics,"[2] (stock #3279) and "Bicycles—Buy Right, Drive Right."[6] for more information.

C. Cycling Skills: If you change from a single-speed bicycle to a 3–5 or 10-speed bicycle, it will take practice to learn to change gears smoothly and accurately while keeping your eyes on the road. "Bike Basics"[2] (Stock #3679) describes activities for testing skills of balance, pedaling and braking, circling, turning and signaling, and control. Once you have developed these skills, practice riding on wet and gravel surfaces away from traffic.

D. Routine Maintenance: All bicycles require routine maintenance to keep them looking good and operating smoothly. Invite a bike dealer to visit your class and demonstrate how to perform minor bicycle repairs and routine maintenance. This will include: how to use a tire gauge, and how to examine tires for cracks, cuts, and bulges; how to adjust the seat and handlebars for a proper fit; how to oil and clean moving parts; and how to tighten and/or adjust loose parts.

E. Discuss bicycle licensing or registration and how to lock your bike securely.

IV. Changing Your Behavior

After studying various aspects of traffic safety, have you become more aware of a certain unsafe habit or behavior of yours that you would like to change?

Directions: In Section A, identify a behavior of yours relating to traffic safety that you would like to change (e.g., not wearing seat belts, not wearing a helmet, jaywalking, etc.). Describe how your present behavior could result in an injury.

In Section B, write out your specific plan to change that behavior.

```
Section A




```

```
Section B




```

Materials

1. Pamphlets: "Defensive Driving—Managing Time and Space,"[2] (stock #3389); "How to go on ice and snow,"[2] (stock #3387) "Freeway Driving Demands Special Skills,"[2] (stock #3396) "Guide to Motorcycling,"[2] (stock #3304) "Bike Basics,"[2] (stock #3279) "Bicycles—Buy Right, Drive Right."[6]
2. Cardboard, Paste and Scissors.

Evaluation

1. Ask students to describe how a driver can stay at least 2 seconds behind the vehicle ahead of them. (Choose an easily visible fixed point—such as a sign—and start to count as the car ahead passes the fixed point. You should be able to count 1,001 . . . 1,002 before you pass the fixed point, if you are maintaining an adequate following distance. A two-second gap will allow you time to change lanes if necessary).

   A four-second gap is needed at highway speeds in order to stop or identify an alternate path of travel if your immediate path is suddenly blocked. Twelve seconds of visual lead time are needed in city drivng (20 to 30 seconds for higher speed driving) to make speed or position adjustments well in advance of possible problems.

2. Prepare a short quiz based on the information found in the pamphlet, "Freeway Driving Demands Special Skills."

3. The value clarification activities mentioned in objective three are discussed under content and procedures.

4. A quiz containing myths about seat belts may be based on the statements contained in Section E—Safety Restraint Systems.

5. Photographs depicting various traffic problems and the best solutions for each problem, may be found in the publication, "10 Traffic Safety Guides For Junior High Teachers," (Guide is rewritten annually), or taken in your community.

6. If possible, ask students to bring their bicycles to school. In small groups, let each student randomly select a simple bicycle maintenance procedure (that has been written on index cards) and evaluate their ability to perform the task.

7. Objective 7 can be met by requiring students to complete the lesson described under Section IV—Changing Your Behavior. Evaluation should be based on the answer given in Section A and if the plan described in Section B is feasible.

First Aid and Safety
Accident Prevention

Objectives

1. The student will demonstrate an increase in his/her knowledge of safety by completing a pre-test and post-test consisting of ten multiple choice questions.

2. The student will be able to identify at least one major causative condition and one major preventive action for each of the nine types of accidents reported in *Accident Facts*.

3. The student will be able to name the three elements that must be present in order to start a fire, and will be able to provide a way each element could be omitted, thus causing the fire to go out or not burn.

4. After studying the reprint: "Fabrics and Fire," the student will be able to determine the flammability potential of various types of wearing apparel.

5. The student will be able to role-play how to control a grease fire that starts in a skillet, and what to do if his clothing should catch on fire.

6. The student will be able to discuss the three distinct classes of home fires and distinguish between the four types of fire extinguishers recommended for home use.

7. After viewing the film, "The Travels of Timothy Trent," the student will recognize common factors leading to accidental poisoning and be able to participate in class discussion and completion of a "One-Word Feeling" activity.

8. The student will be able to recognize potentially hazardous products used daily in the home, that and the kitchen, bathroom, bedroom, and garage/ storage area as the rooms in which accidental poisoning of a small child could most easily occur.

9. The student will be able to identify Syrup of Ipecac, its purpose, its importance in the home, and where it may be obtained.

10. After completion of this unit, the student will be able to define the multiple cause concept, and identify the implications this concept has for safe behavior.

Sources

1. National Evaluation Systems, Inc. "Poison Awareness—A Discussion Leader's Guide." A booklet prepared for the U.S. Consumer Product Safety Commission, Office of Communications, Washington, D.C. 20207.

2. Alton L. Thygerson. *Safety Concepts and Instruction.* Second Edition. Englewood Cliffs, New Jersey: Prentice-Hall, Inc., 1976, pp. 43, 117, 120 reprinted with permission.

3. "Accident Prevention—More than hit or miss," *Current Health 2,* May, 1978, pp. 3–13.

4. National Safety Council. "Fabrics and Fire," 444 North Michigan Avenue, Chicago, Illinois 60611. Reprinted by the Accident Prevention Unit of the Ohio Department of Health.

5. National Evaluation Systems, Inc. "Poison Awareness—A Resource Book for Teachers Grades 7–9." A booklet prepared for the U.S. Consumer Product Safety Commission, Office of Communications, Washington, D.C. 20207.

Content and Procedures

Accidents Are Common

A three-year old boy found a bottle on the table next to his parents' bed. He opened it and swallowed its contents—15 cold tablets. An hour and a half later he became drowsy and wobbly on his feet, and shortly fell asleep—symptoms of poisoning by over-the-counter antihistamines. He was rushed to the hospital. . .[1]

The mother of a four-year old girl stopped waxing the floor momentarily to speak on the telephone in the next room. The girl swallowed three or four mouthfuls from the open container of floor wax. Immediately she gasped, coughed, and turned blue. These symptoms cleared within two to three minutes but within thirty minutes she became drowsy and her breathing became more rapid. She was admitted to a local hospital with a diagnosis of hydrocarbon overdose. . . .[1]

Mike had been swimming in a large, crowded resort pool for about an hour when a girl about 18 years old dived off the low board and began swimming the length of the pool. Neither of them was watching what he or she was doing when they bumped into each other head first. The girl panicked, grabbed hold of Mike around his arms, and pulled him underwater. . .

Three accidents. How could they have been prevented? How would you have responded in each of these examples? What do accidents have to do with teenagers? Accidents are the leading cause of death among all persons aged 1 to 38 years, and account for more deaths each year than all infectious diseases combined. Has someone in your family been injured seriously enough within the last year to require medical attention or to have caused them to restrict their activity for at least one day? According to National Safety Council statistics, one in every four Americans falls into this category.

Activity

How safety conscious are you?

Pre-test/Post-test. Circle the correct answer for each of the following questions:

1. Which type of accident is responsible for the greatest number of deaths among teenagers?
   A. Poisoning B. Drowing C. Falls D. Motor Vehicle E. Fires and Flames

2. Which age group has the highest mortality rate from falls?
   A. One through Four   B. Five through Nineteen   C. Twenty through Forty-four   D. Forty-five through Sixty-four   E. Sixty-five and up

3. What knowledge skill is *least* necessary for safe participation in water activities?
   A. Ability to perform two or more accepted swimming strokes well.
   B. Knowledge concerning the correct use of water tablets.
   C. Knowledge concerning how to help prevent hypothermia.
   D. Ability to perform water rescue techniques, including artificial respiration.
   E. Strength and endurance to stay afloat for a prolonged period.

4. Which statement about fire is *not* true?
   A. Carelessness and lack of knowledge contribute to most fires.
   B. Fire is a chemical reaction involving the rapid oxidation of a combustible material.
   C. Fires are responsible for more teenage deaths than falls.
   D. A fire will not burn without the presence of all three of these elements: fuel, heat and oxygen.
   E. Most fire-related deaths result from suffocation due to hot fumes and smoke, rather than from direct burns.

5. Clothing made out of this fiber is the most noncombustible or flame-resistant:
   A. Wool   B. Cotton   C. Linen   D. Silk   E. Rayon

6. Which type of fire extinguisher is designed only for use against Class A fires?
   A. Standard Dry Chemical   B. Purple K Dry Chemical   C. Water-Type   D. Multipurpose Dry Chemical   E. Carbon Tetrachloride Type

7. Which fact concerning firearms is *not* true?
   A. Half of all fatal accidents involving firearms occur in the home.
   B. A gun should only be cleaned when no one else is present.
   C. A long gun should always be unloaded before placing it in an automobile.
   D. A gun should always be taken out of a car by the muzzle, not by the stock.
   E. The safety should be on, and your finger off the trigger, until you are ready to fire.

8. Which of the following steps should *not* be routinely taken in the case of accidental poisoning?
   A. Immediately induce vomiting.
   B. Immediately call the poison control center, rescue squad, or a physician.
   C. Identify the product and the ingredients from the label and save for the physician.
   D. Save any vomitus.
   E. Estimate how much of the product was taken.

9. Syrup of Ipecac:
   A. is a type of cough medicine
   B. makes a person vomit
   C. neutralizes poisons
   D. is put on burns
   E. is put on pancakes

10. *Accident Facts* lists four principal *classes* of accidents. Which type of accident is not categorized as a principal class?
   A. Motor vehicle B. Work C. Home D. Public E. Recreational

The quoting of accident statistics, use of "scare techniques" and stressing of safety rules are not as effective as the conceptual approach for teaching safety. Full understanding of a concept enables the student to make good decisions in a variety of situations without relying on rote recall of specific safety rules.[2], pg. 95.

Activity

Duplicate the worksheet: "Accident Prevention" and distribute a copy of it to each student in your class. Ask the students to research and identify at least one major causative condition and one major preventive action for each type of accident listed. The sheets may be completed either individually or in small groups.

Motor Vehicles

Since *motor vehicles* account for the greatest number of accident fatalities among teenagers, a separate unit has been devoted to this topic.

Falls

Falls constitute the second *overall* greatest cause of accident fatalities; however, most of these victims are 65 and older. Causative conditions include slipping on ice, loose rugs, spilled liquids, grease, or food. Unsafe climbing practices also contribute to dangerous falls. Activity: Arrange for a lawyer or insurance agent to visit your class and discuss negligence and liability in the home.

Drowning

Drowning was responsible for the death of 240 young females and 2,280 young males in 1976, according to the National Safety Council. Why do you suppose so many more deaths occurred among males? John Fleming of the National Safety Council suggests that males deliberately take more risks and swim in unsupervised facilities more often than females, thereby exposing themselves to greater dangers. Activities: Ben Harris, also of the National Safety Council, advises people to learn two or more accepted swimming strokes and be able to do them well; to develop the strength and endurance to stay afloat for a prolonged period; to know what to do in cold water to help prevent hypothermia (lowered body temperature); to learn water rescue techniques; and to learn artificial respiration and cardiopulmonary resuscitation.[3]

Fires and Burns

Fires and burns result in the annual death of more than 6,000 people and cause millions of dollars worth of property damage.[1] The chief causes of fire include smoking and matches, electrical, overheating, fuel exposed to open flame, and flammable liquids. Carelessness and lack of knowledge contribute to most fires. To prevent and extinguish fire, it is necessary to understand what makes fire burn and the elements of fire.

Fire is a chemical reaction involving the rapid oxidation of a combustible material producing heat and flame. In order to have fire, three elements are necessary—fuel, heat and oxygen. If any one of these elements are eliminated, fire will not burn. *Activities:* Survey your attic and basement for sources of unnecessary combustible fuel—wood, paper boxes, clothes, books, paper, etc. that can be removed in an effort to lessen the possibility of fire.

Distribute copies of the reprint, "Fabrics and Fires,"[4] and divide the class into groups of three or four students. Ask each group to model various types of clothes and have the rest of the class rank the clothing (#1—least flammable) based upon its basic fiber, weight and weave, fabric surface, and garment design.

Discuss how to control skillet fires (cover skillet with a tight fitting lid and turn off heat. Baking soda may be thrown on small flames, but water should not be poured on flaming grease since this will cause the flames to spread). Ask a student to demonstrate what to do in case of clothing fire (never run or remain standing. Wrap yourself in a heavy rug, wool blanket, bedspread, or coat and roll slowly on the floor or grass).

Show students the following types of fire extinguishers and discuss when they should be used:

> *Water-type extinguishers*—These are designed only for use against Class A fires—those involving ordinary combustibles such as paper, wood, fabrics, and common plastics.
>
> *Standard dry chemical extinguishers*—These use sodium bicarbonate and are designed to fight Class B and Class C fires—Class B fires involve flammable liquids, such as paints and solvents, gases, or grease. Class C fires are electrical fires.
>
> *Purple K dry chemical extinguishers*—These contain potassium bicarbonate and may also be used to fight Class B and C fires.
>
> *Multipurpose dry chemical extinguishers*—These use ammonium phosphates and are the only type capable of fighting all three classes of home fires.

Fire extinguishers containing carbon tetrachloride were sold through 1970 until the Food and Drug Administration prohibited their use due to toxicity and ability to produce poison gas under certain conditions.

Firearms

Firearms accidents can be dramatically reduced, as evidenced by the Utah Fish and Game Department when they mandated a gun-safety training program. The incidence of juvenile hunting accidents dropped from 93 annually when the program was inaugurated to as few as three or four in recent years,[2] pg 121. *Activity:* Invite a policeman or other type of gun expert to describe the proper way to clean and handle a gun.

Poisoning

Poisoning by drug overdose is the chief cause of accidental poisoning in teens; however, plants, cleaning substances, aspirin, paint, nail polish remover and a variety of other substances contribute to the large number of poisonings that occur annually. *Activities:* The resource booklet, "Poison Awareness,"[5] and its accompanying "Poison Awareness—A Discussion Leader's Guide,"[1] suggests the following activities as well as many others.

Film—To help students recognize common factors leading to accidental poisoning, show the film "The Travels of Timothy Trent" (available from Modern Talking Pictures, 2323 New Hyde Park Road, New Hyde Park, N.Y. 11040) or "250,000 Ways To Destroy A Child's Life Without Leaving Home" (available from Mar/Chuck Film Industries, Inc., P.O. Box 61, Mt. Prospect, Illinois 60056). At its conclusion, ask each student to think of one word describing the feeling he/she had after viewing the film. Write these words on the chalkboard under a column labeled "One-Word Feeling". As each feeling is volunteered, ask the student to briefly describe what made him/her feel this way and write the response in a column labeled "What Made Me Feel This Way." (See examples)

One-Word Feeling	What Made Me Feel This Way
sad	I felt sad for the parents.
angry	I felt angry that the parents didn't know how to be careful with their medicine.

Looking for Poisons—Compile a list of potential poisons by asking each student to name one household product (cleaning, automotive, gardening, etc.) or medication which is used regularly in his/her home. Instruct your students to take home the list and search their kitchens, bathrooms, bedrooms, and garage or storage areas for each product on the list. Next to each product listed, have the student write down the room or rooms in which the product was found. Compile the results. Ask the students to consider ways to correct the potentially hazardous situations they found. Distribute copies of "Making My Home Safe," and compare the student's list of poison preventive steps against the handout.

Syrup of Ipecac—Pass around an empty bottle of Syrup of Ipecac and ask students to read the label carefully. Initiate a brief question-and-answer or discussion session after you have presented the following information:

1. Syrup of Ipecac is a liquid which irritates the lining of the stomach, causing vomiting.

2. It is a nonprescription product, is inexpensive, and can be purchased in any drug store.

3. An unopened one-ounce bottle is good for several years.

4. Syrup of Ipecac is a valuable first-aid treatment in cases of accidental poisoning, but it should be administered only upon the recommendation of your poison control center or physician.

What Causes Accidents

Accident Causation— "Accidents generally result from a combination of human agent-environmental factors acting in a closely interwoven fashion (multiple cause concept)."[2], pg. 43 Show the film, "The Final Factor," (AAA Foundation for Traffic Safety) and discuss the following type of questions: What are the implications for safe behavior? Does the multiple cause concept apply to all accidents? Does anyone know of an accident for which several known influencing factors existed?[2]

Materials

1. Worksheet: "Accident Prevention." (Sample included)

2. Reprint: "Fabrics and Fire." (Sample included)

3. Skillet with tight fitting lid; baking soda; rug or wool blanket.

4. Various types of fire extinguishers.

5. (Optional) Films—listed under various subheadings.

6. Handout: "Making My Home Safe." (Sample included)

7. Bottle of Syrup of Ipecac.

Evaluation

1. Answers to pre-test/post-test multiple-choice questions: 1-D; 2-E; 3-B; 4-C; 5-A; 6-C; 7-D; 8-A; 9-B; 10-E.

2. Objective two may be met by asking students to complete the worksheet, "Accident Prevention."

3. The student will either describe orally or in writing the three elements that must be present in order to start a fire—fuel, heat, and oxygen—and recommend a way each element could be omitted, thus causing the fire to go out or not burn. Example: It is usually not practical to remove fuel from a burning fire, however, one can remove fuel (wood, paper, boxes, etc.) from an attic to help lessen the possibility of fire. Fuel does not burn. It is the gaseous vapors that burn when exposed to heat. Each kind of fuel requires a different temperature to produce gaseous vapors. To reduce the temperature of fuel below the point at which vapors are produced, it is necessary to absorb the heat. Water is a cheap cooling agent that will cause a fire to go out. Oxygen can be removed by smothering the fire with chemical foam, carbon dioxide—a heavier than air gas—, or dry chemical powders.

4. Objective four is met by the rank-order activity involving the modeling of various types of clothing by students. First permit the students to meet together in small groups and decide who is going to wear what basic fiber and design of clothing to class the next day. Each group of students should determine who will be ranked #1—least flammable, to #3 or 4—most flammable, based on the four factors described on their handout, "Fabrics and Fire." Class members should be given the opportunity to vote for the student they believe is wearing the least flammable clothing.

5. Objective five is self-explanatory.

6. Present the following situations to the students and ask them to determine the *class* of the home fire and which types of fire extinguishers would be

suitable or effective in fighting the fire—*if* the fire is a small one and you have a clear escape route. Choose from the following type of extinguishers:

A. Water-type
B. Standard Dry Chemical
C. Purple K Dry Chemical
D. Multipurpose Dry Chemical

Situation	*Class of Fire*	*Type of Extinguisher*
1. A trash can filled with paper catches on fire.	_____	_____
2. There is a loud crackling noise, then the picture and sound disappear from your television and you see wisps of smoke and little tongues of flame curling up from the TV set.	_____	_____
3. During a party your decorative oil lantern is knocked onto the floor and the liquid suddenly erupts into flames.	_____	_____

(Answers: 1—Class A, Extinguishers A, D
2—Class C, Extinguishers B, C, D
3—Class B, Extinguishers B, C, D)

7. Following the "One-Word Feeling" activity described earlier, ask the class such questions as: What was the message of the movie? What characteristics of children under five may lead to accidental poisoning? What situations were shown in the movie which could potentially have led to poisoning? What type of home situation was used as the background in the movie? Did it remind you of your own home?

8. Objective eight is met by the activity described as "Looking for Poisons," and through use of the handout, "Making My Home Safe."

9. The following quiz questions should be sufficient to determine how well your students have achieved objective nine:
   1. You need a prescription to buy Syrup of Ipecac. True or false?
   2. Syrup of Ipecac can be used when any poisonous substance is swallowed. True or false, and why?
   3. What is Syrup of Ipecac used for?
   4. Why should Syrup of Ipecac be used only when recommended by a physician?

10. Hand out a newspaper account of an accident to each student, or let the students select an accident account that recently appeared. Have the students circle key words, phrases, and/or sentences which might indicate factors affecting the accident. They should write marginal notes if appropriate and turn the article in within one week.

Worksheet: *Accident Prevention*

"Accident Facts," published by the National Safety Council, categorizes accidents into the following nine separate types. Investigate and identify at least one major causative condition and one major preventive action for each type of accident.

Type of Accident	*Causative Conditions*	*Preventive Actions*
Motor-vehicles, both on and off the highway or street:		
Falls (except from motor vehicles):		
Drowning:		
Fires, *Burns*, and accidents associated with fires:		
Firearms:		
Poisoning by solids and liquids. Identify major types of poisonous agents:		
Machinery accidents: (Including in home, farm, and at work)		
Poisoning by gases and vapors—usually involves carbon monoxide:		
Other types: Inhalation of food or other objects; Mechanical suffocation;		

CLOTHING FIRES

Four factors determine the flammability or burning characteristics of wearing apparel and textiles. These four factors are:

Basic Fiber or Fibers

All fibers will burn under certain conditions. Synthetic fibers are usually less flammable than the fibers of cotton, linen, silk and rayon. The property of some synthetics to actually melt and form a syrupy liquid or a sticky, tar-like substance can also produce deep localized burns. Blends of different fibers into one fabric will have varying properties of burning depending on the fibers used.

Weight and Weave of Material

The manner in which fabrics are woven can affect their burning rate. Tightly woven, heavy fabrics will burn more slowly than sheer, lightweight, loosely woven fabrics.

Surface of the Fabric

A napped fabric with air space between loose, fine fibers will ignite much more readily than a smooth surface. Generally speaking, fabrics with shorter pile, greater density, and uncut loop construction will be less likely to burn than fabrics with a high, fluffy pile.

Design of the Garment

Close fitting garments are less hazardous from a fire standpoint than loose fitting ones. Flowing robes, flaring skirts, blousy sleeves, and ruffles and frills on garments are more likely to be ignited in situations involving careless use of fire. Therefore, garments worn by men and boys are usually safer than those worn by girls and women.

REACTION OF FIBERS TO FIRE

Glass This fiber in its natural color is noncombustible, although glass fabrics will burn when treated with certain finishes or blended with some flammable fiber.

Wool The least flammable of the natural fibers, wool is slow to ignite and is naturally somewhat flame-resistant.

Silk Silk in its natural state is not very flammable but materials added to give body as well as its construction affect its burning rate. Sheer silk will burn more readily than a heavy silk yarn.

Modacrylics These synthetics (Verel, Dynel)* burn only when in contact with flame. Once ignition source is removed they are self-extinguishing.

Saran These synthetics (Rovana, Velon)* soften and char when exposed to flame, but will not support combustion.

Nylon The rate of burning varies with the type of weave. Nylon melts before burning. Some forms of nylon (Nomex)* are flame resistant.

Olefins These synthetic fibers (Herculon, Polycrest, Volpex)* do not resist flames, but burn slowly when directly exposed to ignition source.

Polyesters Synthetic fibers (Dacron, Fortrel, Kodel, Vycron)* will burn as long as ignition source is present; self-extinguishing when removed. If blended with a more flammable fiber they continue to burn.

Acrylics (Acrilan, Creslan, Orlon, Zefran)* These synthetic fibers melt and generally burn at a slower rate than either cotton, rayon or acetate.

Acetate Synthetic fibers of acetate and triacetate (Chromspun, Celanese, Acele, Arnel)* are slower burning than cellulose fibers, but are moderately flammable, and melt before burning.

Cellulose Rayon fibers are basically cellulose: therefore rayon has very much the same burning characteristics as **cotton** and **linen**. All burn readily unless treated with chemicals to make them flame-resistant.

*Trademarks

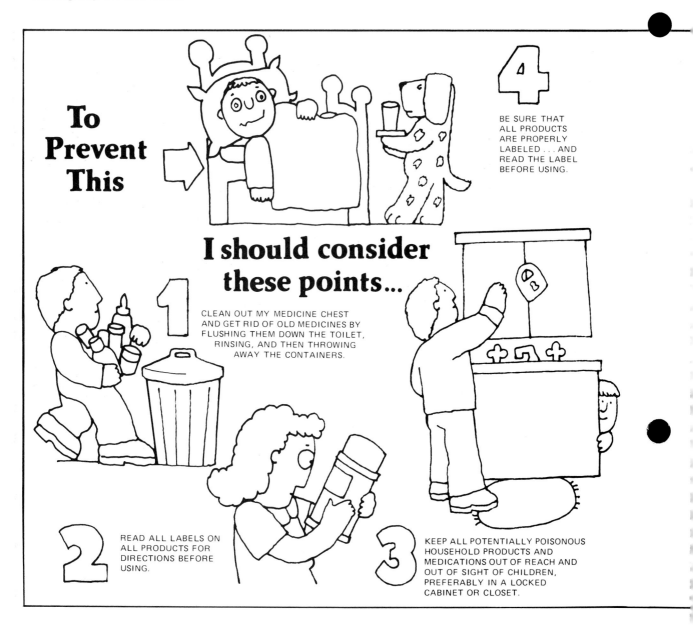

To Prevent This

I should consider these points...

4 BE SURE THAT ALL PRODUCTS ARE PROPERLY LABELED . . . AND READ THE LABEL BEFORE USING.

1 CLEAN OUT MY MEDICINE CHEST AND GET RID OF OLD MEDICINES BY FLUSHING THEM DOWN THE TOILET, RINSING, AND THEN THROWING AWAY THE CONTAINERS.

2 READ ALL LABELS ON ALL PRODUCTS FOR DIRECTIONS BEFORE USING.

3 KEEP ALL POTENTIALLY POISONOUS HOUSEHOLD PRODUCTS AND MEDICATIONS OUT OF REACH AND OUT OF SIGHT OF CHILDREN, PREFERABLY IN A LOCKED CABINET OR CLOSET.

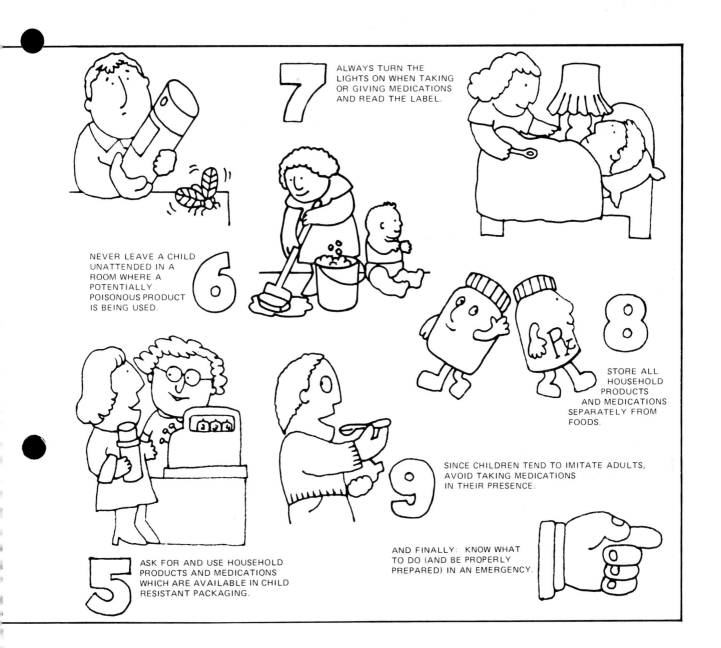

7 ALWAYS TURN THE LIGHTS ON WHEN TAKING OR GIVING MEDICATIONS AND READ THE LABEL.

NEVER LEAVE A CHILD UNATTENDED IN A ROOM WHERE A POTENTIALLY POISONOUS PRODUCT IS BEING USED. **6**

8 STORE ALL HOUSEHOLD PRODUCTS AND MEDICATIONS SEPARATELY FROM FOODS.

SINCE CHILDREN TEND TO IMITATE ADULTS, AVOID TAKING MEDICATIONS IN THEIR PRESENCE. **9**

5 ASK FOR AND USE HOUSEHOLD PRODUCTS AND MEDICATIONS WHICH ARE AVAILABLE IN CHILD RESISTANT PACKAGING.

AND FINALLY: KNOW WHAT TO DO (AND BE PROPERLY PREPARED) IN AN EMERGENCY.

Selected Learning Activities

First Aid and Safety

_____ Invite an insurance agent to speak to your class about negligence and liability in the home.

_____ Sit quietly near a major street intersection for 30 minutes and record the number and kind of traffic safety violations made by both motorists and pedestrians. Compare the results.

_____ Collect recent newspaper articles that describe various types of accidents, then ask students to discuss attitudes and behaviors that may have contributed to the accidents.

_____ Show Medical Self-Help Films available from your public health department or office of civil defense.

_____ Demonstrate what should be done by a person who receives a bomb threat over the telephone.

_____ Discuss ways of protecting yourself from possible attack while at home, walking, or driving.

_____ Share experiences in which class members have used first aid.

_____ Invite the local fire department to demonstrate and discuss CPR.

_____ Make a list of the potential dangers inherent in school-affiliated activities.

_____ Tour the school building and make a list of areas which have potential for accidents.

_____ Discuss the following statement: "Most accidents could have been prevented."

_____ Role play the following situation: At a baseball game, John slides into second base and has severe pains around the ankle. You are two miles away from a telephone and there are no adults near by.

_____ Demonstrate how to lift a person who is unconscious and not bleeding. No stretcher is available.

_____ Prepare a chart showing the causes of injury most frequent among secondary school students.

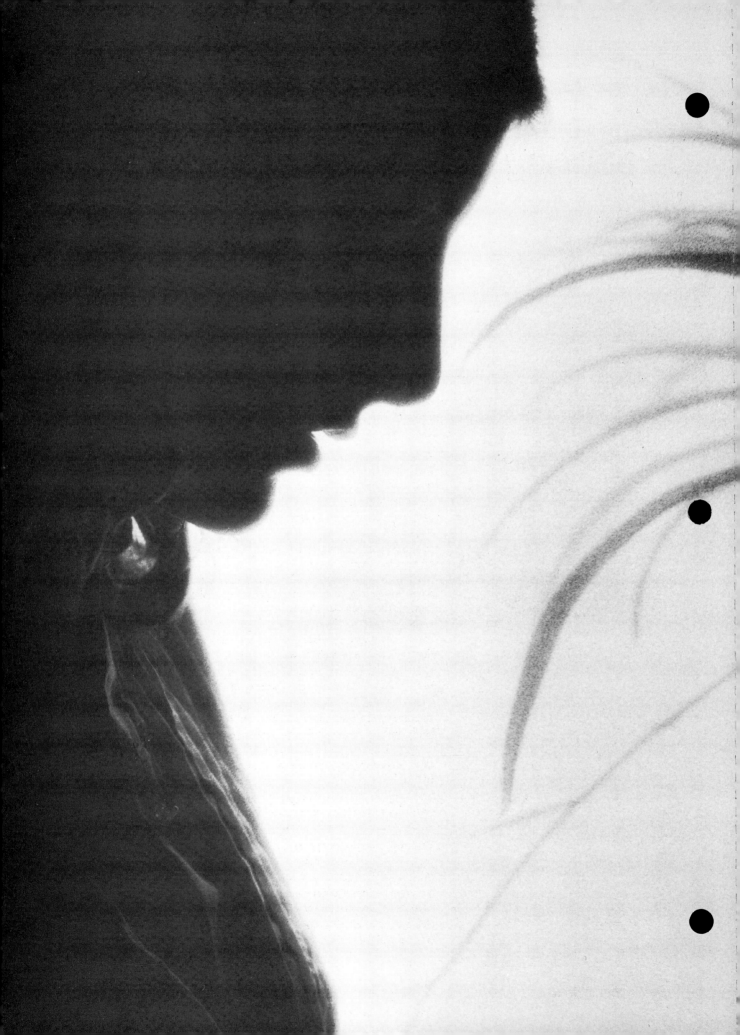

20

Teaching about Human Sexuality

How successful are sex education programs? How do America's youth view the efforts of the schools? A 1978 youth survey by George Gallup reported the following:

America's teen-agers, by their own testimony, aren't necessarily learning all the facts of life on the street, according to the latest Gallup Youth Survey.

The overwhelming majority of teens who have had a class in sex education say these courses have been either "very helpful" (36 percent) or "fairly helpful" (46 percent) in their knowledge of sex. Just 17 percent say the classes were no help at all.

Another Gallup Youth Survey finding may, however, come as bad news to those highly concerned with teenage pregnancy and venereal disease. Fewer than half of all teens—43 percent—have had a course in sex education. On the other hand, a sizeable 72 percent majority say their course included information regarding birth control. About one in four of this group—26 percent—say their class included no such instruction.

One 16 year old girl, who claims the class she took was very helpful, explained that the instruction went beyond mechanics of sex and birth control.

"The class helped me to understand that the methods of birth control are a risk," she said, "and that the maturity of the individual determines his or her understanding of conception."

Another survey respondent a 17 year old boy, claims the class was very helpful but believes gaps remain in his knowledge.

"It helped me because I knew absolutely nothing before this course, and I learned about all the birth control methods," he said. "But I still don't think that I know enough."

And some respondents, though positive in their evaluation of their course, couch their added knowledge in dubious terms.

"At least you know what NOT to do," said a 15 year old girl.

The most distinct demographic differences in evaluation of their sex ed courses are those between the sexes, between younger and older teens, and between those living in different regions of the nation.

An examination of differences by sex reveals that girls are significantly more likely to say the classes they had were very helpful.

Nearly half of all girls who had such a course, 43 percent, label the classes as very helpful while the comparable percentage among boys is just 28.

Similarly, younger teens (13 to 15 years old) of both sexes are more likely to characterize these classes as being very helpful, 42 percent than are their older (16 to 18 years) counterparts, 31 percent.

In fact, among older boys nearly one third, 31 percent, say the classes were not helpful at all.

Among those is a 16 year old who says some of what he learned in his class he had heard before.

"It wasn't too helpful because some things that were taught I had already picked up or learned before the course," he said.

And another boy, an 18 year old, faulted the content of the course.

"They would only talk about the basic material," he said. "They just didn't get deep enough into the subject—it was a real 'once over lightly'."

Regionally, teens living in the South are most apt to call the sex education they have had as very helpful (44 percent), and those in the East least likely (29 percent) to do so.

Regional differences, however, are a matter of degree. Nearly equal percentages in all four regions say the classes were either very or at least fairly helpful.

Clearly, discussion of contraception is a key element in the usefulness of these classes. Among teens whose classes included information pertaining to birth control, 42 percent say the courses were very helpful while just 11 percent call them not at all helpful. Conversely, among those who took a class that did not include birth control as a topic of discussion the comparable figures are 22 and 32 percent, respectively.

Although about equal proportions of boys and girls say they have had a class in sex education, there are again differences by reason of age and region.

Predictably, more of those in the older age group (48 percent) than the younger group (38 percent) report having had such a class.

Regionally, the percentages vary from more than half in the Far West (55 percent) to about one third in the South (30 percent).

However, as high a proportion of those living in the South as in other regions report the class had discussed birth control.

Following are the questions asked in the survey, with the results by important demographic groups.

"Have you ever taken or are you now taking a course at school on sex education?"

Those who replied affirmatively were then asked the following two questions:

"Does (did) this course give information on birth control?" and "All things considered, do you feel that these courses were very helpful to you in your knowledge about sex, fairly helpful, or not very helpful at all."

The findings are based on telephone interviews with 1,174 teenagers, 13 to 18 years old, interviewed during the period Feb. 24 to March 6, 1978.[1]

How helpful was sex education class? (Based on those who have had class)[2]

	very helpful	fairly helpful	not at all helpful	don't know
Nationwide	36%	46%	17%	1%
All boys	28	47	22	3
13–15 years	31	52	13	4
16–18 years	26	42	31	1
All girls	43	45	12	*
13–15 years	52	39	9	*
16–18 years	36	50	14	*
Both sexes				
13–15 years	42	45	11	2
16–18 years	31	46	22	1

1. George Gallup, "Most Teens Say Sex Education Classes Helpful," *Columbus Dispatch*. Wed., Oct. 4, 1978. A-8.
2. *Ibid.*

	very helpful	fairly helpful	not at all helpful	don't know
East	29	50	19	2
Midwest	38	42	19	1
South	44	41	14	2
West	35	49	15	1
Class included birth control information	42	46	11	1
Didn't include birth control information	22	45	32	1

*Less than one percent

The findings of this Gallup Youth Survey are quite relevant to the teacher who is attempting to make the content of instruction for human sexuality relevant and helpful to teenagers.

The following lessons are designed to be meaningful experiences which will be helpful in making decisions as well as in acquiring information. Although there are a number of topics that are important in the area of human sexuality, we decided to focus on teen pregnancy, contraception, dating, and marriage.

The lesson on **Teenage Pregnancy** was included because there is currently an epidemic of teen pregnancies in the United States. Many adults are not aware of the high incidence of such pregnancies, not to mention teen awareness. Because teenagers have an increased risk to mother as well as child it is important for them to understand pregnancy and its social, economic, and health consequences. The important life style decisions that a pregnant teenager can make are discussed in this lesson.

The lesson on **Contraception** was included for a number of reasons. First, the lesson on **Teenage Pregnancy** highlights the incidence and frequency of sexual activity among this age group, as well as their lack of information about pregnancy prevention. We hope that this lesson will encourage those youth who are sexually active to take responsibility for prevention of an unwanted pregnancy. Second, we believe that information about contraception is a part of health prevention information. We do not believe that all youth are sexually active nor do we believe that contraceptive information encourages sexual activity. We do believe that students should have this information, regardless of their involvement in sexual activity. Students have many misconceptions about the use of birth control such as "the first time you have sex, you can't get pregnant." Our task is to replace misconceptions with accurate information.

We also include a lesson on **Dating and Marriage.** We have observed the teaching of this lesson in a rural school. The lesson is activity oriented, with students participating by completing a chart which indicates their feelings about the relationship between commitment and intimacy. Then the students complete the Erotometer which helps them to see different indications of mature love. Lastly, the students write a marriage contract and plan a wedding. The lesson is designed to help students experience some of the decisions that are made while dating, courting, and progressing toward marriage.

We believe that lessons on Human Sexuality are appropriate and meaningful for students who are examining important behavior in an attempt to select behavior that will promote health and happiness.

We also include an outline of Suggested Topics for Teaching About Human Sexuality and additional Selected Learning Activities.

Suggested Topics

Human Sexuality

I. Female Sexuality
  A. Female sexual anatomy
  B. Ovulation and the menstrual cycle
  C. Menopause
  D. Female sexual response
  E. Sex problems
  F. Sex crimes
II. Male Sexuality
  A. Male sexual anatomy
  B. Male sexual response
  C. Sex problems of the male
  D. Sex-related concerns
III. Human Reproduction
  A. Conception
  B. Confirming pregnancy
  C. Prenatal development
  D. Prenatal and post natal care
  E. Labor and delivery
  F. Methods of birth control
  G. Abortion
  H. Infertility
  I. Alternatives to natural conception
  J. Home delivery
  K. LaMaze and other methods of birth
IV. Sexuality and Life Style
  A. Yesterday's and today's mores
  B. Same sex and opposite sex relationships
  C. Forms of sexual expression
  D. Love
  E. Marriage, divorce, and separation
  F. Alternatives to marriage
  G. Alternate sexual preferences
  H. Sex role identity
  I. Preparing for marriage and parenthood
  J. Masturbation
V. Protecting Your Health
  A. Pap tests
  B. Breast self-examination
  C. Feeling comfortable about your anatomy
  D. Rape and incest
VI. Issues in Human Sexuality
  A. The need for sex education
  B. The pregnant teen-ager—To keep or not to keep your baby
  C. Sex and the law
  D. Setting your own standards
VII. Sex Related Problems
  A. Types of assistance available
  B. Methods of sex therapy
  C. Where to get accurate information

Lesson Plans

Human Sexuality
Teenage Pregnancy

Objectives

1. The student will be able to identify at least eight social, economic, and health consequences of teenage pregnancy.

2. The student will be able to complete a ten question quiz on pregnancy testing, prenatal care, prenatal development, labor, and delivery.

3. The student will write a three page essay on the question "Is Teenage Pregnancy a serious Epidemic?" mentioning at least 5 reasons for his/her position.

Sources

1. "Birth Costs Climb," *Columbus Dispatch.* February 16, 1979, C-8.

2. Burt, John and Linda Brower Meeks, *Education for Sexuality: Concepts and Programs for Teaching.* Philadelphia: W. B. Saunders, 1975. (second edition).

3. Carroll, Charles and Dean Miller, *Health: The Science of Human Adaptation.* Dubuque, Iowa: Wm. C. Brown Company Publishers, 1978. (second edition)

4. "Drinking Mother Imposes Damage on Unborn Child," *Columbus Dispatch.* January 31, 1979 (Ann Arbor, Michigan UPI).

5. National Research Council Committee on Maternal Nutrition (1970), "On Recommended Average Weight Gain During Pregnancy," as cited in "Pregnant Weight Watchers Risk Harm to Babies," *Public Health Reports* 85, no. 11 (November, 1970) 74.

6. Planned Parenthood Federation of America. *11 Million Teenagers: What can be done about the epidemic of adolescent pregnancies in the United States.* published by the Alan Guttmacher Institute, New York, 1976. PPFA, 1976.

7. "Teenage Pregnancy: A Major Problem for Minors," *Zero Population Growth.* August, 1977 (prepared by Cynthia P. Green and Kate Potteiger).

8. J. B. Williams Company (makers of ACU-TEST), General Motors Building, 767 Fifth Avenue, 45th Floor, New York, New York, 10022).

Content and Procedures

To the Teacher

The following lesson will make use of overlays, lecture, and a movie of your choice. Before beginning the lesson, check with your local Planned Parenthood or your local health department for films available on teenage pregnancy. One that we especially like is "I'm Seventeen and Pregnant." There are many others, however. Make certain that you preview any film that you use.

You may also want to purchase your own copy of source number 6, Planned Parenthood Federation of America, *11 Million Teenagers: What Can Be Done About the Epidemic of Adolescent Pregnancies in the United States.* published by the Alan Guttmacher Institute, New York, 1976. This booklet has an excellent presentation of statistics which you will find very helpful.

In addition, the authors recommend *Education for Sexuality: Concepts and Programs for Teaching,* available from W. B. Saunders in Philadelphia. This text includes transparencies and additional lessons in human sexuality to augment your program.

Before beginning this lesson, you might also want to check on your local availability of speakers. We have found speakers to be of tremendous value. Our suggestions:

1. Planned Parenthood
2. Home for Un-wed mothers
3. Adoption Agency
4. LaMaze Teacher
5. La Leche League
6. March of Dimes—Better Infant Births
7. Pediatrician

You might also want to demonstrate the use of one of the in-home pregnancy tests.

First read through the lesson carefully and you will be able to incorporate a variety of ideas.

Introduction

Currently, we might say that there is an alarming epidemic of adolescent pregnancy and childbearing in the United States. The consequences of teenage pregnancy are serious and far-reaching.

It is the purpose of this lesson to take a closer look at teenage pregnancy. We can examine why such pregnancies are in epidemic proportions, we can look at ways of preventing unwanted teenage pregnancy, and we can influence the quality of teenage pregnancy by learning about the special health needs in your age group.

Statistics

First, let us examine some statistics about young persons your age so that we will have a better grasp of the problem as it exists. These statistics are reprinted with permission from *11 Million Teenagers: What Can Be Done About The Epidemic of Adolescent Pregnancies in the United States.* published by the Alan Guttmacher Institute, New York, 1976. I have made some overlays from this booklet to share with you.

The first overlay I am showing you portrays sexual activity among teenagers.[6] We can make several statements about teenage sexual behavior with a close look at this overlay.

1. There are about 21 million young people in the U.S. between the ages of 15 and 19 years old.

2. Of these teenagers, more than half, about 11 million, are estimated to have had sexual intercourse,—almost 7 million young men and 4 million young women.

3. In addition, one-fifth of the eight million 13 and 14 year old boys and girls are believed to have had intercourse.

4. In 1976, 30% of sexually active teenagers reported they always used a birth control method. But 44.5% reported only occasional use, and 25.6% never used contraception.

Sexual Activity Among Teenagers

Number of 15-19 year olds* that are sexually
active, United States, 1974-1975 (hundreds of 000's)

■ Sexually Active

*Does not include an estimated 1,290,000 sexually active females under age 15.

Source: Planned Parenthood Federation of America, *11 Million Teenagers*.

Incidence of Teenage Pregnancy

Now we will examine another overlay to relate what we know about sexual activity to rates of teenage pregnancy.[6]

1. Each year more than one million 15–19 year old teenage girls become pregnant.

2. Thus, one out of every ten women aged 15–19 becomes pregnant each year.

3. Two-thirds of these pregnancies are conceived out of wedlock.

4. In addition, some 30,000 girls younger than 15 get pregnant annually.

5. Sixty percent of pregnant teenagers give birth; 30 percent have abortions; 10 percent have miscarriages or still births.

U.S. Births to Teenagers

Because of the high rate of teenage pregnancy and childbearing, 608,000—or one-fifth—of all U.S. births are to women still in their teens; 247,000 are to adolescents 17 and younger; 13,000 to girls younger than 15.[6]

Ninety-four percent of teenage mothers keep their babies at home with them, according to a 1971 study; 2.5% send the child to live with relatives or friends, and 3.5% give the baby up for adoption.[6]

Out-of-Wedlock Births

Five-sixths of the infants born to girls 14 and younger, and more than one-third of those born to all 14–19 year olds, are born out of wedlock; the percentage decreases with each year of age. Between the early 1960s and 1970s, the proportion of children of adolescent mothers who were born out of wedlock doubled, and has risen at every age under 20.[6]

Among those teenagers who give birth out-of-wedlock, 87% send the baby to live with others, and eight percent give the infant up for adoption.[6]

Teenage Pregnancy and Life Style Alternatives

The high frequency of pregnancy during the teenage years has certain consequences for the teenager who is carefully examining and selecting healthy and happy alternatives to life style.

There are several factors that are important for our study related to teenage pregnancy. Let us look at some of the important life style alternatives related to teen pregnancies:

1. The teenager who is sexually active and who does not wish to become pregnant might examine the various forms of birth control available to prevent pregnancy. This topic will be covered in greater detail during our lesson on contraception.

2. The teenager who has not decided whether an adolescent pregnancy is desirable might examine the social, economic, and health consequences of teen pregnancies.

3. The teenager who is sexually active and who becomes pregnant might examine the types of health behaviors and concerns that will enable herself and her child to have optimal health care.

Teenage Pregnancy and Births

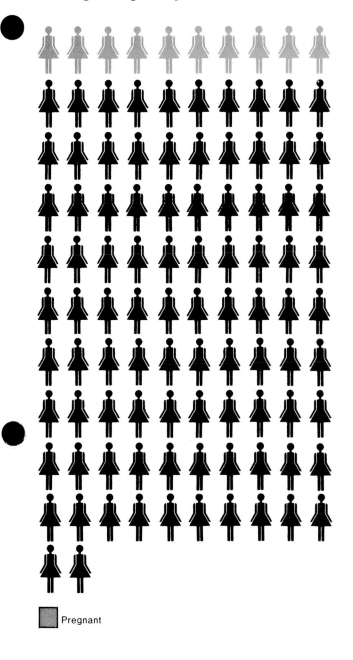

Number of pregnancies to 15-19 year old females, United States, 1974 (hundreds of 000s).

Does not include 30,000 pregnancies to girls under age 15.

Pregnant

Births (in 000s)

3200

3100   2,552.0

3000

2900

2800

2700

2600

2500

2400

2300

2200

2100

1000

900

800

700

600   361.3

500

400

300

200   234.2

100

0

12.5

Number of births, by age group, United States, 1974.

Age of mother   ■ <15   □ 15-17   □ 18-19   ■ ≥20

Source: Planned Parenthood Federation of America, *11 Million Teenagers*, 1976.

Our next lesson will focus on contraception, whereas this lesson will focus more specifically on teen pregnancy. We will look at the social, economic, and health consequences of teen pregnancy and we will discuss the importance of good health care for other and child.

Social, Economic, and Health Consequences of Teen Pregnancy

We can begin by asking "What difference would it make if teens postponed childbearing until their early 20s?" We can begin to answer this question by making some comparisons between teenagers bearing children compared to women ages 20–24, the prime childbearing years.

Infant Mortality

Teenagers are much more likely to lose their babies soon after birth than women who give birth in their 20s. The younger the teenage mother, the more likely that her baby will die. This is referred to as infant mortality.

Low Birth Weight

Babies born to teenagers are much more likely to be premature and twice as likely to be of a low birth rate than infants born to mothers in their 20s.[6]

Low birth weight is not the only major cause of infant mortality; there is a host of other childhood illnesses and birth injuries, such as neurological defects which may involve mental retardation.[6]

Maternal Death

The teenager herself is also subject to risks from a pregnancy at a time in her life when her body is not fully developed. The death rate from complications of pregnancy, birth and delivery is 60% higher for women who become pregnant before they are 15 compared to girls in their early 20s. The rate for 15–19 year olds is 13 percent greater than for mothers in their early 20s.[6]

Hemorrhage, toxemia, anemia

Other risks to teenagers include the risk of dying from hemorrhage and miscarriage. In addition, toxemia has been cited as a "special hazard" of pregnancy among the very young because of lack of development of the endocrine system, emotional stress of such pregnancies, poor diet, and inadequate prenatal care.[6]

The adolescent is more likely to suffer from anemia and from complications at delivery and immediately after birth.[6]

Education

A New York City study of mothers of first borns found that 85% of those who first became mothers at ages 15–17 did not complete high school. This is six and one-half times the proportion of nongraduates among women who became mothers in their early 20s.[6]

Seventy nine percent of the 15–17 year old mothers had no job experience at the time of birth—six times the proportion among women who did not have their first child until they were 20–24.[6]

Pregnancy is the reason most often cited by female dropouts for school discontinuation. The younger the teenager, the more likely she dropped out because of pregnancy.[6]

Unemployment, Welfare

Teenage mothers are less likely to work and more likely to be on welfare than mothers who first gave birth in their 20s. The younger a woman is when she first gives birth, the more likely her family will be in poverty.[6]

Separation and Divorce

An additional social problem for the teenage mother is the risk or rate of divorce. Brides aged 17 and younger are three times more likely and husbands twice as likely to become separated from their spouses than those who marry in their early 20s.[6]

A Baltimore study found that three out of five premaritally pregnant mothers aged 17 and younger were separated or divorced within six years of the marriage. One-fifth of the marriages were dissolved within 12 months, two and one-half times the proportion of broken marriages among classmates of the adolescent mothers who were not pregnant premaritally. Even at the end of three years, the premaritally pregnant teenage brides were nearly twice as likely to have separated as were their classmates. Those teenage mothers who married the father prior to the child's delivery were more likely to stay married than those who did not marry until after the birth.[6]

Summary of Consequences

(Use the overlay social, economic, and health consequences of teenage pregnancy)

Thus far we have focused on the social, economic, and health consequences of pregnancy during the teenage years. Now we are going to focus on the pregnant teenager and the life style alternatives available that will enhance her chances and the chances of her baby being healthy.

Health Care

Some of the factors that will enhance the health of the mother and the baby are:

1. early detection of pregnancy
2. early care of a physician
3. special behaviors during the important prenatal period

Early Pregnancy Tests

Pregnancy tests are based on the observation that the urine of pregnant women contains hormonal substances in greater concentration than would be normally expected in the nonpregnant woman.[2]

The hormone that is measured is called HCG or Human Chorionic Gonadotropin. Pregnancy tests test for the level of HCG. These tests can be done by collecting a sample of the first urine in the morning (it will have the highest concentration of HCG) and taking it to a doctor's office or to a clinic. The test for HCG will be done at the office or clinic and the results will be given.

It is now also possible to do pregnancy testing in the privacy of your own home as well. Pregnancy test kits can be purchased at most pharmacies and range in cost from $10–$12.

How does the in-home pregnancy test actually work? (Use overlay in home pregnancy test) The J. B. Williams Company[8] explains the chemical reaction and directions for the test as on the following page.

In-Home Pregnancy Text

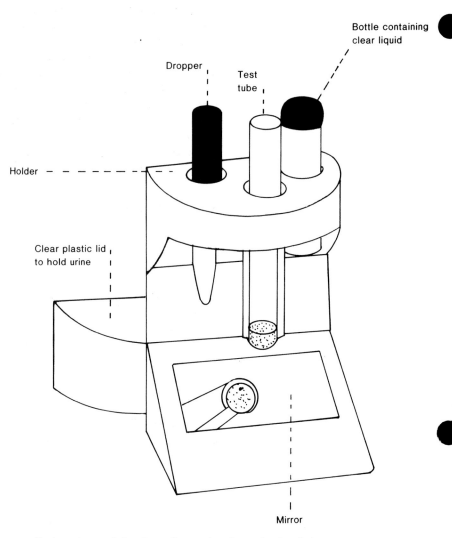

Test can be used nine days after a missed menstrual period.
Simply take the first urine sample in the morning and follow
the test directions, wait two hours, brown ring—pregnant,
no ring—not pregnant. (Repeat in a week, if no ring and no menstrual period.)

"The in-home pregnancy test is a hemagglutination test for the detection of the HCG hormone. The chemicals in the test kit include HCG hormone (coupled to sheep red blood cells) and anti-HCG serum—present so that there is an optimum amount of each to react with the other, with no excess of either. When the urine of an *un*pregnant woman is added to this mixture, the HCG cells and the anti-HCG serum clump together and form a smooth mat on the bottom of the test tube. The clumping together is called hemagglutination."[8]

"But if the woman is pregnant and her urine contains HCG this process will be disturbed—inhibited and the cells will fall to the bottom of the test tube in a brown ring pattern. Thus the phrase hemagglutination inhibition."[8]

"While the chemical reaction may sound complicated, using the test is very simple. The woman simply mixes a few drops of her first morning urine with the test ingredients and lets the mixture stand undisturbed for two hours. At the end of the two hours she reads the results. Brown ring, pregnant. No ring, not pregnant."[8]

The in-home pregnancy tests are designed to be used nine days after a teenager or any woman has missed her period. Sometimes a girl cannot remember when her last period occurred and she uses the test early and she gets a "false negative." A "false negative" test means that a girl is pregnant but that the test does not yet show the positive signs of pregnancy.

Why do "false negative" tests occur? Sometimes early in pregnancy, the level of HCG may be too low for the test chemicals to detect. If this is the case, the HCG level will have risen enough in a week to be detectable, and a second test will produce a positive, pregnant, result.

Just how reliable or accurate are in-home pregnancy tests? There are a number of different tests available at the pharmacy. The tests are generally field tested on large populations. Major medical studies have shown these tests to be estimated at 95% accurate, with some 97–98% accurate.

Saxena Blood Test

"A new test to determine pregnancy is the Saxena blood test. Developed by Dr. Brij B. Saxena of Cornell University Medical College, this test, like the self diagnostic test, measures levels of HCG. The Saxena test makes it possible to ascertain pregnancy as early as six to eight days after conception. Most previously developed and presently used blood tests for pregnancy do not give reliable results until the second week after a missed menstrual period."[3]

"In addition to identifying whether the woman is pregnant, the Saxena test gives warning of imminent spontaneous abortion, ectopic pregnancy, and other abnormalities. Low levels of HCG during the first trimester of pregnancy often result in spontaneous abortion. Early diagnosis may offer opportunity for needed therapy."[3]

"Presently the Saxena test is performed only in laboratories or hopspital clinics. This is because the procedure requires the use of a gamma counter. Dr. Saxena hopes that eventually the test may be conducted in a physician's office."[3]

Early Care

Regardless of the type of pregnancy test used, it is important for every teenager (and every woman) who suspects a pregnancy to confirm the pregnancy as early as possible.

Doctors and other health experts know that the first trimester, or the first three months of pregnancy, are very important to the development of a child. During these first three months, the unborn actually develops a brain, spinal cord, nervous system, the beginnings of eyes, arms, legs, hands, feet, and tiny fingers and toes. The sexual features are distinguishable and there is evidence of a heart beat.

With all these important developments happening during the early stages of pregnancy, it is very important for the mother to make wise and healthy life style decisions. The mother affects the quality of her unborn child through her behavior.

Each year 250,000 children are born in the United States with birth defects. The percentage is even higher for births to teenage mothers. The teenage mother needs to: (1) have her pregnancy confirmed as early as possible; (2) begin or continue healthy behavior.

We are going to discuss the different ways that a teenage mother can effect the quality of her unborn baby.

Decisions, Behavior Affect Offspring

Nutrition

The National Research Council Committee on Maternal Nutrition (1970) recommends "an average weight gain during pregnancy of twenty to twenty-five pounds. The recommended daily calorie intake should be only 200 more than the woman consumes when she is not pregnant."[5]

But the critical question, is the quality of the diet and not the quantity. Doctors frequently examine the teenager's diet and recommend vitamin and mineral supplements. They also make suggestions as to the types and quantity of foods eaten. After all, the pregnant teenager is not only carrying a baby but is herself still growing.

The important reason for good nutritional care is related to the development of the baby. Low birth weight is related to a number of problems in new born babies.

Blood Tests

When the pregnant teenager seeks the care of a physician he will automatically do a blood test for the early detection of Rh incompatibility.

"Rh is a protein found in the red blood cells of 85% of all adults; that is, they are Rh positive. The remaining 15% are Rh negative. Rh incompatibility occurs in approximately one out of every eight marriages. When the factor does not exist in the mother and does exist in the father, it is possible that the baby is Rh positive. If some of the fetus's Rh positive blood finds its way into the mother's bloodstream, it acts as an antigen, and the mother's blood produces antibodies to combat the foreign Rh factor. Should these antibodies reach the fetus, hemolytic disease may develop, causing the destruction of the child's red blood cells. Without treatment, the child could die from jaundice or anemia."[3]

Fortunately, doctors know what to do for this condition, called erythroblastosis fetalis or hemolytic disease. In 1969 there were 10,000 fetal or newborn deaths from this condition. However, early prenatal care from a physician will avoid this unnecessary problem.

Smoking

When a teenager learns early in her pregnancy that she is carrying a child, she can also make the decision early whether or not to smoke.

Smoking has several effects which combined together have unhealthy impacts on the unborn child. First, smoking decreases the appetite and affects metabolism. Babies born to teenagers who smoke generally are of lower birth weight, an increased risk that we discussed previously.

The nicotine in cigarette smoke causes the blood vessels to constrict, affecting the blood supply to the uterus. In addition, there is an increase in uterine contractions. Thus, smoking is related both to miscarriage and to a threefold increase in premature birth.

Marijuana

Another substance that the pregnant teenager needs to consider seriously is the smoking of marijuana. There are 16 million regular users in the United States, according to a recent study. The smoking of marijuana tends to have many of the same effects as that of smoking cigarettes.

There are things that we do not know about marijuana as yet. The ingredient in marijuana, THC or tetrahydrocannabinol, does cross the placenta. The effect on the fetus is unknown.

Drugs

Doctors generally advise the pregnant teenager against all drugs without first consulting them. Different drugs affect the fetus in different ways and may depend upon the stage of fetal development.

For example, a teenager who uses an opium drug may give birth to a child that is dependent on that drug.

Radiation

During pregnancy the doctor will also offer advice to the pregnant teenager about radiation, whether or not she should have medical and dental x-rays. Radiation may change tissue division in the fetus, therefore, it is important to check with a physician before such exposure.

Alcohol

"Alcohol abuse specialists see the problem of excessive drinking by expectant mothers as a potential epidemic in the United States. It already is cited as the third most common cause of mental retardation in infancy."[4]

"Abnormalities in offspring have been classified as the Fetal Alcohol Syndrome, or FAS. These include growth, weight and cardiac deficiencies, lower IQ and malfunctions of the brain."[4]

"You really have to think of this situation that when a mother drinks during her pregnancy her unborn baby is drinking too," pediatrician Kenneth Lyons Jones said at a recent FAS conference at the University of Michigan."[4]

"So, if you will, the baby is being pickled in alcohol during the entire time that the mother is drinking during her pregnancy."[4]

Infections

The pregnant teenager will also receive the kind of attention she needs for various infections if she is under the care of a physician early in her pregnancy. Her doctor will discuss the advisability of certain innoculations as well as treat her should she be infected with syphilis, German measles, hepatitis, etc.

Summary of Prenatal Decisions

In summary, we can understand that the teenager who seeks medical attention early in her pregnancy can make several important decisions for herself and for her baby. We have discussed some of the healthy decisions that a pregnant teenager might make:

1. She can decide to eat well balanced meals in the right quantity.

2. She can have a blood test for the Rh factor.

3. She can decide not to smoke during the remainder of her pregnancy.

4. She can decide not to smoke or ingest marijuana during the remainder of her pregnancy.

5. She can consult her doctor for advice before using any drugs or other forms of medication.

6. She can consult her doctor before having any medical or dental x-rays.

7. She can avoid drinking alcohol during the remainder of her pregnancy.

8. She can be under the care of a physician should she contract any infections while pregnant.

Growth of the Baby

We have discussed the important prenatal care that the teenage mother needs to receive. Now let's talk about the growth of the baby.

(The source for the month by month growth of the baby is Burt, John and Linda Meeks, *Education for Sexuality: Concepts and Programs for Teaching.* Philadelphia: W. B. Saunders, 1975, second edition).

By the end of the *third or fourth* week after conception, the embryo is a quarter of an inch long, has a heart beat, a two-lobed brain, and a spinal cord.

After *two months* the embryo has started to form fingers, toes, and ears, and the beginnings of eyes and facial features are present. It weighs 1/30 of an ounce and is about 7/8 of an inch long.

After eight weeks, or the beginning of the *third month,* the embryo is called a fetus and is about 3 inches long.

By the end of the *fourth month,* ears, toenails, and teeth have developed. If it were possible to see inside the uterus, the sex of the child could be determined. At the end of the fourth month the fetus is about 6 1/2 inches long and weighs about 4 ounces.

By the *fifth month* movement may be detected by the expectant mother. The physician may be able to detect a heart beat at this time, but an infant born at this time would not be likely to live.

From six to eight months. At the end of eight months the fetus weighs about 5 pounds and is about 18 inches long. If the baby is born during the seventh or eighth month, there is a 50 to 90 per cent chance that it will survive.

Full term (approximately *nine months*) girls weigh about 7 pounds, whereas full term boys average about 7 1/2 pounds. The range is between 5 and 9 pounds. Full term babies usually are 19 to 21 inches in length.

Labor

We have just discussed the growth of the baby inside the uterus. Now we will consider labor and delivery. Most teenagers ask questions about "How would a woman know that labor had begun?"

First stage

There are different signs that the first stage of labor has begun. One of these is the breaking of the bag of waters. This gush of water from the vagina is the rupture of the amniotic sac that has cushioned the baby during the pregnancy. Sometimes this occurs before and sometimes it is the onset of labor.

Another sign that labor has begun is the discharge of the mucous plug. The mucous plug seals the cervix during pregnancy. When it is discharged down the vagina as a blood tinged discharge it is a sign that labor is going to begin. It is termed the "show."

The most obvious labor sign is the onset of contractions in the muscles of the uterus. At first these muscular contractions last 45 seconds and are 15–20 minutes apart. The doctor will tell his/her patient when to notify him/her depending on frequency of contractions and distance from the hospital.

Associated with the previously mentioned happenings during the first stage of labor, is the dilation or widening of the cervix. The cervix is the lower part of the uterus next to the vagina. The cervix needs to widen or open so the baby can pass into the vagina. At the beginning, the opening of the cervix is about an 1/8 of an inch.

Second Stage

When the cervix widens to about four inches the second stage of labor begins. This widening takes an average of 8–24 hours (usually 16) for the first baby but may be less for a second birth.

In this stage the fetus is pushed down the vagina by the muscular contractions of the uterus. The mother can help this movement by bearing or pushing down.

In most deliveries the head of the fetus is expelled from the vagina first. The doctor uses a syringe and removes any fluid, mucous, or blood from the baby's mouth and nose. The doctor helps to guide or deliver the baby.

Two practices sometimes used to aid in delivery are worth noting:

1. An *episiotomy* is a surgical incision made in the vaginal wall to make the delivery easier on the baby and to prevent stretching and tearing of the tissues around the vaginal area.
2. *Forceps* are sometimes used to help guide the baby's head during delivery.

After the baby is expelled from the uterus, the doctor cuts and ties the umbilical cord.

Third Stage

The final stage of delivery involves the contraction of the uterus and the separation of the placenta. The separated placenta is expelled with a small amount of blood. This is called the "afterbirth."

Teenagers usually have many questions about labor and delivery. Two of the most frequent involve: (1) types of delivery, and (2) anesthesia.

Types of Delivery

With regard to types of delivery usually the baby enters the birth canal posterior head first (95%). In one per cent of the cases the brow or face is first.

Three percent of the time the baby presents the buttocks, knee, or foot first. These are referred to as *breech births*.

In about one per cent of births, the shoulder or shoulder blade enters the birth canal first.

In a small number of deliveries (one out of fifty), it is necessary for the baby to be delivered by making an incision through the abdominal wall and through the uterus. This becomes necessary when the baby is abnormally positioned, the pelvic area is small, or other problems exist. This is referred to as a *Cesarean birth*.

Anesthesia

There are many different ideas about labor and delivery, and what a pregnant woman (father) and doctor might consider as alternatives. It is best to discuss these alternatives with your doctor. A brief look at some of the alternatives available:

1. The mother may select a light, gaseous anesthesia which produces a sleepy effect.

2. The mother might select complete consciousness and use a low spinal anesthesia which blocks pain. These are known as a "spinal" or "saddle-block."

3. The mother (and father) may desire what is commonly referred to as "natural childbirth." In the Lamaze Method of Childbirth the mother learns a series of exercises to relax and to relieve pain. If the father is present he is trained in the method and assists her in relaxing, massaging her, and helps her progress through the delivery.

4. The mother may also desire what is known as the Leboyer method (although this method is not accepted by all U.S. doctors at this time). Dr. Frederick Leboyer believes that we traumatize the baby in delivery and we should make the birth much less violent. In the Leboyer method, the lights are lowered, sound levels are minimum, and there is a delay before cutting the umbilical cord. The baby is bathed in warm water to once again feel the warmth similar to being inside.

There are important life style decisions that each of us can make about pregnancy. The life style decisions that we make in this area have an effect on us, upon the family unit, upon the baby, and upon society.

Let us review some of the points that have been made during our lesson:

1. Half of teenagers 15–19 have had sexual intercourse; one fifth of 13–14 year old boys and girls have had sexual intercourse.

2. Of those who are sexually active, 30% say they always use birth control, 44.5% occasionally use birth control, and 25.6% never have used birth control.

3. Twenty percent or one-fifth of all U.S. births are to teenagers.

4. Teenagers who are pregnant versus women in their 20s have increased risks of infant mortality; low baby birth weight; maternal death risk; incidence of hemorrhage, toxemia, and anemia; loss of life development skills, education, and employment; higher rates of separation and divorce.

5. For the teenager, prenatal care is especially important. An early confirmation of pregnancy either at a doctor's office or clinic or by the new in-home pregnancy tests is important.

6. After the early confirmation of pregnancy and the early care of a doctor, the pregnant teenager can make many decisions which will affect her health and the health of her baby. These decisions focus on nutrition, blood tests for Rh, smoking, marijuana drugs, radiation, alcohol, and care for infections.

7. We have discussed what happens during the baby's development inside the mother.

8. We have discussed what can be expected during normal labor and delivery and some of the alternatives available during the birth of a child.

9. We have examined the cost of having a child.

I am certain that you may have other questions about teenage pregnancy, teenage behavior and the kinds of facts that you need to examine for you to have the healthiest, happiest life style possible. Some of your questions will be answered in other lessons in this unit. Please ask any questions that you would like answered about teenage pregnancy that I haven't covered, or that you would like explained again.

Evaluation

1. In the first objective, the student was asked to identify at least eight social, economic, and health consequences of teenage pregnancy. You might want to simply ask the students to list these eight consequences. Another way to complete this objective, would be to divide the class into eight groups. Ask each group to make a skit assigning them one of these consequences. For example, one group might deal with the consequence of the pregnant teenager not finishing high school. They might role play this teenager trying to find a job without educational skills. Then the class can discuss the skit.

2. In the second objective, the student is asked to complete a ten-question quiz on pregnancy testing, prenatal care, prenatal development, labor, and delivery. This test is included on separate sheets in this text so that you might simply run it through a copy machine for class use. Remember, if you plan to use this lesson with the accompanying test again, you will need to collect and keep the students' tests.

3. In the third objective, the student is asked to write a three-page essay on "Is Teenage Pregnancy a serious epidemic?" The student supports his/her position with at least five reasons. This assignment is to ascertain the values the student holds regarding teenage pregnancy. After the papers are completed, you can ask students to share some of their ideas and reasons with the class. We like to ask students which was the most important reason they wrote about in their paper. Of course, in class discussion, it is appropriate for a student to not want to share what he or she has written. We simply allow a student who is uncomfortable with sharing his or her position to pass.

Answers to Quiz
1. C
2. D
3. B
4. C
5. B
6. A
7. A
8. B
9. D
10. B

Quiz on Pregnancy

Your Name _____

Directions: Circle the letter of the correct answer on your paper. Each question has only *one* answer.

1. The *prime* child-bearing years are:
   A. 12–14
   B. 15–19
   C. 20–24
   D. 25–29

2. Toxemia is a "special hazard" of pregnancy for teenagers because:
   A. poor diet
   B. inadequate prenatal care
   C. lack of development of their endocrine system
   D. all of the above

3. The reason *most* often cited for females dropping out of high school:
   A. marriage
   B. pregnancy
   C. bad home environment
   D. job opportunity

4. Teenagers who marry between the ages of 15–19 are likely to:
   A. build a close relationship because of the number of years ahead
   B. have smaller families due to lack of educational skills
   C. be separated or divorced within six years
   D. return to school after the birth of the baby

5. Which statement *best* describes *in-home* pregnancy testing:
   A. These tests are currently highly unreliable in the United States.
   B. These tests are easily made by taking a few drops of morning urine and mixing with the contents of chemicals contained in the test kit.
   C. These tests are easily done by taking a small blood sample and mixing the blood with HCG.
   D. These tests can only be purchased by someone twenty-one or over.

6. What is the *most* likely reason that a girl would have a "false negative" test (a test saying she is not pregnant when, in fact, she is)?
   A. Sometimes early in pregnancy, the level of HCG may be too low for the test chemicals to detect.
   B. A girl using an IUD will have a reaction to the test chemicals.
   C. "False negative" generally means that a girl will have twins and this throws the test results off.
   D. Girls below the age of 14 rarely secrete HCG during pregnancy.

7. When does the brain and spinal cord develop in the fetus?
   A. during the first trimester
   B. during the second trimester
   C. during the third or final trimester
   D. three weeks prior to labor

8. What statement best describes the nutritional needs of a pregnant teenager?
   A. She should gain one tenth of her normal weight.
   B. She should gain an average of 20–25 pounds during pregnancy.
   C. She should diet as much as possible to assure low birth weight for the baby.
   D. She should "eat for two" doubling her caloric intake at each meal.

9. Smoking during pregnancy increases the risk of:
   A. miscarriage
   B. premature birth
   C. low birth rate
   D. all of the above

10. Drinking alcohol during pregnancy:
    A. helps to control pain during delivery
    B. is related to mental retardation in infancy
    C. affects the mother but not the baby
    D. is a good source of carbohydrate

Human Sexuality
Contraception

Objectives

1. The student will demonstrate his/her knowledge of contraception by accurately completing the Contraceptive Word Scramble.

2. After the lesson on contraception, the student will express his/her attitudes, beliefs, and values by completing unfinished sentences.

3. The student will be able to complete a ten-question quiz on contraception.

Sources

1. Burt, John and Linda Brower Meeks *Education for Sexuality: Concepts and Programs for Teaching*. Philadelphia: W. B. Saunders Company, 1975. (second edition)

2. Family Planning Methods of Contraception. U.S. Department of Health, Education, and Welfare, Public Health Service, Health Services Administration, Bureau of Community Health Services, 5600 Fishers Lane, Rockville, Maryland, 20857.

3. Kaplan, Robert and Linda Brower Meeks and Jay Scott Segal. *Group Strategies in Understanding Human Sexuality: Getting in Touch*. Dubuque, Iowa: Wm. C. Brown Company Publishers, 1978.

4. Planned Parenthood Federation of America. *11 Million Teenagers: What Can Be Done About the Epidemic of Adolescent Pregnancies in the United States?* Published by Alan Guttmacher Institute, New York, 1976.

5. "Teenage Pregnancy: A Major Problem for Minors," *Zero Population Growth*. August, 1977, (prepared by Cynthia P. Green and Kate Potteiger).

Content and Procedures

To the Teacher

The following lesson on contraception can be presented in a variety of ways. We are including a lecture outline appropriate for the methods that you decide are most suitable. The lecture outline contains material which we have found helpful in our teaching of contraception to junior and senior high school students. It is important to read through this lesson carefully before beginning and to make any changes that would better meet your needs. We have, at times, made statements that reflect our views on the teaching of this subject matter.

In terms of the methods, once again there are a variety of means to reinforce the lecture material. First, you might want to call your local health department or Planned Parenthood for a film to use. We like the film, "Hope Is Not A Method," available from Planned Parenthood. Always preview the film. It would also be possible to preview the film yourself the first time and then have a small group of students preview the film, then make up discussion questions for the class.

To cover the lecture material, we have included an overlay so that students can visualize what the different contraceptives available look like. You could also bring a sample of each of the contraceptives to class. When we have had a display of contraceptives we have been careful to keep the display in full view and anticipate ways that students could possible "borrow" from the display.

In most localities, Planned Parenthood as well as local health departments have speakers who deal with the topic of contraception. When using a speaker, always clarify exactly what information that you want covered. Also, if there are certain guidelines in your school district about teaching about contraception you will want your speaker to clearly understand these guidelines.

Introduction

As we discussed in our last lesson, the rate of teenage pregnancy is very high. About 20% of the live births in the United States are to teenagers. One out of six teenage girls who are sexually active become pregnant.[4,5]

This is not to say that all teenagers are having sexual intercourse. But of the teenagers who are, pregnancy is a reality that needs to be examined. Just as we have examined the reality of a teenage pregnancy and birth in our last lesson, in this lesson we will discuss another possible reality—the prevention of pregnancy.

Conception and Contraception

Conception is the fertilization of the egg by the sperm. Conception usually results when the man deposits semen inside the woman and the sperm reach the egg in the fallopian tube. This is not always the case. It is possible although not frequent for the male to ejaculate or deposit the semen near the vaginal opening, and the sperm might still reach the egg in the fallopian tube and effect fertilization. And, of course, artificial insemination is another means of depositing semen inside a woman.

But we are going to discuss the most frequent occurrence—a pregnancy resulting from sexual intercourse with penetration of the penis into the vagina and the ejaculation of the semen.

When normal sexual intercourse takes place it is highly likely that conception will occur. In fact, statistics are worked out for the probability of pregnancy. This statistic is called the pregnancy rate.

Pregnancy Rate

The *pregnancy rate* is established by determining how many women out of 100 would get pregnant (conceive) if they participated in sexual intercourse for one year without using any preventive measures or forms of birth control. The pregnancy rate using no means of contraception is 80. So you see the chances of becoming pregnant when you are sexually active and using no means of prevention are 80 out of 100.

In our previous lesson we said that "in 1976, 30% of sexually active teenagers reported they always used a birth control method. But 44.5% reported only occasional use, and 25.6% never used contraception."[4,5]

Why Teenagers Do Not Use Contraceptives

Many teenagers who are sexually active have been asked why they use no method of contraception. What reasons would you think that others would give for not using contraception while sexually active. Let's list as many as we can think of:

1. _____
2. _____
3. _____
4. _____
5. _____

Some of the reasons that teenagers have given are as follows (state each that has not already been listed and then discuss each reason on the list).

1. Some teenagers say that they did not understand how conception related to a girl's menstrual cycle. Their major handicap was ignorance.

2. Other teenagers believe that you cannot have a baby unless you want to.

3. Many teenagers believe that it is not possible for a girl to become pregnant the first time that she has intercourse.

4. Other teenagers believe that intercourse must be frequent for a pregnancy to occur.

5. Interestingly, other teenagers believe that you must be "really in love" to get pregnant and that the risk is "ok."

6. Teenagers often complain that they don't know where to get contraceptive counseling, who to see, what to purchase, etc.

7. And many believe that if contraceptive counseling is desired or contraceptives are purchased, that parents will find out.

8. There is also the feeling among some teenagers that contraception will take the enjoyment out of sex.

9. Then there are teenagers who say that if they take precautions then they are admitting that they desire sex rather than that it just "happened." They feel this is more promiscuous than unplanned, unprepared for sexual activity.

10. And as in many behaviors there is the belief "It just can't happen to me."

With these misconceptions operating, it is difficult to make wise decisions with regard to the responsibility that surrounds sexual behavior. Our following discussion on contraception is intended to inform you about the many different contraceptives available and how they work.

As I mentioned before, some teenagers are sexually active and some teenagers are not sexually active. It is not the purpose of this lesson to deal with your decision as to whether you should be sexually active or whether you should not be sexually active. But rather the purpose is to discuss contraception so that you will be an informed person, having more information about your health and how your body works.

Contraception: A Definition

Contraception is the prevention of pregnancy and may be accomplished by a variety of chemical, physical, and surgical means. Interception is the prevention of implantation of the fertilized egg, usually by morning after pills.[1]

The effectiveness of any contraceptive method is dependent upon several factors:

1. theoretical effectiveness;
2. motivation to use the method;
3. knowledge and understanding of the method;
4. availability at the needed time;
5. personal acceptability;
6. values—such as religion, etc.

By theoretical effectiveness we mean the pregnancy rate for a contraceptive method when the directions are followed carefully. Taking the pill as an example, the pill is theoretically 100% effective. This means that when a woman takes the pill and she takes one every day, on the right days, this method is theoretically 100% effective. Sometimes persons do not use a contraceptive method as directed, and the effectiveness will be lowered. For example, skipping pills or taking pills on the wrong day will change the rate of effectiveness when using the pill.

This is one of the many reasons for contraceptive education. With greater knowledge and understanding about how each method works, hopefully persons will achieve an effectiveness rate that is as high as possible. We will discuss several different methods of contraception.

The Pill

The pill (oral contraceptive pill) is the most commonly used method of contraception among teenagers. Most pills contain a combination of estrogen and progesterone. These are two female hormones. Some pills contain only progesterone. But the pills which combine estrogen and progesterone are the most popular.

A woman begins to take the pill on the fifth day of her menstrual cycle (five days after her period has begun) and takes the pills for 21 days. A couple of days after she stops taking the pills her period will begin. Usually menstruation is light and will last about three to five days. Then on the fifth day after her period has begun she begins a new pill pack.

The pill is theoretically 100% effective; this means if it is taken as directed and no pills are missed. If one pill is missed, a woman should take the missed pill as soon as she remembers. The pregnancy rate does not increase a great deal. However, if two or more pills are missed a woman should also use another means of contraception for the remainder of the month. Also, the first month that a teenager takes the pill it is *essential* to also use another method of contraception such as the condom. The pills need a month to begin before they are completely effective in preventing ovulation.

What are the pros and cons of using the pill? The pill's beneficial assets to the adolescent are: helping her periods to become more regular and decreasing the chances of menstrual cramping. Also, the pill has been helpful for girls with acne.

The disadvantages of the pill have been publicized a great deal. When a woman first takes the pill (since it blocks the release of the egg) her body will actually respond in some ways as if she were pregnant. She might experience some of the signs that pregnant women have. These are nausea with possible vomiting, a slight weight gain, tender breasts, and some fluid retention. Usually after three months of taking the pill these side effects will disappear.

There are some other possible side effects that warrant a woman discussing the use of the pill with her doctor. Women who have a family history of thromboembolism (blood clots), diabetes, and hypertension (high blood pressure) need a more thorough look at the benefits and risks of pill use.

In some adolescents, headaches, nervousness, and depression result from pill use. These symptoms should be reported immediately to a doctor, clinic, or wherever the woman has received her prescription. She may need to select another form of contraception.

Intrauterine Device

The intrauterine device is more popularly known as the IUD. The IUD is a small plastic device with a nylon string attached that is inserted into the uterus. Some IUDs have a copper wire wrapped around them and are the shape of a 7. They are called the "Copper 7." Other IUDs give off the hormone progesterone.

It is not completely clear how the IUD works. Many researchers believe that it causes an inflammation of the lining of the uterus and that this does not make possible the implantation of the egg in the uterine wall. In the case of the Copper 7, the addition of copper is believed to act as a spermicide increasing the effectiveness of the IUD.

The major advantage of the IUD is that once it is placed in the uterus it can be left there for about 3–5 years. Of course, the length of time that the IUD is left in the uterus depends on the type of IUD and on the doctor's or recommending clinic's recommendation.

What disadvantages might occur from IUD usage? Some women will experience cramping, spotting, and uterine infections. Any time that a woman has pain in the abdomen, fever, or a discharge she should notify her doctor immediately.

The IUD is about 97–99% effective when used properly.[2]

Condom

A condom is a thin sheath that is placed over the penis to collect the man's semen. The condom is 97% effective when used with the following precautions:

1. There is some room left at the tip of the condom to collect the semen.

2. It is used with foam and the foam is inserted into the vagina not longer than thirty minutes prior to sexual intercourse.

3. The condom is not removed until the penis is withdrawn from the vagina.

There are some other important things to know about condoms. They should always be bought at a reputable store to insure their quality. A pharmacy is better than a "friend." Condoms should not be stored more than two years. A condom should never be used more than once.

An additional benefit of the condom is a fair degree of protection from disease with its use. Also, condoms are an excellent back-up method. Since they are readily available, condoms can be used when a woman forgets to take her pills, a diaphragm has a tear, and IUD has been expelled.

Diaphragm

A diaphragm is a shallow rubber cup that is placed inside the vagina as a barrier to the uterus.

The diaphragm is 97% effective[2] when used as follows:

1. It must be used with spermicidal cream or jelly that is placed inside the cup. This acts to provide further protection.

2. The diaphragm can be used up to six hours before intercourse.

3. The diaphragm should not be removed for at least 6 hours after intercourse. If it is removed the sperm could still travel through the uterine opening and eventually reach the egg.

If intercourse occurs more than once, an additional application of foam is necessary for more spermicidal protection.

When the diaphragm is removed it can be rinsed with warm water and examined for tears. The diaphragm should never be boiled.

A diaphragm needs to be fitted by a doctor or qualified person. The diaphragms available come in many different sizes and shapes and each girl's body is different. When a woman is fitted for her diaphragm, she learns how to use it correctly. It is important to practice inserting the diaphragm in the vagina and checking with a finger to see if the diaphragm has sealed off the opening to the uterus. When a woman is not sure that she knows how to insert her diaphragm she should make another appointment and make certain that she knows how. It is not an infrequent question.

Withdrawal or Coitus Interruptus

Coitus interruptus really means interrupting coitus or intercourse. Another term is withdrawal. Both of these are descriptive as this form of contraception relies on the male removing his penis prior to ejaculation.

Withdrawal is not really a safe means of preventing conception. When a male becomes sexually excited his penis becomes erect and he secretes a small amount of lubricating fluid. There may be sperm in this fluid, so although he withdraws or "pulls out" before ejaculation he has deposited some sperm inside the vagina.

The other drawback to withdrawal besides its lack of safety is its lack of satisfaction to many couples. It requires some skillful planning on the part of the male who might not be totally aware of the exact timing needed. Many couples also say that it takes away from the completeness of the sex act itself.

Douche

The douche is a contraceptive method where the woman rinses out her vagina with water or another substance right after intercourse in an attempt to rinse out the sperm.

Sperm, however, can be found in the cervical opening as soon as 90 seconds after intercourse. It is highly unlikely that a girl might douche that quickly and even if she did it is generally not effective. The douche is not an effective contraceptive.

Spermicidal Agents

A variety of spermicidal preparations are available without prescription[1]:

1. Contraceptive cream
2. Contraceptive jelly
3. Vaginal foam
4. Foaming tablets
5. Suppositories

Spermicidal contraceptives consist of an inert base to hold the preparation in the vagina and against the cervix. Additionally, they include spermicidal chemicals, usually nonylphenoxypolyethoxy ethanol, which kills the sperm.[1]

Use of spermicidal agents increases the effectiveness of both the condom and the diaphragm.[1]

The following suggestions will maximize the effectiveness of spermicidal agents[1]:

1. Foams are generally more effective than creams or jellies.

2. Spermicidal preparations should not be applied more than 30 minutes before sexual relations, and they should not be removed for six to eight hours.

3. Spermicidal agents should be reapplied if intercourse occurs again.

Despite all of these devices for increasing the effectiveness of spermicidal agents, they do not represent a safe means of birth control unless used with the diaphragm or condom.

The Rhythm Method

The rhythm method is based on the idea of rhythm or cycle and that if no sexual relations occur during the part of the woman's cycle when it is possible for an egg to be fertilized, then pregnancy will not occur.

Thus, the most important information that a woman needs in order to use the rhythm method is her exact day of ovulation. Unfortunately, in single women and in childless women the cycle is very irregular and it is difficult to predict ovulation. In addition, many persons find it difficult to abstain from intercourse.

There are three basic ways that the rhythm method is used and that the date of ovulation is determined:

1. Calendar Method;
2. Basal Body Temperature Method;
3. Saliva-litmus test.

Calendar Method

The *calendar method* is based on predicting the time of ovulation by keeping a record or calendar of the length of a menstrual cycle for at least one year. This record is then used to predict the time of ovulation and then to estimate the days that are safe to have intercourse and the days that are not safe to have intercourse.

This is done by taking the cycle with the longest number of days between menstruation and the cycle with the shortest number of days between menstrual flows.

The formula is as follows:

1. number of days in the shortest cycle- 18= the first unsafe day.

2. number of days in the longest cycle- 11 = the last unsafe or fertile day.

Let's take the following example and we will work out the calendar method of rhythm. First, a woman keeps a record of the length of her cycles for one year and they turn out to be: 25, 24, 31, 24, 26, 26, 27, 30, 28, 26, 24, 26

We could predict the fertile days for her with our formula:

1. (shortest cycle) 24- 18 = 6
2. (longest cycle) 31- 11 = 20

Her unsafe time for intercourse is from day 6 after she menstruates until day 20. As you can see there are very few days left during the month for intercourse. This is one of the reasons that the calendar method is generally not very effective.

Basal Body Temperature Method

The *Basal Body Temperature Method* is based on the slight rise in temperature that occurs with ovulation. This slight rise in temperature is due to the secretion of progesterone.

To use this method of predicting ovulation a woman needs a special basal body thermometer that is marked with smaller intervals. The temperature is taken every morning after eight (at least six) hours of sleep *and* before rising. The temperature will be fairly consistent and then will rise at the time of ovulation.

When is it safe to have intercourse? From day one of menstruation until three days after the rise in temperature it is unsafe to have intercourse.

Once again, this method of contraception means abstinence for many days of the month. Other complications would be any event that would alter being able to closely watch for a slight rise in temperature: illness, stress, infection. However, if this method is followed *exactly* it is a reliable means of contraception.

Saliva Litmus Test

The *saliva litmus test* detects the chemical changes in the saliva that signal that ovulation has occurred. The test is currently in the testing and marketing stage but it works as follows—the girl puts a piece of treated paper in her mouth every day. When ovulation has occurred, the treated paper (called "litmus" paper) turns blue.

Once again, the woman needs to abstain from intercourse from day one of her period until three days after the turning "blue" of the paper. This test is not finalized yet, however. We will probably be hearing more about the test, its effectiveness, and use.

Sterilization

Sterilization is a procedure by which an individual, male or female, is made incapable of reproduction. Sterilization is usually accomplished by surgery.

Male Sterilization

Male sterilization is usually by means of a *vasectomy*. A vasectomy is the cutting of the vas deferens or sperm ducts. This prevents the passage of sperm from the testes through the vas deferens. When the male ejaculates, his semen is lacking sperm.

A vasectomy is a simple procedure that can be done with a local anesthetic in a doctor's office or clinic. The actual surgery should not impair or change the normal sexual functioning of the male. The male will still get an erection and have his same sex drive. Some men actually report a higher sex drive because pregnancy is no longer a fear.

The man will not notice any difference in the quantity of semen, the ejaculate. Sperm are so small that their absence in the ejaculate goes unnoticed. Also, there is no change in the size of the testes or in hormones secreted by the testes after a vasectomy.

A vasectomy is not likely to be reversible. A vasovasotomy or reversible vasectomy has not been very successful. When a man decides upon a vasectomy he needs to recognize and accept the likelihood that he will be permanently sterile. Many doctors require that their patients have counseling prior to a vasectomy and then sign a form stating that they realize that they are most likely rendered permanently sterile.

Although most men do not report psychological problems after having a vasectomy, a slight percent report difficulty dealing with their masculinity and their inability to reproduce.

Female Sterilization

Female sterilization involves cutting or severing the fallopian tubes and closing off the cut ends. The term for this procedure is called *tubal ligation.* The two most common techniques for tubal ligation are laparoscopy and culdoscopy.

A *laparoscopy* is a 30-minute procedure done with a laparoscope. This instrument has a high intensity beam and a magnifying lens to aid the doctor. The doctor inserts this instrument through a small incision in the abdominal wall to locate the fallopian tubes. Then the doctor makes another small incision and with another instrument he cauterizes part of each tube and then cuts or severs the tube. After this procedure, scar tissue forms in the tubes and the tubes are blocked.

A *culdoscopy* is another means of female sterilization. It requires a local anesthetic and lasts about 20 minutes. The culdoscope is inserted through the vagina. The fallopian tubes are located and cut.

Female sterilization does not interfere with ovulation nor does it change the menstrual flow. The hormones secreted do not change either. The physical experience of sterilization should not change sex drive, however, some women experience such relief from fear of pregnancy that there is an increase in their drive. Once again, it is important to note that female sterilization is likely to be permanent. Although there are researchers working with valves that will be able to be switched "off and on" currently there is no foolproof method of reversing either male or female sterilization.

Summary of Lesson

We have discussed several alternatives to contraception for sexually active persons. Let's summarize some of the things that we have said:

1. We defined *conception* as the fertilization of the egg by the sperm.

2. We discussed the *pregnancy rate,* the percentage of women who will get pregnant using a particular type of contraception for one year.

3. We discussed the *reasons* that many teenagers who are sexually active do not use contraception. And we mentioned a study that was done in 1976 that found that "30% of sexually active teenagers reported they always used a birth control method. But 44.5% reported only occasional use, and 25.6% never used contraception."[4,5]

4. We defined *contraception* as the prevention of pregnancy by chemical, physical, or surgical means. And then we discussed each of the different contraceptives.

5. The *pill* is a combination of estrogen and progesterone (or progesterone alone) and is used to prevent the release of an egg. The pill is the most commonly used method of sexually active teenagers.

6. The *IUD* is a small plastic device with a nylon string attached that is inserted into the uterus. It is about 97–99% effective.[2]

7. The *condom* is a thin sheath of rubber that looks like the shape of a finger. It is worn over the penis to prevent the sperm from being deposited in the vagina.

8. The *diaphragm* is a shallow rubber cup that is placed inside the vagina as a barrier to the uterus.

9. *Withdrawal or coitus interruptus* involves the male withdrawing his penis prior to ejaculation.

10. The *douche* is a contraceptive method where the woman rinses out her vagina with water or another substance right after intercourse in an attempt to rinse out the sperm.

11. *Spermicidal agents* (contraceptive cream, jelly, vaginal foam, foaming tablets, suppositories) are used to kill the sperm. They are most effective when used with the diaphragm or condom.

12. The *calendar method* is based on predicting the time of ovulation by keeping a record or length of a woman's cycles for one year and using this record to predict the time of ovulation, the safe and unsafe days for intercourse.

13. The *basal body temperature* method relies on predicting ovulation from a slight rise in temperature early in the morning after at least six hours of sleep.

14. The *saliva-litmus test* detects the chemical changes in the saliva that signal that ovulation has occurred.

15. *Sterilization* is a procedure by which an individual, male or female, is made incapable of reproduction.

16. A *vasectomy* is the cutting of the vas deferens or sperm ducts to prevent passage of the sperm from the testes through the vas deferens.

17. A *tubal ligation* is a method of female sterilization involving cutting or severing the fallopian tubes and closing off the cut ends.

18. A *laparoscopy* is a method of tubal ligation done with a laparoscope and through an abdominal incision. Scar tissue forms and the tubes are blocked after being cauterized and severed.

19. A *culdoscopy* is another means of tubal ligation only the incision is made through the vagina and then the tubes are severed.

Evaluation

We have already stated that many sexually active teenagers do not use any form of contraception or use contraception only occasionally. I would like for us to discuss some questions:

1. Do you think sexually active teenagers should discuss contraception with a sexual partner?

2. Unfinished sentences are also included with this lesson to accomplish the second objective.

3. To reach objective three, have the students complete the quiz. Quiz answers:
   1. A
   2. B
   3. D
   4. D
   5. C
   6. D
   7. C
   8. C
   9. D
   10. B

Contraceptive Word Scramble[3]

Directions: Unscramble the words below to form words which are contraceptive methods. Next to each scramble is a clue relating to the identity of the hidden words(s). For example:

Scramble	Clue	Answer
LAME	Female	Male

Fifteen minutes is the time limit.

Scramble	Clue	Answer
1. LIPL	hormones	1. _____
2. RITNA TEENIRU EVCIDE	plastic	2. _____
3. ASETMYVCO	sperm duct	3. _____
4. BATUL GLIOATNI	cut	4. _____
5. OEHCUD	rinse	5. _____
6. OTPNCCEINO	fertilization	6. _____
7. GERNANPYC ATRE	number	7. _____
8. DMOCNO	rubber	8. _____
9. IRLATWDHAW	pull out	9. _____
10. VALSAI LITMSU STET	blue	10. _____
11. NDRLACAE	length	11. _____
12. MIAPGRADH	cervix	12. _____
13. LSAAB DYOB PMRAURTETEE	thermometer	13. _____
14. CORMSPEIIAL NEGAT	kill sperm	14. _____
15. PITACECTRONON	birth control	15. _____

Unfinished Sentences

Directions: Finish each sentence with your own feelings.

1. The most effective contraceptive _____

_____

_____

2. The most important thing I learned in this lesson _____

_____

_____

3. Teenagers who are sexually active _____

_____

_____

4. Talking about contraceptives _____

_____

_____

5. My parents _____

_____

_____

6. When it comes to sex _____

_____

_____

7. I don't understand _____

_____

_____

8. A girl _____

_____

_____

9. A guy _____

_____

_____

10. Teenagers who use contraceptives _____

_____

_____

Quiz on Contraception

Directions: Circle the letter that is the correct answer. Only circle one letter for each answer.

1. Which of the following statements about the pill is *not* true?
   A. The pill is 100% effective the first month it is taken.
   B. Some women who take the pill will have headaches.
   C. The pill may be helpful for girls with acne.
   D. The pill is the most widely used form of contraception among teenagers.

2. Which of the following statements about the IUD is true?
   A. The IUD can not be used by women who have had a child.
   B. Another form of contraception should be used the first month that the IUD is inserted.
   C. Women who have an IUD have a higher incidence of venereal disease.
   D. It is best to check for the IUD string at least once every six months.

3. Which of the following statements about the condom is *not* true?
   A. The condom should not be removed until the penis is withdrawn from the vagina.
   B. The condom should be placed on the erect penis prior to any contact with the vagina.
   C. It is safer to use the condom with foam than to use the condom alone.
   D. Condoms should be bought at a drug store and may be kept for up to four years.

4. The diaphragm is 97% effective when:
   A. Used with a spermicidal agent such as cream or jelly.
   B. Used not more than 6 hours before intercourse
   C. Not removed for at least 6 hours after intercourse
   D. All of the above

5. Withdrawal:
   A. Is the most common method of contraception among teenagers.
   B. Is more effective as a contraceptive than the pill.
   C. Is highly risky in terms of effectiveness as a contraceptive method.
   D. Is another term for vasectomy.

6. Which of the following is a spermicidal agent:
   A. vaginal foam
   B. contraceptive jelly
   C. contraceptive cream
   D. all of the above

7. A method of rhythm based on the length of a female's cycles for at least one year:
   A. saliva litmus
   B. basal body temperature
   C. calendar
   D. counting

8. When using the basal body temperature method the *unsafe* time for sex is:
   A. the three days that the temperature has risen
   B. from after the temperature rise till the next menstrual period begins
   C. from the first day of the menstrual period until three days after the temperature rise
   D. from the last day of the menstrual period until three days after the temperature rise

9. A vasectomy:
   A. is the surgical removal of the testes
   B. requires a general anesthetic and 3-day hospital stay
   C. lowers the sex drive
   D. is most likely permanent

10. The following is *not* a method of sterilization:
    A. laparoscopy
    B. spermatogenesis
    C. vasectomy
    D. culdoscopy

Human Sexuality
Dating and Marriage

Objectives

1. After the lesson on dating and marriage, the student will write a paper which: 1. describes the double funnel theory about intimacy and commitment, and 2. discusses typical male and female attitudes and responsibilities about intimacy and commitment.

2. After completing "The Rules of the Game," the student will express his/her feelings, attitudes, and values about the relationship between intimacy and commitment by completing 5 unfinished sentences.

3. After completing the Erotometer, the student will rank order five feelings, attitudes, or desires appearing on the Erotometer that are the greatest indication of heterosexual love and will write at least two sentences to comment on each.

4. The student will be paired with another student and will plan a wedding, write a marriage ceremony, and a marriage contract.

Sources

1. Bardis, Panos D., "Erotometer," *International Review of Sociology.* 1 (1971): p. 71-77.

2. Broderick, C. B., "Going Steady: The Beginning of the End," in *Teenage Marriage and Divorce.* eds. S. Farber and R. Wilson, San Francisco: Diablo Press, 1967.

3. Burt, John and Linda Brower Meeks. *Education for Sexuality: Concepts and Programs for Teaching.* Philadelphia: W. B. Saunders Company, 1975. (second edition)

4. Hayes, John P., "Marriage Contracts: Why Couples Want Them and How to Write Your Own," *Glamour Magazine.* January.

Content and Procedures

Introduction

Dating and marriage are important topics in a health class devoted to the development of a healthy, happy lifestyle. The closeness of being with a member of the opposite sex as a friend, date, steady partner, and/or spouse offers many challenges as well as many personal satisfactions.

The success of a relationship and the ability to be close is related to the kinds of learning experiences each of us has and how we use these experiences. The more that we know about relationships and about closeness the easier it will be to learn from experiences and to use our learning to promote better relationships.

Each person has expectations about dating, about what is expected in dating, and about where dating will or will not lead. Mutual understanding of expectations and differences is important in the development of healthy relationships.

Double Funnel Theory

With this in mind, I want to begin by discussing some ideas about commitment and intimacy and the different expectations held by males and females when dating.

A man named Broderick developed some ideas about intimacy and commitment and he called it the "Double Funnel Theory of Commitment."[3] His ideas are interesting and might help us clarify some points in our discussion of dating and learning about our expectations and how they differ from or are similar to the expectations of others.

First, let us take one of the funnels in the double funnel theory. This is the commitment funnel. In our society, the commitment funnel begins very casually. It might mean a coke after school or sitting next to someone at a basketball game. The commitment funnel moves through a series of stages where deeper and more meaningful commitments are made. In our society, the final step in the commitment funnel is marriage.

The other funnel Broderick mentions in the double funnel theory has to do with intimacy. The intimacy funnel begins with light embracing or fond holding of hands and moves to greater intimacy, with full sexual experience as the final step.

Thus, there are two funnels operating in dating relationships—intimacy and commitment. Each of us has an idea of how these two funnels relate to each other. Our ideas about the relationship between intimacy and commitment influence how we behave and how we expect others to behave.

We are going to complete a chart, "The Rules of the Game,"[4] to see how each of us feels about the relationship between intimacy and commitment. There are instructions with the chart to explain how to fill it out.

(Note to the teacher: Prior to the class make a copy of "The Rules of the Game" for each student. It is probably best to go over the directions. Make certain that you tell the students that they do not need to share their answers with the class and that they will learn more if they write down their true feelings.)

Now that you have completed "The Rules of the Game" do you have any insights or new feelings about what intimacy and commitment mean to you or to other people that you know? How does commitment affect a relationship?

I will give you some more of the ideas of Broderick's Double Funnel Theory and we can talk about how his ideas relate to "The Rules of the Game."

The Rules of the Game[3]

Every basketball player learns early in his career to abide by the rules of the game. He knows that if he does, the game will move along more smoothly, and he'll get more chances to play. He also knows that his opponents have learned the same rules. Because basketball players are all committed to play by rules, each basketball player can predict and evaluate his behavior and the behavior of others in the game. There is much value to be gained from abiding by the rules; it makes the game more meaningful and gives direction to its outcome.

Direction and meaning are essential to all human experience if the outcome is to be favorable. Rules or standards are essential to guide behavior according to the purpose of the game. Male-female dating is not meant to be a game, but it does possess some of the same ingredients. The first common ingredient is purpose. The purpose of male-female dating is to prepare oneself and one's companion for the deepest relationship known to man—married love. The depth of genuine married love is not reached haphazardly. It begins in much the same way that a coach approaches the team for the first time. First, the rules of the game are set for the players. In the preparation for love, first, we set standards for ourselves. These standards are called commitments— commitment to what we believe is the appropriate type of sexual behavior for a particular human relationship. Neither the basketball game nor the human relationship should begin without commitment and a sense of direction.

After a commitment has been made to a given set of standards, the game can begin, the players always abiding by the rules. Of course, at times it's most difficult to abide by the sexual standards to which one commits himself. It's difficult to keep from fouling in a basketball game, too. But what happens when we break the rules? Let us suppose that a basketball player fouls his opponent and his opponent is badly injured as a result of this infraction of the rules. Can the consequences of rule breaking be brushed off lightly? Certainly not. The player who was injured suffers unnecessary injury. And what about the player who committed the foul? If he has compassion for his fellow man he aches inside from his mistake. This aching is a form of guilt—we have guilt feelings when we deviate from our standards. The effects of the mistake do not end with the two players involved; rarely does any mistake affect just the individual. There is what we call a "social mistake," a mistake that affects the members of society. In this case, the entire team of the injured player was hurt; his friends were hurt and his family. So you see one person's action can have quite an effect on society.

Sexual mistakes have the same consequences. When we deviate from a standard of behavior we have set for ourselves, and when we cause another person to deviate from his standards, who is hurt? Both persons; each person has deviated from set standards and each person will suffer guilt feelings. Society, or the so-called social team, suffers too. The social team in this case is composed of your friends, your family, his or her friends, and his or her family.

How can a social mistake be avoided? Suppose that there is a basketball player standing under the basketball hoop. Another basketball player, not looking ahead, drives hard under the basket. He sees the player he is about to crash into, but it's too late to stop. BAM! Now we both know that the basketball player would like to have avoided the painful crash. If only he had stopped to look and to think ahead. But it was just too late.

Sexual behavior works much in the same way. Teenagers can begin their dating years without looking and thinking ahead. Soon they become engaged in sexual activity that leads to full sexual activity quite different from what they had originally intended. For this reason it is necessary for young people to do some thinking and to adopt some personal standards, limits, or guidelines to assist them in disciplining their sexual activity.

The chart that follows has been designed to help you make some preparation for the future. (Look at the chart). It will help you to set standards for yourself concerning your sexual behavior as it relates to another person. This relationship of yourself to another person is in the form of a commitment. When you make a commitment, you agree to take personal responsibility for your sexual behavior and for the rights and feelings of another individual.

In the center of the chart is an inverted triangle listing sexual behavior beginning with "light embracing or fond holding of hands" and ending with "sexual intercourse." It is represented by an inverted triangle to show that as we progress in sexual behavior, our relationship becomes more meaningful and we are more selective in choosing a partner. At the bottom of the chart is a code for indicating the depth of the relationship. "A" symbolizes casual attraction. "B" symbolizes good friends. "C" symbolizes going steady. "D" symbolizes tentative engagement (engagement that is not formally announced). "E" symbolizes official or announced engagement. "F" symbolizes marriage.

On the left side of the triangle is a column entitled "Male Commitment"; males will fill in this column. On the right side of the triangle is a column entitled "Female Commitment"; females will fill in this column. You are ready to begin filling in your personal commitments. Begin on the line that says "light embracing or fond holding of hands." Decide what type of relationship is appropriate for this type of sexual behavior—this will be your commitment. Remember that whenever you decide upon this commitment it means that each time that you engage in this behavior this is how you feel about the other person—you are committed to him or her on the relationship level you indicate. Find the proper code (A,B,C,D,E,F) and mark it in the code box. There is a Column to indicate any additional meaning this relationship might have to you. Now move down to the item "casual goodnight kissing." Find and record the proper code letter for the relationship and any additional criteria you feel are appropriate for the relationship. Continue these steps throughout the entire range of sexual behavior.

When you have completed half of the chart, you are ready to begin the other half. Males should now fill in the female half of the chart and females the male half. Begin again at "light embracing and fond holding of hands." This time decide the commitment you would like the other person who is dating you to have. Think of yourself, if this boy or girl embraces me or holds my hand, how should he or she feel about me in our relationship. Look at the code and choose a relationship (A,B,C,D,E,F) and mark it in the code box. Add any additional criteria you want. Continue these steps throughout the entire triangle of sexual behavior.

Source: John Burt and Linda Meeks. *Education for Sexuality: Concepts and Programs for Teaching.* Philadelphia: W. B. Saunders Co., 1975.

SEXUAL BEHAVIOR CHART

Code	Male Commitment / Additional Criteria		Female Commitment / Additional Criteria	Code
		light embracing or fond holding of hands		
		casual good-night kissing		
		intense (French) kissing		
		horizontal embrace with some petting but not undressed		
		petting of female's breast from outside her clothing		
		petting of female's breast without clothes intervening		
		petting below the waist of the female under her clothing		
		petting below the waist of both male and female under clothing		
		nude embrace		
		sexual inter course		

Personal Commitment	Code
casually attracted	A
good friends	B
going steady	C
tentatively engaged	D
officially engaged	E
married	F

(To the teacher: Ask the students how they felt most females responded to matching levels of sexual intimacy with degree of commitment. Ask the students how they think that most males responded to matching levels of sexual intimacy with degree of commitment).

Broderick believes that males and females assume different roles in the commitment and intimacy funnels.[2] Let me explain what he says and you can comment as to whether you see the roles and responsibilities in the same way.

With regard to roles, he says that:

1. the male role in our society is to move the relationship through the different levels of intimacy;

2. the female role in our society is to move the relationship through the different levels of commitment.

Interestingly, the role of moving the relationship through the different levels of intimacy is different than the role for placing controls on the movement from one level to another. Broderick says:

1. the male usually controls the pace of commitment;

2. the female usually controls the pace of intimacy.

Do you agree with his observations? Some people have suggested that his observations about roles in relationships are changing and that males are tending to take on more responsibility for commitment and females are taking on more responsibility for intimacy. Do you think that this is true? If you do not, why? If you do feel that this is true, why do you think that there is such a change? Are you able to decide for yourself what the relationship between intimacy and commitment in a dating situation means to you?

Engagement

As a relationship progresses in commitment one of the stages that it may go through is the period of engagement. During this time, the couple can: (1) ask themselves how serious their commitment is and how likely they are to meet each others needs in a marriage; (2) plan the marriage itself.

In asking about the seriousness and intent of the commitment, the couple can look closely at mutual needs meeting. The divorce rate is one divorce for every two marriages. This is evidence of a lack of meeting of needs or misunderstanding.

How do you know if you are in love? How do you know if you are working at meeting each others needs? We are going to complete the Erotometer[1] so that you can experience one technique that someone has developed to measure love and commitment between a man and a woman.

(Give each student a copy of the Erotometer to complete. We usually allow the students to keep this handout, as many will share it with someone special).

Did you learn anything from completing the Erotometer? What questions or statements did you find were the most important indications of love to you?

Erotometer

Directions: Below is a list of items concerning heterosexual love. Please read all statements very carefully and respond to all of them on the basis of your own actual feelings without consulting any other person.

Do this by reading each item and then writing, in the space provided at the left only one of the following numbers: 0, 1, 2. The meaning of these figures is:

0 absent

1 weak

2 strong

In other words, each of the following statements refers only to your own actual feelings, attitudes, desires, wishes, and the like regarding only a specific person of the opposite sex. So always keep that person in mind and answer every item with 0, 1, or 2, depending on how you feel about that person only. For instance, if your willingness to accept responsibility for the other person's actions is absent, write 0; if it is weak, say 1; and if it is strong, reply 2.

Please check here who that person is: spouse _____, fiance _____, dating partner _____, other (indicate relationship) _____ .

Remember: Each statement refers only to your own feelings about that person only!

_____ 1. Willingness to accept responsibility for the other person's actions.

_____ 2. Feeling as if we were one person.

_____ 3. A sense of loyalty.

_____ 4. A desire to be together forever.

_____ 5. Loneliness when separated.

_____ 6. A desire to make the other person a source of my security.

_____ 7. Putting the partner's welfare before mine.

_____ 8. Helping the partner financially when possible.

_____ 9. A feeling of intellectual closeness to the other person.

_____10. A desire to share religious convictions.

_____11. Longing to experience things together.

_____12. Making the other person secure.

_____13. Making financial decisions together.

_____14. A general feeling of dependence on the partner.

_____15. Sacrificing for the partner.

_____16. Longing to do things together.

_____17. Realizing financial limits and accepting what is possible.

_____18. Helping the partner improve.

_____19. Sharing the partner's unhappiness.

_____20. Acceptance of the partner's ideas about family size.

_____21. Sharing the partner's opinions.

_____22. Acceptance of the other person's ideas about child rearing.

_____23. Efforts to make our relationship grow.

_____24. Unselfish giving.

_____25. Sharing the partner's interests.

_____26. Sharing a philosophy about dividing labor between male's and female's.

_____27. Finding joy in the partner's happiness.

_____28. Helping in sickness.

_____29. Enjoying just being together.

_____30. Pride in the partner.

_____31. Giving moral support.

_____32. Avoiding things that hurt our relationship.

_____33. Doing things for the other person's friends and relatives.

_____34. Helping solve the partner's problems.

_____35. Enjoying just talking with the partner.

_____36. Patience when problems arise.

_____37. Forgiving faults and weaknesses.

_____38. Speaking about my daily experiences.

_____39. Acceptance of the other person's goals.

_____40. Lifting the other person's ego.

_____41. Willingness to settle differences constructively.

_____42. Willingness to share responsibilities.

_____43. Willingness to plan together.

_____44. Sharing a philosophy of family life.

_____45. A sense of trust.

_____46. Expressing my feelings openly.

_____47. Enjoying listening to the other person.

_____48. Respect for the partner's actions.

_____49. A need to be wanted by the partner.

_____50. Making the other person feel important.

Source: Panos D. Bardos, "Erotometer," *International Review of Sociology.* 1 (1971): p. 71–77.

Planning A Wedding

When a couple decides to make the final step in commitment—marriage—they decide on the type of wedding and the kind of marriage that they will have. The couple can do some planning:

1. The couple can examine their needs and talk about the kind of marriage that they want. Some couples work through their needs by writing a marriage contract that outlines the expectations of each.[4]

2. The couple can plan a wedding.

We are going to simulate or pretend that you are in this stage of commitment and that you are working through your needs and planning a wedding with someone. I am going to assign you a partner and you will do these two things. As you work on these, we will be having class discussion and speakers to assit you in this project.

First, I would like you and your "mate" to write a marriage contract and clearly state what your expectations are of each other. You can examine different sources that deal with writing marriage contracts.

Second, I would like you to plan a wedding. You can agree to any kind of wedding that you want. I am giving you a handout on Planning A Wedding to use for the project. We will also have a variety of speakers. Before each speaker comes to class, you and your mate will want to write down any questions that you need answered in order to plan your wedding. The following speakers will share with the class:

1. minister,
2. rabbi,
3. priest,
4. jeweler,
5. bridal registrar,
6. reception hall director,
7. wedding gown—bridal consultant,
8. tuxedo or formal wear,
9. florist,
10. travel agency,
11. organist,
12. bakery—cake,
13. stationer,
14. photographer,
15. insurance man,
16. banker,
17. realtor.

At the end of our project, we will have a mock wedding. For the mock wedding, you and your mate will need to write your own wedding ceremony. I will make copies of some of the different ceremonies that our class writes for the whole class, and we can pick a couple for the mock wedding.

(The project was developed by Hazel Augsburger for her students in Hamilton Township Schools. Local personnel came to the school to assist the students. They enjoyed talking about the cost of wedding cakes, etc. and even had a sample cake. In addition the students enjoyed and learned a great deal by writing the marriage contract and completing "Planning A Wedding" handout).

Summary of Lesson

In our lesson on dating and marriage, we have discussed the following:

1. A couple needs to be able to state their expectations of a relationship and of each other for mutual needs meeting.

Planning a Wedding

1. Estimated Budget

   Bride and bride's family _____

   Groom and groom's family _____

2. Date of wedding

   Time of day

3. Schedule of events

   Date and job to be done, etc.

4. Type of wedding

   Number in wedding party, ushers, number of guests, etc.

5. Write an engagement announcement for the paper

   Date of paper

6. Rings

   Approximate cost, describe, draw or have a picture

7. Wedding dress—tuxedo or suit

   Draw or a picture, design, color, sample of material, etc.

8. Attendants

   How many, color and design of dresses or suits, draw or a picture, sample of material, etc.

9. Reception

   Explain—decorations, food, receiving line, music, etc.

10. Cake

    Size, decorations, design, draw picture, etc.

11. Invitations

    Color, type of print, fold of paper, etc. make a sample with envelopes, date of mailing

12. Sample of thank you note for a gift

13. Flowers

    Kinds, colors, arrangement, etc.

14. List of music for wedding

15. Ceremony

    Vows, length, etc.

16. Honeymoon plans

    Where, how long, how travel, etc.

17. Banker

    Where, type of accounts, etc.

18. Residence

    Where, realtor, expense, etc.

19. Insurance

    Agent, type, amount, etc.

Budget

Bride and Bride's Family Budget

_____ Invitations (number _____)

_____ Postage

_____ Thank you notes

_____ Postage

_____ Gown and trousseau

_____ Flowers for attendants

_____ Flowers for church and reception

_____ Picture

_____ Church fees (janitor, etc.)

_____ Fees for organist, soloist, etc.

_____ Rental of aisle carpet or other equipment
Reception

_____ food

_____ cake

_____ beverages

_____ music

_____ hall rental

_____ decorations

_____ Groom's ring

_____ Gift for groom

_____ Gifts for attendants

_____ Medical examination

_____ Other (bridesmaid's lunch, etc.)

_____ TOTAL

Groom and Groom's Family Budget

_____ Rental of tuxedo and other clothes

_____ Bride's engagement and wedding rings

_____ Marriage license

_____ Blood tests

_____ Clergy's fee

_____ Bride's flowers

_____ Boutonnieres

_____ Mother's corsages

_____ Gift for bride

_____ Gifts for best man and ushers

_____ Rehearsal dinner

_____ Wedding trip

_____ Other

_____ TOTAL

The Rules of the Game

1. COMMITMENT IS _____

_____

_____

2. I FEEL THAT INTIMACY _____

_____

_____

3. WHEN IT COMES TO COMMITMENT, MEN _____

_____

_____

4. MOST WOMEN FEEL _____

_____

_____

5. REGARDLESS OF WHAT ANYONE ELSE THINKS, I _____

_____

_____

Erotometer

Directions: Look at the statements made on the Erotometer. Find five statements which in your opinion are the most important measure of love between a man and a woman. Write them below beginning with the most important. Then make two statements about each one.

1. _____

_____

_____

2. _____

_____

_____

3. _____

_____

_____

4. _____

_____

_____

5. _____

_____

_____

Selected Learning Activities

Human Sexuality

_____ Ask students to identify positive or negative feelings related to their sexual responsiveness that has evolved from their childhood conditioning.

_____ Collect pictures or develop a slide show that illustrates the use of sexuality to sell a product.

_____ Develop a poster that depicts at least one factor that influences sexuality (parents, peers, media, church, school).

_____ Arrange to visit the birth and reproductive area of a health and science museum.

_____ Develop a panel discussion concerning the advantages and disadvantages of parenthood.

_____ Research and report on the new tests and treatments that are offering new hope to infertile couples who want to become parents.

_____ Invite a speaker from Lamaze to discuss childbirth.

_____ Have students do outside projects to determine the expenses associated with giving birth to a baby (doctor, hospital, etc.).

_____ Have students write letters to Dear Abby. The letters are anonymous. Read the letters and ask the class for suggestions and how to respond to the different questions asked.

_____ Make a family tree to trace the heritage of your family. Depict genetic characteristics in some artistic fashion on the tree.

_____ Make a collage that has at least three factors that you think contribute to healthy sexuality.

_____ Design a crossword puzzle using at least ten words that have to do with pregnancy and childbirth.

_____ Make a poster that says "Love Is." Share the poster with the class.

_____ Bring records to class to play that have to do with intimate relationships. What are some of the titles of these records? What is the message in each? Do you agree with the message in each record? Are any of the lyrics misleading?

_____ Role play a married teenage couple who are expecting a baby. What feelings does the male have? What feelings does the female have? What difficulties will they each face? What are the positive aspects of teenage pregnancy?

_____ Make a list of the places that an adolescent might seek help with problems in relating with others.

_____ Plan a social function for the class. The purpose of the function is to mix with one another. What ideas can be brainstormed for making everyone feel comfortable meeting others? dancing with others?

_____ Write an essay on "the ideal couple."

_____ Compile a list of reasons for studying human sexuality in the secondary school.

_____ Compile a list of places that adolescents receive sex instruction.

_____ Develop a questionnaire on the dating habits in your school. What questions would you like to include? Give the questionnaire out. Tabulate the results. What did you learn from this questionnaire?

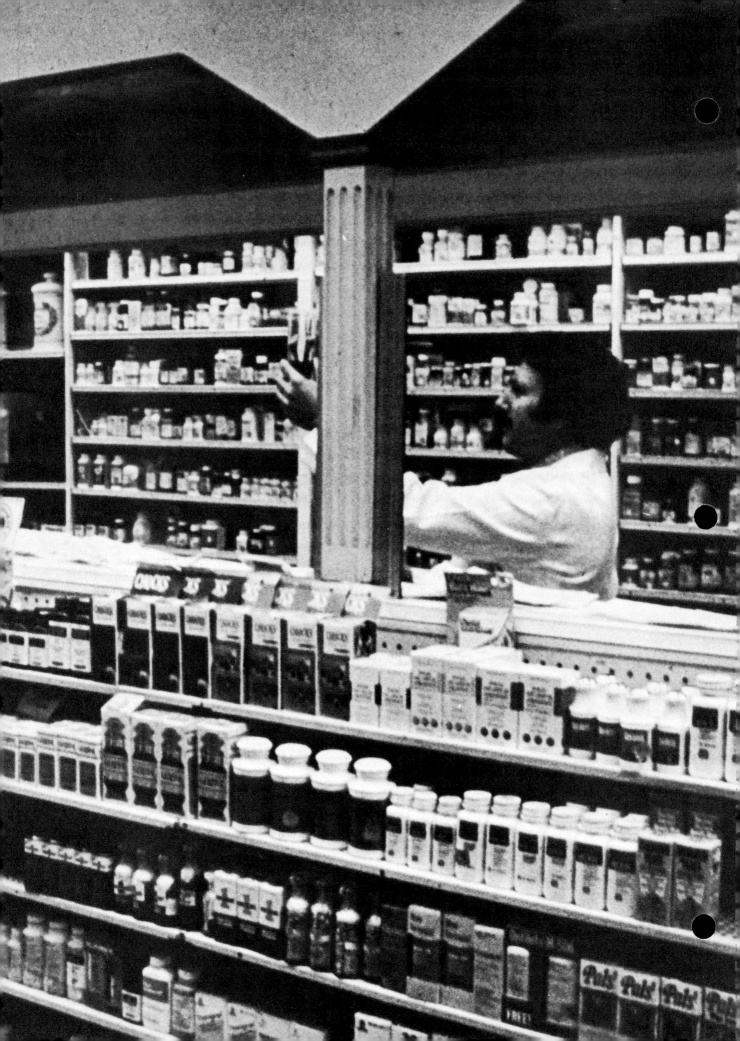

Teaching about Consumer Health and Medical Care

Today's consumer is faced with numerous alternative products from which to make a selection that will promote and protect health. Certain background information will be useful in making wise selections and in avoiding the deceit and fraud that is prevalent. This chapter includes an outline of Suggested Topics for Teaching About Consumer Health and Medical Care, Three Detailed Sample Lessons, and additional Selected Learning Activities.

The first lesson, **The Informed Consumer,** familiarizes the student with quackery. What are the common gimmicks that quacks use? How can you easily spot fraud? What consumer protection resources are available? These questions and many others are dealt with in this lesson.

The second lesson deals with **Selecting the Right Physician and Medical Facility.** The student is given some criteria for selecting a physician, and then examines the criteria for identifying. The student then examines the different types of medical care—primary, secondary, and tertiary. Also included is a discussion of medical specialities and of hospitals.

The third lesson, **The High Cost of Medical Care,** examines the different medical plans available. Often young persons are not given this information. A discussion of the following terms is helpful for the student in planning for the future: Blue Cross, Blue Shield, cash indemnity, Health Maintenance Organization, Independent Plan Insurance, Medicaid, Medicare, and National Health Insurance. The student evaluates critically the various plans designed to pay for health care, evaluating them according to their services, benefits, costs, advantages, and disadvantages.

Suggested Topics

Consumer Health and Medical Care

I. Major Areas of Quackery
   A. Chronic and Disabling Diseases (Arthritis and Cancer Quackery)
   B. Energy "Restorers" (Promise to Increase Energy Level/Sexual Ability)
   C. Beauty Aids (Wrinkle Removers; Lost Hair Restorers; Breast Developers)
   D. Weight Reducing and Food Quackery
   E. Mental Health and Psycho-quackery
   F. Mechanical Quackery (To Diagnose or Cure Disease)

Drug Enforcement
Administration Photo

II. Quackery and Health Care
    A. Characteristics of Health Quacks
    B. Unethical Medical Practices
    C. Issues in Treatment: Acupuncture, Naturopaths, Chiropractors
    D. Licensing and the Medical Profession
    E. Nursing Home Abuses
III. Selecting Health Care
    A. Selecting a Physician
    B. Types of Medical Specialists
    C. Professional Training of Physicians
    D. Selecting a Hospital
    E. Alternatives to Traditional Medical Care
    F. Possible Results of Self-Diagnosis
    G. Patient Rights
IV. Paying for Health Care
    A. Voluntary Types of Health Insurance Protection
        1. Loss of Income
        2. Hospital Expenses
        3. Surgical Expenses
        4. Regular Medical Expenses
        5. Major Medical Expenses
    B. Governmental Medical Care Programs
        1. Medicaid
        2. Medicare
V. Evaluating Prescription and Over-the-Counter Drugs
    A. Safety and Effectiveness
    B. Brand vs Generic Drugs
    C. Manufacturing Controls
    D. Drug Labeling
    E. Need for Supplementary Vitamins
    F. Drug Pricing
    G. Possible Results of Self-Medication
VI. Scrutinizing Health Advertisements
    A. Propaganda Strategies
    B. Claims and Emotional Content
    C. Valid Facts
    D. Is the Product Really Necessary?
VII. The Teen-age Consumer
    A. Buying Power
    B. Type and Quality of Products Purchased
    C. Influence on Family Buying Patterns
VIII. Consumer Protection Agencies
    A. Governmental Agencies
    B. Non-governmental Agencies

Lesson Plans

Consumer Health and Medical Care
The Informed Health Consumer

Objectives

1. Given an advertisement of a health product, the student will be able to evaluate its worth on the basis of its claims, cost, emotional content, and propaganda strategies.[2]

2. The student will be able to identify three characteristics of health quacks.

3. The student will demonstrate an understanding of medical quackery by listing five reasons some people turn to quackery.

4. The student will be able to identify five major types of quackery, and repeat a claim that is often used for each type.

5. The student will be able to distinguish between the various consumer-protection resources available to him/her.

Sources

1. Lee Ann Larson. "The Teenage Consumer," *Health Education,* January/February, 1976, pp. 20-21.

2. Robert H. Kirk and Michael Hamrick. *Focus on Health and Nutrition—A Comprehensive Health Education Curriculum Guide For Grades 9-12.* Rosemont, Illinois: National Dairy Council, 1977.

3. Miriam L. Tuck and Arlene B. Grodner. *Consumer Health.* Dubuque, Iowa: Wm. C. Brown Company Publishers, 1972.

4. Orvis Harrelson, M.D., Elenore Pounds, Wallace Ann Wesley. *Consumer Health.* Glenview, Illinois: Scott, Foresman and Company, 1973.

5. Jacqueline Seaver. *Fads, Myths, Quacks—and Your Health,* Public Affairs Pamphlet #415 (1968)

Content and Procedures

Introduction

You are already a consumer, but are you an *informed* health consumer? A wise consumer needs to know how to appraise the quality of things he/she buys and how to evaluate advertisements. The consumer must learn to be wary of medical quackery, special "treatment" centers, and items that sound "too good to be true." The informed consumer is also aware of the many agencies that exist to help protect us from unscrupulous persons. ACTIVITY: Introduce this unit by giving students health books and asking them to find definitions for the following words:[1]

bait and switch	media
code-dating	nostrum
comparison shopping	patent medicine
consumer	product
cosmetic	proprietary compound
dentifrice	quack
fraud	trademark
indirect lie	

This activity may be followed by an investigation of propaganda strategies used in advertising today, compared with past claims of the "medicine man" and his cure-all drugs. Examples of propaganda strategies include the "Band Wagon," "Plain Folks," and "Famous Personality" techniques. They may make use of door-to-door sales, promotion by sensational magazines, faith healing groups, crusading organizations, scare techniques, and testimonies; or may offer a quick cure or secret remedy.[2] Create a bulletin board display illustrating various propaganda strategies. Activity: List on the chalkboard all the items your students say they buy (e.g. food, gifts, records, cosmetics and other grooming products). Ask students to explain why they buy a certain product rather than another one. The following rank or order of activity may help students clarify their buying habits and determine what is most important to them.

Directions: Rank order the following items, placing #1 by the reason most important to you when buying a product:

_____ Promises to alter appearance.

_____ Promises to give extra energy.

_____ Promises extra strength.

_____ Largest quantity for the least money.

_____ Most fragrant scent.

_____ Most effective, according to scientific research.

_____ Information obtained from label.

_____ Other.

Bring in advertisements or tape radio and television commercials. List the claims made for each advertisement and analyze its emotional appeal. Identify the techniques which convinced you the most. Consider the following points when determining an advertisement's validity:

_____ Are claims about the product supported by valid facts?

_____ Does the advertisement describe the type of group and what percentage of people have been polled when they claim that their product is the public's choice?

_____ When research is described, was it conducted by an unbiased, scientific organization, or did the manufacturer hire a team or do the research himself?

_____ Is the language clear, concise, and simple?

_____ Does the advertisement avoid scare techniques?

_____ Is the advertisement attractive to the eye and pleasing to the ear?

_____ Does the advertisement call upon an individual to diagnose and treat his/her own family's illnesses?

_____ Does the advertisement avoid belittling the consumer?[2,3]

Bring in several comparable products and perform experiments in class to test commercial claims. Compare a product label to an ad pertaining to the product and to a synopsis of a commercial for the product.

What are three benefits of advertising?

1. _____

2. _____

3. _____

Advertising is an effective way of introducing the consumer to new products; it attempts to show differences between products; and encourages competition between producers to develop a product that is pleasing to consumers.[2]

Ask students to keep track of the commercials they watch over several days and to identify those commercials they think are directed to their age group. Why are companies interested in the teenage consumer?

Health Quackery

Americans spend more than a billion dollars each year on worthless treatments for physical ailments, useless gadgets, devices sold as "cures" for various illnesses, and for many other types of ineffective "health aids." *Health quacks,* or someone who practices medicine without the proper qualifications, are responsible for many of these worthless treatments.

How can a health quack be identified? It's not as easy as it used to be. Today's quack looks professional. He/she may wear a white coat and use multisyllable technical terms. "Diplomas" may hang on the walls of their offices. The health phony is often kind, patient, and sympathetic, but there are clues that may give him/her away: The quack often uses a *special machine* that he claims can cure a disease; or promotes *"cure-all"* drugs and treatments. Often his product will contain a "secret" formula, that will "pep you up" or provide a quick and easy cure. The quack advertises, using "cure histories" and testimonies from his satisfied customers or ex-patients. Although the quack constantly clamors for recognition of his work by the medical profession, he avoids tests and refuses to supply the information needed for scientific evaluation of his product. He may say that other physicians are jealous of his discoveries and are persecuting him. The health phony does not have the educational background and training recognized by the medical society, but this does not keep him from promising medical miracles.[2,3,4,5]

A fear of pain, surgery, and death persuades many people to abandon traditional medicine for medical quackery, while the promise of good looks, youth, vigor, popularity, sex appeal, and sexual potency attracts other people. Many indivduals do not know the differences between a licensed medical doctor and a quack; they are ignorant of what ethical medicine can and cannot do; they are anxious about their health and are gullible. Some people are faced with a serious or terminal illness and wish desperately to accept a false statement or half-truth from a quack, rather than believe their physician.[2]

Divide the class into small groups and assign each group one of the following major areas of quackery to investigate and summarize for the rest of the class. Encourage students to bring in advertisements or pictures to supplement their presentation.

1. *Chronic and disabling diseases*— Quacks are often drawn to chronic and disabling diseases such as arthritis, or to those which fill many people with fear (e.g. cancer). They prey upon people who seek painless alternatives to surgery and radiation and who want a guaranteed cure. Some of the better known "treatments" for cancer include Krebiozen, Mucornicin, and the Koch Cancer Treatment.[3] Arthritis sufferers have been duped into drinking mineral oil "to lubricate aching joints"; wearing copper bracelets or "radioactive" gloves, and swallowing a combination of hormones produced by a doctor in Canada. Epilepsy and diabetes are other medical conditions that are often exploited.

2. *Beauty aids*—Like disease, many people fear growing old. They want to be young, beautiful, and sexy forever. Losing weight is difficult and requires a reduction in calories and an increase in physical activity. "Miracle, wonder methods" involving devices, pills, formulas, and easy diets, offer an attractive alternative to changing one's habits. The desire to have lost hair restored or to have wrinkles removed, has led many people to purchase special creams, lotions, and massage devices. Some people now have permanently scarred faces because they let a quack apply a caustic solution to their skin in an effort to burn and peel off their wrinkles. Many women throw money away on massage machines, mechanical exercisers, cream "developers," and products said to contain hormones, all in the pursuit of larger breasts.

3. *Energy "restorers"*—Closely allied to the fear of lost youth, is loss of energy and loss of sexual ability (impotence). Impotence in young men often has a psychological basis and requires psychological help in order to eliminate the underlying cause. It is not cured through a topical application, mail-order medicine, or an injection made from human testicles and ovaries. Similarly, vitamins and other diet supplements will not rebuild sexual powers or lead to increased feelings of energy. When unusual fatigue persists, the individual should consult a physician and not rely on "pep" pills, which can be harmful when misused.

4. *Mental health and psychoquacks*—The intense fear, shame, or embarrassment that sometimes accompanies mental illness makes this type of problem a perfect environment for quackery. Everyone is subject to mood shifts; but frightened, lonely, anxious, and unhappy people are particularly susceptible to charlatans who are medically unqualified to comprehend fully the seriousness of a person's problems. Hypnosis performed by amateurs can result in depression, panic states, and a general deterioration of a person's mental state. Sensitivity sessions may be led by a person whose only training consists of having once attended a session or consulted a person with advanced degrees in psychology. They can be either enlightening or dangerous, depending upon the safeguards provided. ACTIVITY: Some students may be interested in constructing a mood chart (with gradations from ecstasy to severe depression) on an hourly basis for three days, and discussing the possible reasons for the variations in their mood.[3]

5. *Mechanical quackery*—Mechanical quackery includes the misuse of legitimate medical equipment and the invention of fake machines either to diagnose or to cure diseases. "Studded with switches, meters, flashing and moving lights, these marvels of pseudo-science also may emit heat and electrical impulses, or have vibrating parts."[5] Phony devices may often look like legitimate medical equipment and have scientific sounding names. Pictures of mechanical quackery can be found in *Consumer Health*.[3,4]

   As an informed consumer, be wary of anyone who claims he or she alone possesses the knowledge of a certain therapy or has a machine that is capable of diagnosing or treating different kinds of diseases simply with the turn of a dial. Question the need for routine x-rays and strive to investigate medical resources in your community before an emergency arises.

6. *Food quackery*—Since food faddism and fraud represents one of the most lucrative kinds of quackery, we devoted an entire lesson to it in our nutrition chapter. Nevertheless, it is important to stress that reliance on special foods, diets, or extra vitamins, is "not only a waste of money but prepares one psychologically for acceptance of other, more dangerous procedures."[3] Furthermore, diets which emphasize fats can cause serious damage to the liver; diets emphasizing protein may lead to kidney damage; and diets which call upon the use of vitamins to prevent or relieve certain conditions are asking us to indulge in self-diagnosis and self-medication.[3] An old but true fact remains: You are likely to be well nourished if you simply include moderate portions of a wide variety of foods from each of the four basic food groups in your daily diet.

Consumer Protection Agencies

After investigating some of the major areas of quackery, "students may become pretty outraged about what quacks are getting away with."[1] This is an ideal time to introduce them to some of the following organizations working to protect the consumer from fraud and to discuss the individuals responsibility in reporting an incident or complaint:[3]

A. Community level
   1. (Local) Better Business Bureau
   2. City Health Department
   3. Family physicians and dentists
   4. Local medical and dental societies
   5. Voluntary health agencies, e.g. Arthritis Foundation and American Cancer Society

B. State level
   1. Attorney General—Department of Law
   2. Department of Agriculture
   3. State Health Department
   4. State Medical and Dental Associations

C. National level
   1. American Cancer Society, New York, New York
   2. American College of Radiology, Chicago, Illinois
   3. American Dental Association, Chicago, Illinois
   4. American Dietetic Association, Chicago, Illinois
   5. American Medical Association, Chicago, Illinois
   6. Arthritis Foundation, New York, New York
   7. Consumers Union of U.S., Inc., Mt. Vernon, N.Y.
   8. The Federal Trade Commission, Washington, D.C.
   9. The Food and Drug Administration, Washington, D.C.
   10. National Better Business Bureau, New York
   11. Pharmaceutical Manufacturers Association, Washington, D.C.
   12. U.S. Department of Agriculture, Ithaca, New York
   13. U.S. Postal Service, Washington, D.C.
   14. U.S. Public Health Service

Materials

1. Various health books and consumer health pamphlets.

2. Advertisements from newspapers and magazines.

3. (Optional) Tape recorder—to record radio and television commercials.

4. Several comparable products (e.g. aspirin bottles, toothpaste, shampoo, vitamin tablets).

Evaluation

1. Objective One can be achieved by taping a variety of radio and TV commercials and assigning a number to each advertisement. Ask students to evaluate each commercial, using the eight questions listed under content and procedures or to identify the type of propaganda strategy used.

2. Show students three or four brands of several products and ask them to rank the products, assigning #1 to the product they would buy. Students should base their decisions upon the ingredients listed on the label, the products uses, its potential for possible harm, advertising available to them, price comparison, etc.

3. Ask students to design a product label containing all of the information they believe it is important for a consumer to have.

4. Select four students to portray various types of quacks and two students to portray "real" physicians. Permit the students adequate time to discuss and investigate their roles before presenting themselves as realistically as possible to the rest of the class. It is up to the remaining students to cull out the various types of quacks and to explain the characteristics that made them suspicious. Students may also be asked to identify a consumer protection agency they would contact for reliable information.

5. The following matching activity may be used to evaluate a student's awareness of various consumer-protection agencies.

Directions: Place the letter of the protective agency next to the function it most closely performs.

Agency Function	Protective Agency
_____ 1. Sets standards to prevent fraudulent advertising in the mass media.	A. American College of Radiology
_____ 2. Sets nutritional standards for human beings and inspects wholesomeness of meat and poultry products.	B. American Dental Association
_____ 3. Especially interested in exposing cultists who misuse X-ray.	C. American Medical Association
_____ 4. Concerned with the quality and legitimacy of advertising and the general promotion of health products, devices, and services to the public.	D. The Federal Trade Commission
_____ 5. Maintains Department of Investigation and Health Education to supplement the role of governmental agencies in exposing quacks, cultists, and harmful or worthless devices.	E. The Food and Drug Administration
_____ 6. Sets national standards for health; educates through publications.	F. The National Better Business Bureau
_____ 7. concerned with truthful labeling of consumer products with promoting purity, safety, and effectiveness through testing and surveillance.	G. U.S. Dept. of Agriculture
	H. U.S. Postal Service
	I. U.S. Public Health Service

(Answers: 1–D; 2–G; 3–A; 4–F; 5–C; 6–I; 7–E.)

Consumer Health and Medical Care
Selecting the Right Physician and Medical Facility

Objectives

1. The student will be able to identify at least five criteria that should be considered when selecting a physician.

2. Given a list of criteria, the student will be able to rank order (beginning with #1 as most important) the qualities he/she believes to be most important when selecting a family physician.

3. Given a particular health problem, the student will be able to identify the specialist most likely to be consulted.

4. The student will be able to list and discuss at least three services that have been approved for their efforts to develop a more meaningful health care system for youth.

5. The student will be able to describe five characteristics of hospitals that often are associated with high quality physicians.

6. The student will be able to distinguish between primary, secondary, and tertiary medical care.

Sources

1. Stephen P. Strickland. "Choosing a Doctor," *Saturday Review of the Sciences,* March 24, 1973, pp. 34–36.

2. Donald M. Vickery, M.D., and James F. Fries, M.D. *Take Care of Yourself—A Consumer's Guide To Medical Care.* Massachusetts: Addison-Wesley Publishing Company, 1976.

3. G. Timothy Johnson, M.D. *What You Should Know About Health Care Before You Call a Doctor!* New York: McGraw-Hill Book Company 1975.

4. David Mechanic. *Medical Sociology.* New York: The Free Press—A Division of Macmillian Publishing Company, Inc., 1968.

5. John Burt, Linda Meeks, Sharon Pottebaum. *Toward a Healthy Lifestyle Through Elementary Health Education.* Belmont, California: Wadsworth Publishing Company, 1980.

6. Betty Klarnet. "One of Their Own," *Family Health,* November, 1969.

7. "Teen-Age Patients: Their Legal Rights—And Yours," *Medical World News,* May 14, 1971.

8. Theodore Irwin. "The Rights of Teenagers As Patients," Public Affairs Pamphlet #480. 1972. Available from Public Affairs Committee, Inc., 381 Park Ave. South, New York, N.Y.

Content and Procedures

How Would You Choose a Physician?

Do you think competence is the prime criterion when choosing a doctor? Physicians and their patients often do not agree. If you live in a small, semi-rural community, perhaps the sometimes difficult problem of selecting a physician that is right for you is nonexistent, for there may only be one medical practitioner. (People living in those 134 counties in the 24 states in this country where no physician presently practices would probably say that the real issue of physician choice is having a doctor choose their community.)[1] (p. 34) On the other hand, you may live in a large city but be limited in your choice of health care because of poverty or ignorance. Nevertheless, this lesson is directed to those in our society who are fortunate enough to assume the responsibilities associated with many alternatives.

How should you begin your search?

1. The section of the Yellow Pages in your telephone directory that lists physicians, also lists physician referral services. Operated by the county medical society, a referral bureau can help narrow your choice and provide you with the names of three physicians who are located relatively near you. Upon request they will also provide you with information concerning the physician's training and qualifications and with what hospital he/she is affiliated. However, it is important to remember that the county medical society will only provide information—they will not make recommendations.[1,2]

2. Select a hospital which has a good medical reputation based on the quality of its staff doctors, then choose an appropriate doctor on its staff. This approach has an advantage, in that the best kind of control exerted on physicians today is by their peers in the hospital.[3]

3. Carefully evaluate the advice of friends and neighbors. Testimony from people you trust that a doctor seems to know his business, is personally pleasant, and charges reasonable fees, is not without merit. However, friends may also base their advice solely on a physician's personality or appearance and not his knowledge and technical skills.

4. Before moving to a new locale, ask your present physician for recommendations. He/she may be familiar with medical personnel in that area.

5. Go the library. The *American Medical Association Directory* describes the educational background of physicians licensed in the United States, and The *Directory of Medical Specialists* provides information about physicians who are certified in various specialties. You may also inquire about a specific physician's training and expertise by calling his/her office, the local or state medical society, or the hospital where he/she practices.

6. Other important considerations include geographical convenience; the physician's personality—do you prefer a doctor of few words who acts with "silent authority" or who is willing and available to answer all of your questions; and the physician's age. A young person may be interested in forming a long-range association with his/her physician and may prefer a younger doctor. Another person may value an older doctor for his experience.

Suppose you have selected a physician and he/she does not answer your questions or perform any kind of physical exam. What if nearly every visit results in a new medicine or injection even though you were not aware of the need? "Vote with your feet."[2] In other words, seek another physician. Although physicians do not like patients who engage in frequent "doctor-hopping," sometimes a discreet change can bring satisfaction. Any competent physician will be happy to arrange for a second medical opinion whenever major surgery is recommended. This is especially important when you do not know the primary surgeon.

Activities: In small groups, compile lists of the things that make one doctor better than another, and then compare lists.

Using class-developed criteria or the following items, ask students to individually rank order the qualities, beginning with #1 as the most important.

Qualities of a Good Physician[1,4]

_____ Affiliated with a good hospital.

_____ Available on short notice.

_____ Aware of latest medical developments.

_____ Best possible education and training.

_____ Can treat most illnesses.

_____ Explains things so patient understands.

_____ Gives each patient plenty of time (thorough)

_____ Has good reputation in the community.

_____ Has his own equipment.

_____ Interested in preventive care.

_____ Knows how to use a specialist.

_____ Listens to the patient and looks directly at him/her.

_____ Makes house calls.

_____ Takes personal interest in patient.

_____ Tells patient the whole truth.

_____ Will treat patient regardless of ability to pay.

When 1,000 U.S. physicians were asked to identify the two or three items they thought were most important in a physician, they valued knowledge and capacity—knowledge based on educational training and experience, and capacity including technical support and personal skill. Most physicians believe that a person is best advised to select a doctor who has the background and ability to treat "the whole patient", who knows when to call in a specialist for assistance, and who is affiliated with a good hospital. While most patients want a "good family practitioner," they tend to value a doctor who is available on short notice, takes a personal interest in them; and who will take care of them regardless of their ability to pay.

Rank in order the following reasons which would cause you to change doctors.[4]

_____ Does not meet your expectation for professional competence.

_____ Not thorough enough.

_____ Does not talk with you—lack of personal interest.

_____ Made a wrong diagnosis.

_____ Poor personality.

_____ Sloppy or unhygienic personal habits.

_____ Other.

Specialists

The five major clinical specialties are: internal medicine, obstetrics and gynecology, pediatrics, psychiatry, and surgery. There are other specialties such as anesthesiology, clinical pathology, and radiology, but patients seldom go directly to them.[2] Assign each student a specialty, and then have him or her submit a report concerning the education and training involved and the primary functions and services performed by each specialist. A listing of specialists and a brief description of each can be found in the book _Doctor!_[3] _Toward a Healthy Lifestyle Through Elementary Health Education_[5] describes several activities pertaining to medical specialists and hospitals that can also be used with middle and Senior High School students e.g. "Children's Hospital" game; "Health Specialists Concentration"; and the _Malpractice_ card game. Teenagers may be especially interested in learning more about specialists in adolescent medicine and the rather new type of health care that is becoming increasingly available for this particular age group. Encourage students to read "One of Their Own,"[6] "Teenage Patients: Their Legal Rights—and Yours,"[7] and "The Rights of Teenagers as Patients."[8]

History of Adolescent Health Care

1759–1777—De Montbeillard measured own son

1776—50% chance of survival by age 21.

1810—Massachusetts passed "Cow Pox Act"

1857—Abraham Jacobi lectured on infant diseases

1872–1911—Compulsory medical inspection in the schools

1888—First chair of pediatrics, Harvard Medical School

1892—Nathan Straus started milk stations to control infection

1904—G. Stanley Hall publishes *Adolescence: Its Psychology, etc.*

1909—First White House Conference on Children

1912—Children's Bureau established. Later called Division of Maternity and Infant Care

1920—B.K. Rachford started pediatrics in Cincinnati

1930—American Academy of Pediatrics established

1930–1945—Significant improvement in infant/child nutrition.

1935—Social Security Act passed by Congress

1941–1945—Three babies die for every two G-Is killed

1945—Antibiotic era began

1951—First Adolescent Clinic in Boston, founded by Dr. J. Roswell Gallagher (considered "the father of Adolescent Medicine")

1955–1969—Salk-Sabin polio vaccine; measles vaccines

1960—Birth control era begins

1960—Cincinnati Adolescent Clinic established

1967—First Free Clinic (San Francisco)

1968—Society for Adolescent Medicine established

1970—Legislation allowing self-consent for treatment of minors

1977—25% of U.S. medical schools teach adolescent health care

Discuss which of the following services your students would most like to see in existence:[7] pg. 57

_____ "A network of adolescent service centers staffed and directed by highly trained and experienced professionals.

_____ Revision of existing health department standards to guarantee that a minor in need of medical service can obtain it with a minimum of red tape and without the prerequisite of parental consent.

_____ A citywide telephone, information and referral service specifically for adolescents and their medical and health problems.

_____ A qualified personal service counselor in every junior and senior high school to provide health information.

_____ Trained counselors in public welfare center to give guidance and encouragement to adolescents whose families are on welfare.

_____ A group education program to assist adolescents with health problems.

_____ A training program for teachers and staff at all city schools, particularly in drug and sex education.

_____ Various information programs to encourage young people to enter the health field as a career.

_____ State reimbursement to physicians and medical service facilities treating adolescents."

How to Choose a Hospital

Like most things in life, hospitals can not usually be regarded as entirely good or bad, but rather strong in some areas and weak in others. However, there are some general guidelines which may be useful in selecting a hospital for the specific purpose of selecting a doctor on its staff.[3]

_____ Is the hospital accredited by the Joint Commission on Accreditation of Hospitals? (You can ask the hospital administrator or write to JCAH, 875 N. Michigan Avenue, Chicago, Illinois 60611). Accreditation implies that at least minimal standards of care—as determined by an investigating team, usually every two years—are being met.

_____ Does the hospital have a formal affiliation with a medical school? One sign of a teaching hospital is the presence of interns and residents, who often serve to keep other staff physicians "on their toes." Some teaching hospitals, however, are large and impersonal despite their often higher standards.

_____ Is the hospital "nonprofit, community," rather than privately owned and run for profit? Hospitals run for profit are not always synonymous with concern for quality care.

_____ Does the hospital have a high percentage of "board-certified" or "board eligible" physicians on staff? Each specialty has a "board" which supervises training and certifies competency.

_____ Does the hospital maintain high quality education programs for its staff? Is attendance required to maintain staff privileges? Do the doctors actively participate in the continuing education of nurses and other hospital health personnel?

_____ Does the hospital have ways of identifying the physician who has become incompetent?

After obtaining all of the "official" information available to you, try to get some "inside" information from a friend who works in the hospital, such as a technician or therapist. Nurses are a good source of information because they work closely with many doctors. Operating-room technicians have the opportunity to view many surgeons. Whatever your source, you will have to evaluate the worth of the information. Obviously the best time to make such an investigation is before an illness strikes.

Activity: Have students make a list of the various medical facilities that exist in your community—hospitals, emergency rooms, convalescent homes, clinics and private physician offices. Such facilities usually offer "primary" care— care that is provided by a physician and which may be obtained without the referral of another physician. Does the facility offer _"secondary"_ care? Secondary care usually requires referral from a physician and is often care by a specialist in a typical community hospital. Does the facility offer _"tertiary"_ care? Tertiary care includes special and extraordinary procedures such as kidney dialysis or open-heart surgery. This type of care is found at university affiliated hospitals and regional referral centers. It may never be needed during your entire life.

Perhaps several students can arrange to visit a "free clinic" and then lead a class discussion regarding the advantages and disadvantages of this type of medical care compared to more traditional settings.

Materials

1. Telephone directory
2. Optional—"Children's Hospital" game board and cards.[5]

Evaluation

1. Objective one may be evaluated by presenting the following situation to your class and requiring them to respond in no more than one written page: You have just learned that you will be moving to another city next month. Your family will need to change their pediatrician, gynecologist, and dentist. Knowing that you have studied about consumer health and medical care in school, your parents ask you what would be the best ways to locate "good" physicians and a dentist in your new community. What would you suggest? What qualities would you want medical practitioners to possess?

2. A rank-order activity is included under content and procedures that can be used to fulfill Objective Two. After the activity is completed on an individual basis, you may wish to have the students form small groups and try to reach a consensus regarding the three most important qualities a physician should possess.

3. Attainment of Objective Three may be evaluated by asking students to match the following health problems with the medical specialist most likely to be consulted:

Health Problem	*Medical Specialist*
1. Heart Disease	A. Allergist
2. Removal of Enlarged Prostate	B. Dermatologist
3. Acute Skin Problem	C. General Practitioner
4. Disease Affecting Female Reproductive System	D. Cardiologist
	E. Neurosurgeon
5. Desensitization Shots and Skin Tests	F. Obstetrician—Gynecologist
6. Spinal Cord Injury	G. Ophthalmologist
7. Rectal Growth	H. Orthopedist
8. Cataract Surgery	I. Otolaryngologist
9. Ear, Nose, and Throat Surgery	J. Pediatrician
10. Chronic Low Back Pain and Problems with Joints	K. Urologist
	L. Proctologist

Answers:
1–D; 2–K; 3–B; 4–F; 5–A; 6–E; 7–L; 8–G; 9–I; 10–H

4. Objective four is self-explanatory.

5. Answers to objective five: 1. JCAH accreditation; 2. formal affiliation with a medical school; 3. nonprofit, community hospital; 4. high percentage of "board-certified" or "board-eligible" physicians on staff; 5. Regular, high quality education programs; 6. Procedure for identifying incompetent physicians.

6. Objective six may be evaluated through the use of several multiple-choice or matching-type questions. The student may also be asked to discuss how a patient suffering from heart failure could receive primary, secondary, and tertiary care.

Objectives

1. The student will be able to distinguish between the following terms: Blue Cross plan; Blue Shield plan; cash indemnity; Health Maintenance Organization; Independent Plan Insurance; Medicaid; Medicare; and National Health Insurance.

2. "The student will critically evaluate various plans designed to pay for health care according to their services, benefits, costs, advantages and disadvantages."[3]

3. The student will be able to describe at least three ways medication costs can be reduced.

4. The student will be able to discuss both the pros and cons involved with the trend towards increased "Do-It-Yourself Doctoring" as a means of reducing the high cost of medical care.

Sources

1. G. Timothy Johnson, M.D. *What You Should Know About Health Care Before You Call A Doctor!* New York: McGraw-Hill Book Company, 1975.

2. David Kotelchuck (Editor). *Prognosis Negative: Crisis in the Health Care System.* New York: Vintage Books, 1976.

3. Robert H. Kirk and Michael H. Hamrick. *Focus on Health and Nutrition.* Rosemont, Illinois: National Diary Council, 1977, p. 75.

4. Earl Ubell. "Unraveling the Mysteries of Health Insurance," (Part I) *Family Health,* October, 1978.

5. Earl Ubell. "The Great American Health Insurance Machine," (Part 2) *Family Health,* November 1978.

6. "The Financing of Health Care" by Herbert F. Klarman found in John H. Knowles, M.D. (Editor). *Doing Better and Feeling Worse—Health in the United States.* New York: W.W. Norton & Company, Inc., 1977.

7. Donald M. Vickery, M.D. and James F. Fries, M.D. *Take Care of Yourself: A Consumer's Guide to Medical Care.* Reading, Massachusetts: Addison-Wesley Publishing Company, 1977.

8. Ralph Nadar. "The Overprotective Doctor," *Family Health,* August, 1978, pg. 20.

9. John Grossmann. "Do-It-Yourself Doctoring". *Family Health,* February, 1979, pg. 20.

Content and Procedures

Introduction

In trying to understand the American Health Care system, one must traverse a tangled web of government-financed programs, regulatory measures, national health insurance proposals, and a conglomeration of health personnel and facilities. One must try to view health care through both the eyes of the sick consumer "unable to gain easy entry into the health care system and the harried professional trying to respond via traditional patterns."[1], pg. 387.

Dr. Timothy Johnson suggests three guiding principles for all of us, whether we are public consumers, responsive government officials, or concerned professionals:[1], p. 388

1. Health Care is a right;
2. Health Care is costly; and
3. Health Care is personal.

Activity: Discuss the following questions:

—Do you believe that health care is a basic human right that must be provided if the society is capable of doing so? _____

—Do you believe that without good health it is possible to pursue life, liberty, and happiness? _____

—Do you believe that health care is a very special concern to most people? _____

—Do you think that every health care professional (whose training is increasingly subsidized by public money) should be required to serve two years in a medically deprived area in place of military service?

_____

—Do you think that the basic costs of health care should be removed from the direct responsibility of the individual and moved into the sector of public financing by means of tax revenues? _____

—Do you think it is a *right* or a *privilege* to be cared for by a physician? _____

—Do you think Americans should be willing to pay the cost of health care, *whatever it is?* _____

—Do you think a reduction in *personal care* by health professionals is acceptable if medical costs can be decreased through efficiency techniques and management expertise? _____

Ask students to investigate the health status of Americans (e.g. infant mortality, life expectancy, illness and disability, distribution of health services). Why do they think the quality of our health-care delivery system is uneven and often inadequate when we pay far more than any other country? (In fiscal 1975, Americans spent $104 billion for health care).[2]

Private Health Insurance

Invite several health insurance sales representatives to present various types of private health insurance plans to your class and to compare their costs and benefits. Discuss the following types of health protection:

a. *Hospital expenses*—How long does the policy cover room and board in a semi-private room? Does it cover nursing services; laboratory fees; X-ray; and drugs?

b. Does the insurance policy cover *maternity bills,* or is it listed as an option? Does the policy cover extensive hospitalization for the baby if it should be born prematurely or with a congenital defect?

c. Are *physicians' fees* covered, both inside and outside the hospital? (Does this include the anesthesiologist's bill?) Office visits are frequently not covered, unless they are part of a postoperative follow-up.

d. *Major Medical* insurance is supposed to take care of your medical bills when other basic policies run out. Since premiums are high, try to obtain as much protection as possible while leaving no gaps you can't handle financially. (Learn what the terms exclusion, deductible, and co-insurance mean).

e. Does the policy provide compensation for *loss of income* incurred during an extended illness?[3,4]

Since there are over 1,500 different health insurers in this country, it is difficult to determine which company offers the best plan. Students may wish to examine some of the following sources of information in addition to relying on insurance sales representatives:

—Health Insurance Institute, 1850 K Street, N.W., Washington, D.C. 20006. Ask for "Our Family's Health Insurance: Do You Know The Answer?" which is a quiz and record of family's health care and insurance costs. Also available is "The New ABC's of Health Insurance."

—Sylvia Porter's Money Book (Doubleday and Company, Inc.) carries a chapter on "The High Cost of Good Health."

—American Dental Association, 211 East Chicago Avenue, Chicago, Illinois 60611. Ask for "Dental Insurance, Your Dentist and You" and "Understanding Dental Prepayment."[4]

Health Maintenance Organizations (HMOs)

Unlike most basic and major medical insurance policies which limit the portion of the medical bills that they cover and often do not cover routine services, HMOs are more all-purpose. They comprise a group of doctors who, for a fixed monthly sum, provide everything from routine checkups to major operations to 24-hour emergency service. They may be sponsored by the government, private individuals, medical schools, hospitals, employers, labor unions, consumer groups, private insurance companies or Blue Cross and Blue Shield.[5]

HMOs have their own staff of generally full-time physicians who are salaried employees. Although you cannot select an outside doctor, you can choose your doctor from among the staff physicians and change doctors if necessary. For information about HMOs in your area, write to The Group Health Association of America, 1717 Massachusetts Avenue, N.W., Washington, D.C. 20036. Or write to the Director, Division of HMOs, Department of HEW, Park Lawn Building, 5600 Fishers Lane, Rockville, Maryland 20857. Additional information may also be obtained from the article, "The Great American Health Insurance Machine,"[5] and Chapter 9 of *Prognosis Negative*.[2]

Medicaid and Medicare

Critics of HMOs point out that this form of health care (which has been suggested as an alternative to nationalized medicine) is often only available to employed and relatively healthy individuals—not to the elderly and indigent, who are hardest hit by illness. That is where Medicaid and Medicare come in. They are government sponsored medical care programs that care for people who have low or no incomes (Medicaid), or are elderly and disabled (Medicare). Investigate the advantages and disadvantages of Medicaid and Medicare programs. For Medicaid information, contact your local Department of Social Services listed in the telephone book or write to Medical Service Administration, Social and Rehabilitation Services, U.S. Department of HEW, Washington, D.C. 20201. For information on Medicare, again from the Health Insurance Institute, ask for "What You Should Know About Health Insurance When You Retire." Or write to the Social Security Administration, Bureau of Health Insurance, East Highrise, Baltimore, Maryland 21235. Students may also wish to read Chapter 8 of *Prognosis Negative*[2] for another viewpoint.

National Health Insurance

National Health Insurance of various types has been promoted as another way of providing high quality medical care to all individuals. However, "it is generally believed that enactment of national health insurance would lead to further increases in healthcare expenditures. The reason is that the scope and depth of health insurance exert a major influence on the utilization of services and price per unit and therefore on the total amount spent."[6], p. 224 Students may be interested in comparing the major health plans that have been presented to Congress and reading Chapter 11 of *Prognosis Negative*[2] and Herbert E. Klarman's essay on "The Financing of Health Care."[6]

Reducing the Cost of Health Care

Have students try to determine how much Federal money was spent on the following items for a given year: medical care, dental care, nursing services, health products, hospitalization, health insurance, health education, disease prevention, and medical research. Develop a pie-graph to illustrate the findings.

Medications provide one way of saving money. When drugs are prescribed, take them regularly and as directed, but do not expect to receive a prescription every time you go to a doctor. In other words, don't urgently request relief for every minor symptom that appears or a "shot of penicillin" for your cold. You should, however, expect to have your medication program thoroughly reviewed every time you see your doctor. When your physician prescribes a drug you may wish to inquire if (s)he is familiar with the relative cost of alternative drugs. By requesting a drug by its "generic" name rather than its "brand" name, the physician can save you money. When selecting a pharmacy, it pays to do comparison shopping. Select the store that is least expensive and most convenient. Pharmacists are not required to give you the cheapest equivalent alternative even though your physician has written a prescription by its "generic" name. If they have stocked only one manufacturer's formulation of each drug, you will probably not know it.

Review your home pharmacy. Does your stock only include the most inexpensive and the most frequently needed medications? Are all of your medicines less than three years old?

Another contributing factor to the high cost of health care is the practice of "defensive medicine" by American physicians. In this age of "Sue the Doctor," physicians have sought to protect themselves by ordering more tests than are clinically necessary for each patient. One official of the Department of Health, Education, and Welfare (now called Health and Human Services) estimated that the practice of defensive medicine costs the American public $5 billion a year.[8] What do you think can be done about this practice? If you were a physician, how would you try to protect yourself? The fear of law suits has also pervaded surgery, causing some doctors to decline performing certain operations and to cease publishing case reports in medical journals that detail adverse effects of diagnostic and therapeutic procedures. On the positive side, consumers may now be receiving improved Emergency room treatment and more thorough examinations and explanations from their physicians.

Activity: Ask students to debate whether defensive medicine is worth its immense cost. Would the money be better spent on medical research, outpatient clinics, or a range of other medical services of a more certain benefit to the patient? Can we place a price tag on health issues?

"Do-It-Yourself Doctoring" is another area that is steadily gaining both support and criticism. A "self-care" revolution is taking place that is reducing the number of unnecessary doctor visits that are made annually, while increasing the individual's role in caring for him/herself. The ramifications of medical equipment in the hands of lay people are profound. Ask students to read the article "Do-It-Yourself Doctoring,'" and any other similar articles that you can find.

Materials

1. Various health insurance policies.
2. Optional—stethoscopes, otoscope, sphygmomanometer, pregnancy test kit, home cholesterol test.

Evaluation

1. Ask students to answer the questions in Column A by selecting the best answer in Column B. The same answer may be used more than once.

Column A

_____ 1. This plan only covers your *hospital* expenses.

_____ 2. This prepaid plan covers routine checkups, major operations, and 24-hour emergency service.

_____ 3. If you only have a very low income, you will probably qualify for this plan.

_____ 4. This plan would probably rely heavily on the existing combination of independent health insurance plans.

_____ 5. This plan uses its own staff of full-time physicians.

_____ 6. You qualify for this plan if you're 65 or older or entitled to Social Security disability benefits.

_____ 7. This plan would focus on the 24 million Americans not now covered by other insurance plans.

_____ 8. This private insurance plan will pay a fixed sum to cover doctor's bill connected with a hospital stay.

_____ 9. This plan grew out of the Great Depression and pays the hospital directly rather than the insured individual.

_____10. This plan guarantees equal coverage for every citizen.

Column B

A. Blue Cross

B. Blue Shield

C. Cash indemnity

D. HMO

E. Medicaid

F. Medicare

G. National Health Insurance

2. Objectives two and three are self-explanatory.
3. Bring in examples of stethoscopes, otoscopes, sphygmomanometers, pregnancy test kits, and home cholesterol tests. Ask students which tools they feel are probably safe for home use. Check to see whether they know how to properly use the tool or test. Which devices do they think may be dangerous if improperly used? What could happen? Ask students to rank the devices, beginning with the one they would be most apt to purchase and use.

Selected Learning Activities

Consumer Health and Medical Care

_____ Discuss why some medical specialists (chiropractors and naturopaths) are not universally recognized. Should they be?

_____ Play "Medical Specialists Concentration." Make matching cards. On one card print the name of the specialist and on the other card describe his service. Place all cards face down and play the game as you would play the card game of concentration. Whoever has the largest number of matches at the end of the game is the winner.

_____ Make a Medical Specialists Bulletin Board. The bulletin board could be a medical building with many windows. Each student could be in charge of a window, placing the name of a particular kind of specialist in the window.

_____ Play Medical Specialist Charades. Act out a speciality and your group must guess.

_____ Identify and discuss some of the possible dangers associated with self-medication and self-diagnosis.

_____ Prepare an exhibit or bulletin board display showing both traditional and nontraditional sources of medical care.

_____ Investigate the importance of laughter and a positive mental attitude for preventing or alleviating ill health.

_____ Research and report on health programs designed to promote high level wellness on the job.

_____ Role play techniques used by health quacks to sell or promote products to the public.

_____ Identify the different consumer protection groups and write a pamphlet describing one in detail (Better Business Bureau, Consumer Reports, etc.).

_____ Identify a product that you are interested in owning. Read Consumer Reports and outline some of the points that will help you in making a wise selection.

_____ Visit three drug stores and compare their layout, design, and appeal.

_____ Select a product that is produced by several different companies. Compare and contrast the price of different brands, the packaging, the advertising, etc. What have you learned about yourself and about your consumption of products?

_____ Examine magazines for advertisements for health products. What kinds of health products do consumers buy through the mail?

_____ Visit a nursing home or other medical facility and donate two hours of time.

_____ Select a health topic of interest and write a three page report using five resources that are reliable.

22

Teaching about the Environment

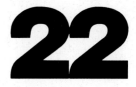

The current interst in the shortage of gas has prompted the American public to focus on the need for conservation. What is our personal role in conservation and our personal responsibility in making decisions that enhance the environment? These questions require careful examination in the 80's. This chapter includes an outline of Suggested Topics for Teaching About The Environment, Three Detailed Sample Lesson Plans, and additional Selected Learning Experiences.

The first lesson, **Major Pollutants,** identifies the different pollutants which exist in the environment and relates the existence of these pollutants to problems with our physical health. The student also learns about the Pollutant Standard Index.

The second lesson on **Saving the Environment,** is an affective lesson in which students examine their personal role in energy conservation. The lesson is based on changing attitudes and behaviors.

The third lesson, **The Energy Crises,** examines the problems associated with energy depletion. The student examines the inherent dangers associated with nuclear power plants. The lesson should raise some important questions about public morality and the right to have good health.

Suggested Topics

The Environment

I. Air Pollution
   A. Causes of air pollution
   B. Temperature inversions
   C. Principal air pollutants
   D. Legal efforts to control pollution
   E. Temperature changes

II. Water pollution
    A. Causes of water pollution
    B. Common water pollutants
    C. Diseases related to water pollution
    D. Water purification systems
    E. Legislation and water pollution
III. Solid Wastes
    A. Why it is a problem
    B. Waste disposal procedures: incineration, recycling, landfill, dumps.
IV. Noise Pollution
    A. Why it is a problem
    B. Pitch and loudness as characteristics of sound
    C. Effects of noise on the ear
    D. Sound levels of common noises
V. Pesticides
    A. Uses of pesticides
    B. Kinds of pesticides
    C. Pesticides and cancer
    D. Pesticides as an aid
VI. Flurocarbons
    A. Its use in aerosols
    B. Its effects on the upper atmosphere
VII. Radiation
    A. The relationship to leukemia and cancer
    B. X rays and radiation
    C. Radioactive fallout
VIII. Reasons for Environmental Problems
    A. Failure to obey the laws
    B. Poor law enforcement
IX. Agencies Dealing With Pollution
    A. Federal agencies
    B. State agencies
X. Solutions to Environmental Problems
    A. Community action programs
    B. Incentives—i.e. cash for aluminum cans

Lesson Plans

Environment
Major Pollutants

Objectives

1. The student will be able to explain how water and air pollution, pesticides, noise, and solid waste debris affect physical health.

2. The student will be able to identify the components of the different types of pollutants.

3. The student will be able to explain the Pollutant Standard Index.

Sources

1. Arthur Boughey, *Man and the Environment,* New York: Macmillan Publishing Co., 1971.

2. George Waldbott, *Health Effects of Environmental Pollutants,* St. Louis: C.V. Mosley Co., 1973.

Content and Procedures

Introduction

As human beings have triumphed over "natural" enemies to the environment, they have created new problems which have introduced new hazards. While humans have sought to reach a high level of wellness, their adaptations to the obstacles of environmental pollutants, such as air, noise, water, pesticide and solid waste, have provoked concerns about the impact on health. To determine the effects of these pollutants, it is important that we examine each as a separate entity.

Air Pollution

Air pollution is contamination by waste products of the air we breathe. Each year, we pollute the air with 200 million tons of "aerial garbage." The damage caused costs $12 billion each year in clean-up and health related expenses. This means that the cost to each man, woman and child is $65 annually.

Air pollution is caused by power plants, factories, and most of all, automobiles. The major pollutants include:

1. *Sulfur oxides*—colorless gas which results from the burning of *fossil fuels* such as oil and coal. When sulfur oxides combine with moisture in the air, *sulfuric acid* is formed. Exposure to sulfur dioxide can cause considerable irritation in the throat and lungs as well as bronchial constriction.

2. *Carbon monoxide*—colorless, odorless, highly toxic gas emitted from automobiles. Carbon monoxide limits the blood's oxygen-carrying capacity, a deficiency which can cause dizziness, blurred vision, headaches, distorted perception of time, and fatigue. People with heart conditions and respiratory ailments are especially susceptible to the effects of gas.

3. *Hydrocarbons*—emitted from automobile exhausts can react with sunlight to form photochemical pollution which, in turn, cause damage to crops. Hydrocarbons also can cause noses and throats to burn as well as eyes to water.

4. *Ozone*—is formed when nitrogen oxides ard certain hydrocarbons combine in the presence of sunlight. Produced mainly from automobiles, ozone is one component of photochemical smog. It can affect the tissues in plants and is irritating to the eye, nose and throat.

5. *Particluates*—small solid or liquid particles in the air that can aggravate respiratory diseases. The major sources of particulates are iron and steel operations, as well as electric power generation plants. Particulates are carriers for other pollutants by enabling these substances to be absorbed by them or stick to them. The pollutants can then be breathed deeply in the lungs.

At this point the teacher can discuss the Pollutant Standard Index (PSI). Although the PSI is mentioned during weather forecasts, very few people understand its meaning. The PSI was designed to make it easier to understand air quality from state to state and region to region.

Although one or more pollutants may be measured each day, the pollutant with the highest reading is given as the PSI. Particulates, sulfur dioxide, carbon monoxide and ozone are the pollutants measured. The following chart adopted from the Ohio Environmental Protection Agency indicates the meanings of PSI numbers;

		HEALTH EFFECTS	HEALTH WARNINGS
0 ——————— Good 50 ———————	Moderate		
100 —— Air Quality Goal ——	Unhealthful	Mild aggravation of symptoms in susceptible persons, with irritation symptoms in the healthy population.	Persons with existing heart or respiratory ailments should reduce physical exertion and outdoor activity.
200 —— 1st Stage Alert ——	Very Unhealthy	Significant aggravation of symptoms and decreased exercise tolerance in persons with heart or lung disease, with widespread symptoms in the healthy population.	Elderly and persons with existing heart or lung disease should stay indoors and reduce physical activity.
300 —— 2nd Stage Alert ——	Hazardous	Premature onset of certain diseases in addition to significant aggravation of symptoms and decreased exercise tolerance in healthy persons.	Elderly and persons with existing diseases should stay indoors and avoid physical exertion. General population should avoid outdoor activity.
400 —— 3rd Stage Alert —— 500	Hazardous	Premature death of ill and elderly. Healthy people will experience adverse symptoms that affect their normal activity.	All persons should remain indoors, keeping windows and doors closed. All persons should minimize physical exertion and avoid traffic.

Ask your students to make a log of the PSI's each day and interpret its significance according to the chart.

Noise Pollution

Sixteen million people in the U.S. suffer some hearing loss due to exposure to excessive sounds. Among the loud sounds to which one may be exposed are airplanes, TV's, radios, power tools, and household appliances. In addition to the health detriments of noise to hearing, the following can also result:

1. muscle tension;
2. increased blood pressure;
3. nervous tension;
4. constriction of blood vessels;
5. an increase of hormones entering into the blood, due to greater activity in the endocrine glands.

Noise is measured in decibels. Most sound humans encounter range between 50 and 90 decibels, i.e., a two-person conversation may be around 60 decibels. Examples of other noises may be around 60 decibels. Examples of other noises and their corresponding decibels are:

a jet plane 100 feet away	=	140 decibels
loud disco music	=	120 decibels
lawn mower	=	110 decibels
noisy kitchen	=	100 decibels
heavy truck passing	=	90 decibels
alarm clock	=	80 decibels

freeway traffic	=	70 decibels
ordinary conversation	=	60 decibels
light auto traffic	=	50 decibels
quiet office	=	40 decibels
soft whisper	=	30 decibels

Between 10–20 decibels, sound is just audible.

Using the chart as a base, the teacher can ask students to list the sounds they heard for a 24 hour period and determine the sound levels.

Water Pollution

As many as 500,000 different chemicals have found their way into water. It is estimated that 8.1 million Americans are served questionable water from public suppliers. Polluted waters have revealed an increase in sodium levels, which in turn can damage the circulatory system of susceptible people. A number of carcinogenic chemicals from industrial waste have been found in drinking water. Many fish have been killed due to oil spills in water.

However, the government is placing stricter controls on industries that pollute our waters. Although this is only a beginning, it indicates a concern about our preservation of water as well as the fish living in it.

Pesticides

While pesticides have improved human health by killing the insects that kill our crops, it has also presented another health problem. Pesticides have been transferred to humans, and are suspected of causing cancer. Concerned about this, the government has banned the use of various insecticides such as aldrin and dieldrin.

Solid Waste Debris

Solid waste is everything man produces, uses, and discards. It includes food scraps, plastics, glass, clothing, automobiles, chairs, buses, etc.

The usual composition of solid waste by weight is:

paper	59%
wood, lawn and garden waste	10%
food waste	9%
glass and other ceramics	8.5%
metal	7%
clothes, plastic, rubber	6%
other	.5%

Each year we dispose of enough solid waste to fill 5 million large truck trailers.

Some of the common methods used to dispose of waste is to:

1. use the city dump;

2. through incineration, although this may increase air pollution;

3. through sanitary landfill, which is considered the most practical since one acre, eight feet deep can accommodate solid waste for a city of 10,000 for one year.

Apparently solid waste is not as much of a problem as the other pollutants mentioned previously.

Evaluation

Through examinations and assignments, the teacher will be able to determine the degree to which the objectives were met.

Environment

Saving the Environment

Objective

Students will discuss how each can play a role in energy conservation.

Sources

Paul Ehrlich, *Population Bomb*, New York:
Ballantine, 1971

Content and Procedures

Introduction

Students must become convinced that a change in lifestyle is needed if they are to begin to conserve our energy. If people can begin to see the impact which each and every one can make upon energy consumption, the results will be satisfactory.

Many things can be done on a day to day basis to help save the environment. For example, if people would ride bicycles or walk to nearby places, less gasoline would be wasted and less pollutants would be released into the atmosphere, not to mention the health benefits of physical activity.

Energy Activity Sheet

List five things you do daily which wastes energy.

1. _____
2. _____
3. _____
4. _____
5. _____

List five things you do or can do daily that will conserve energy.

1. _____
2. _____
3. _____
4. _____
5. _____

Recycling

It has been estimated that more than 80 percent of solid wastes produced annually can be recycled. Many cities have sites where newspapers, aluminum, etc. can be returned and sold for recycling. Some states have passed laws which require deposit bottles—that is, a fee is charged on all bottled beverages, so that disposable bottles are outlawed.

Another step being taken by auto makers to conserve energy is the increase in the production of small cars. Small cars use less gasoline and therefore also emit less pollutants in the air.

To help save gasoline, the Federal government has supported the maintainence of 55 mile per hour speed limits. This has aroused controversy in some states where the feeling exists that the speed limit should be increased to accommodate the driver who is on a long, open stretch of road.

If you had the power to enforce rules, what would you impose as the speed limit on highways? Why?

If you had the power, would you mandate small cars for everyone? Would you make exceptions? What would be your exceptions?

Evaluation

The student will make a list of ten ways that he or she can conserve energy and will keep this list (on an index card) in his or her wallet. After two weeks, each student will write an essay listing at least five observations about his or her behavior.

Environment
The Energy Crisis

Objectives

1. Students will discuss the implications of energy depletion.

2. Students will describe the inherent dangers associated with nuclear power plants.

Source

John Phillips, *Environmental Health: A Paradox of Progress,* Dubuque: William C. Brown Company, 1971.

Content and Procedures

Now more than ever before, the United States is concerned about the rapid depletion of energy. With the increase in the price of crude oil necessary for gasoline and the increased consumption of energy due to an increase in population, the "energy crisis" has surfaced. The possible impact of the increased use of energy on our environment and health has been discussed in theory. One theory states that all energy will be dissipated and spread throughout the atmosphere in the form of heat. This, in turn, can cause the earth's temperature to rise and the polar ice caps to melt. Thus, all major coastal cities can be flooded. The second theory states that because of the increase in particulate matter, solar radiation will be reflected away from the earth, causing a decrease in temperature. This can cause another "ice age."

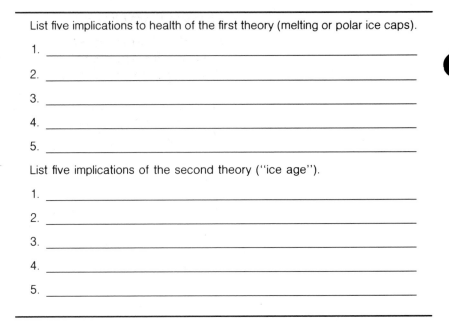

List five implications to health of the first theory (melting or polar ice caps).

1. _____
2. _____
3. _____
4. _____
5. _____

List five implications of the second theory ("ice age").

1. _____
2. _____
3. _____
4. _____
5. _____

Nuclear Power

Nuclear power has been on the minds of many individuals. While nuclear power plants are regarded by many as an energy producing source, they have many inherent dangers. Among these are meltdowns, leaks in cooling pipes, and core cooling-system failure. The release of radioactive wastes into the environment poses a serious threat to health. The 1979 incident in Harrisburg, Pennsylvania, causing a mass evacuation of individuals from that city, has resulted in second thoughts about the feasibility of nuclear power plants.

Although we may be exposed to low levels of radiation, whether it be from nuclear power plants or X-ray, no low level is considered safe. It is generally accepted that increases in radiation exposure lead to increases in the frequency of cancer.

Many people have concerns about the use of x-rays. It should be noted that x-rays are valuable medical aids serving to diagnose disease, broken bones, and other serious physical conditions.

Although a single x-ray will probably not cause damage, all exposures involve some risk. This means that a person who *needs* an x-ray should not be afraid to have it, since the potential benefits of a necessary x-ray far outweigh the possible damage from radiation exposure. Among the points to be aware of are:

1. Dental X-rays—Although many people feel their teeth should be x-rayed on a regular basis, the American Dental Association contends that x-ray examinations should not be standard at each examination but only when necessary. Let the dentist be the judge.

2. Chest X-ray—Since the detection by use of x-rays of T.B. and other chest diseases is not as effective as are other means, the Food and Drug Administration has discouraged this process.

3. X-ray During Pregnancy—Unless postponement will be detrimental to the mother's health, x-rays should not be taken during pregnancy.

Alternate Energy Sources

A steadily increasing number of American's are building solar homes. Solar energy is being used to heat and cool homes. This type of energy can save half of the cost of electric for a house.

Ask students to compute their home or apartment electric bills for a year and then have them compute the savings per year by having a solar home.

Evaluation

1. Ask students to describe the energy conservation methods they use in their house. Have them list the steps they or their family take—i.e. turn off all lights when leaving a room, use less hot water, etc.

2. Examination based upon objectives.

Selected Learning Activities

The Environment

_____ Working in small groups, ask students to 1. create a new product, 2. design a TV commercial or magazine advertisement to promote the product, and 3. develop a chart describing what natural resources would be affected by their product.

_____ Invite a speaker from the State Highway Department to discuss the problems involved in clearing an area for a super highway and how they are solved.

_____ Make a list of all the environmental agents which you can discover that contribute to birth defects in animals, including humans. Contact the March of Dimes for assistance.

_____ Collect algae from a nearby pond and use it in a study of green plants in the food pyramid and their response to increased amounts of nutrients such as phosphorous.

_____ Write to the U.S. Department of Agriculture, Soil Conservation Service, for their publication _Outdoor Classrooms on School Sites_, PA-975.

_____ Write an essay on the following topics: "Our planet could become unfit for human habitation if people continue to blithely ravage the delicately balanced environment."

_____ Investigate the campaigns that have been held in different states concerning disposable bottles and cans versus returnables. What were the pros and cons? What were some of the issues raised? Where do you stand? Why?

_____ Take a litter walk around the school, picking up pieces of litter and trash. Make a poster or a collage out of the things that you have collected.

_____ Make an environmental pledge card for your wallet. On the card identify one thing that you will pledge to do to make our environment a better place to be.

_____ Make a bulletin board depicting the parts of an ecosystem. Have each student identify and describe the parts.

_____ Make jingles that promote the environment. Put a different jingle on the board each day.

_____ Develop an environmental check list to take home.

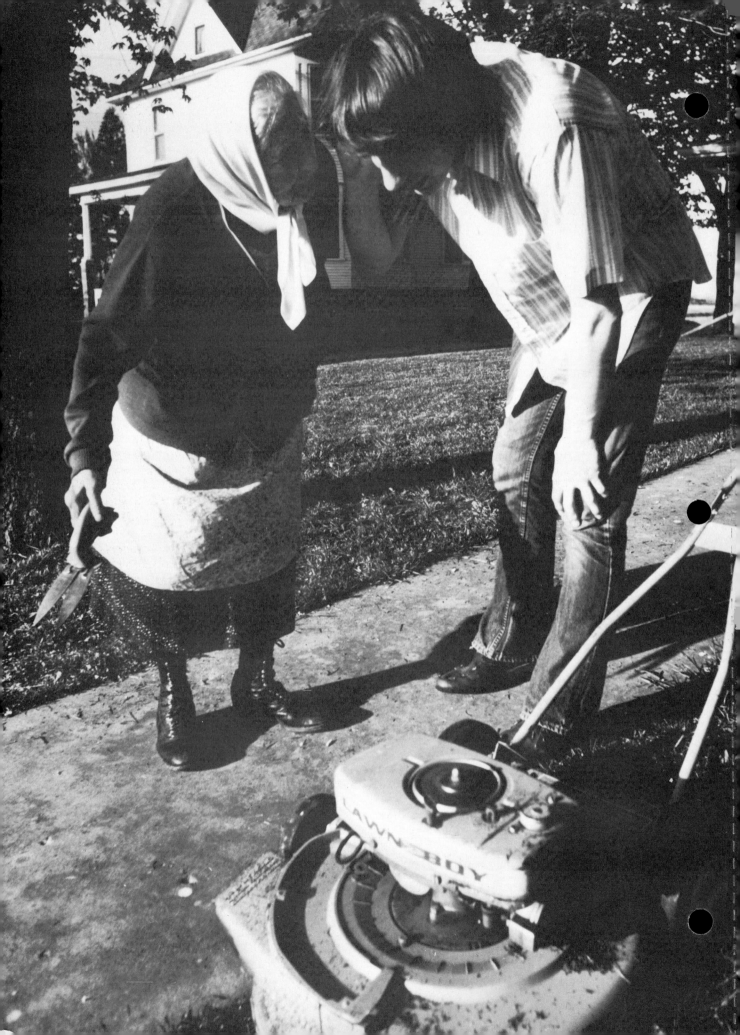

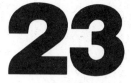

Teaching about Aging, Dying, and Death

In a curriculum focusing on the development of a healthy lifestyle and examining the possible alternative behaviors from which to choose, the discussion of aging, dying, and death is of paramount importance. Its relationship to quality living can not be underestimated. Accepting aging and ultimately death may increase the possibility for making life meaningful and for viewing one's decisions as important. In addition, aging, dying, and death signify our final adaptation. In this chapter, we include an outline of Suggested Topics for Teaching About Aging, Dying, and Death, Three Detailed Sample Lessons, and additional Selected Learning Activities.

The first lesson, **The Aging Process,** identifies and discusses the varied physiological changes that take place when one reaches the later years of life. Through simulations, the students will be able to experience physiological changes that take place during the aging process.

The second lesson, **Preparing for Death,** examines the different alternatives available to a person who is preparing for death. Practical information about arranging a funeral and writing a will are covered.

The third lesson, **Stages of Dying,** carefully covers the steps or aspects of death identified by Elizabeth Kubler Ross. The student becomes familiar with each stage. Hopefully, with adequate information the student will be able to deal more comfortably with death of a family member.

Suggested Topics

Aging, Dying, and Death
I. The Aging Process
   A. Longevity
   B. Physiological changes occurring with aging
   C. Psychological changes related to aging
II. Coping With Getting Old
   A. Understanding and accepting aging
   B. Maintaining a healthy self concept
   C. Psycho-social theories
   D. Relating to and with others

Photo Courtesy of the
Environmental Protection Agency

III. Dimensions of Death and Dying
   A. Types of death: functional, brain, cellular
   B. Stages of death: denial, anger, bargaining, depression, acceptance
IV. Prolonging Life
   A. The will to live
   B. Euthanasia
   C. Life support systems
V. Grief and Mourning
   A. Stages of grief
   B. The funeral
   C. Alternatives to the traditional funeral
VI. Suicide
   A. Suicide as a leading cause of death for young and old
   B. Suicide and the terminally ill
   C. Causes of suicide
   D. Prevention of suicide
   E. Issues related to suicide
VII. Aging and Economics
   A. Housing needs
   B. Medicare and Medicaid
   C. Social security
VIII. The Youthful Science of Aging
   A. Kinds of age (physiological, chronological, sociological and psychological)
   B. Current research
   C. Retarding aging

Lesson Plans

Aging, Dying and Death
The Aging Process

Objectives

1. The student will be able to identify and discuss the physiological changes that take place when one reaches the later years of life.

2. Through simulations, students will be able to experience physiological changes that take place during the aging process.

Sources

1. James E. Birren (Ed.), *Handbook of Aging and the Individual,* Chicago: University of Chicago Press, 1971.

2. P.S. Timiras, *Development Physiology and Aging,* New York: Macmillan Publishing Company, 1972.

Content and Procedures

Introduction

At the age of 15, most adolescents do not appear concerned about old age. With 59 years living ahead of them, students are not thinking about the physiological changes that will occur later in life. Yet, in a society where people are living longer than ever before younger people are becoming intimately exposed to older people. For example, many students in the teenage years are faced with the prospect of having their grandparents live with them, so that mother and father can be readily available to help when they are needed.

Due to a variety of reasons, young people are often reluctant to understand the physiological changes that take place with their grandparents. As a result, the adolescent may become irritable when the elderly, living in the same household, drop dishes, ask statements to be repeated, or request assistance with physical tasks.

To help the teenager better understand the behaviors exhibited by older people, both now and in the future, it is important that a comprehension of physiological changes of aging be understood.

Physiological Changes of Aging

Aging begins at birth. From the day we are born, the body changes. Up to the age of 15, rapid growth takes place. The peak of physiological strength and skills take place during the late teens. From there we begin to witness a tapering off. Up to age 50, this decline is gradual, but after age 50 many individuals begin to notice changes indicative of greater age. Among these changes may be:

1. Less efficient functioning of oil glands, which can cause wrinkling skin.

2. Changes in hair color as well as loss of hair on the head and other parts of the body possibly due to changes in the sebaceous glands.

3. Stiffening of the joints, which can cause poor body posture.

4. Changes in muscle fibers, which can cause poor muscle tone and loss of muscular strength.

5. Arteriosclerosis, which can cause high blood pressure and restricted blood flow to the extremities.

6. Deterioration of different parts of the eyes which takes the form of *cataracts* (clouding of the lens) and thus creates difficulty in seeing. Also, presbyopia (far-sightedness) or the inability to see objects close by may be a common occurrence.

7. *Presbycusis* (hearing loss) may take place due to aging.

8. Reduced sensitivity in the olfactory nerves and taste buds will cause a loss of sense of taste and smell.

9. Difficulty digesting food.

10. *Polyuria* (excessive urination).

11. Pain in the joints, which in turn would make movement difficult and painful—a condition known as *arthritis*. The pain in the joints is caused by an inflammation of the connective tissue.

12. *Diabetes Mellitus,* which is a metabolic disorder in which the pancreas is unable to produce sufficient insulin which, in turn, can convert sugar to energy.

In addition to the items mentioned, the aging process in older adults increases the incidences of *malignant neoplasms* (cancer), influenza, pneumonia, and accidents.

If the younger person can understand the aforementioned conditions which are characteristic of aging, he will be more sensitive to the needs and concerns of older people—more especially, the concerns of his or her grandparents as well as parents. Besides this, he can develop an understanding of physiological changes of aging as it relates to himself.

An Exercise

The following exercise can be used with classes to enable students to have the opportunity to "experience" some of the physiological changes mentioned previously.

Losing Our Senses and Coordination
Experiencing Loss of Sight

1. Have students bring a pair of regular glasses or sunglasses to class.
2. The teacher can supply a petroleum jelly which is to be placed over the glasses.
3. Students will then be asked to read a page from their text.

Experiencing Loss of Hearing

1. Students will place cotton or earplugs in their ears.
2. They will need to listen to directions from their teacher and take part in a task the teacher deems appropriate.

Experiencing Loss of Touch and Dexterity

1. Students will wrap tape around each joint of each finger.
2. Teacher will then ask students to turn pages of their textbook one at a time without damaging pages.

Experiencing Losses of Taste and Smell

1. Teacher will ask students to pinch their noses so they cannot smell.
2. Healthy foods such as apples and oranges will be consumed while noses are pinched.

Experiencing Arthritis

1. Using supplies from a first aid kit, the teacher will demonstrate how to wrap a bandage around a student's knee (while sitting). The bandage should be wrapped so as to prevent the knee from bending.
2. The student (or student's depending upon existing supplies) will then be asked to take a five minute walk around the school, making sure to use the stairs.

After students have performed the exercises, the teacher can have the class share experiences. Among the questions that may be asked are:

1. What did it feel like to have a limitation?
2. How did you feel about your friend's limitations?
3. What did you learn from the experience?
4. What similarities do you think people close to you have (older relatives)?
5. What are your feelings now as opposed to before the exercise?

Note—The teacher can combine some or all of these exercises, so that, for example, a student can experience loss of hearing, sight, and arthritis simultaneously.

Evaluation

1. Teacher can ask students to identify physiological changes that take place during the later years.

2. Teacher can ask students to write a reaction paper about their experiences with the simulations.

Aging, Dying and Death
Preparing for Death

Objectives

1. The student will differentiate between functional death and brain death.

2. The student will be able to examine alternatives within the funeral process.

3. The student will write his own will based upon a sample model.

Source

Jessica Mitford, *The American Way of Death,* Connecticut: Fawcett Publications, 1963.

Content and Procedures

What Does It Mean "to Be Dead?"

The last experience for a living person is death. Yet, controversy exists concerning the actual occurrence of death, since a universally accepted definition of when death begins has not been formulated. Is a person dead if his heart stops beating? What if a person's heart stops beating but his brain waves are still recorded?

Let us look at two definitions of death. *Functional* death is characterized by the absence of a heartbeat and voluntary breathing. However, modern medicine, with its resuscitation equipment can often revive the absent heartbeat. Therefore, many medical authorities will now include *brain* death as the termination of life. Brain death is characterized by the absence of electrical impulse activity in the brain as indicated by an EEG (electroencephalogram). The latter is the commonly accepted definition of death in the United States.

Seven Facts to Realize about Death

Before one can rationally think about the alternatives related to decision-making and death, one must come to the realization that eventually, he will die. In his book *Explaining Death to Children,* Earl Grollman includes a chapter by Robert Kastenbaum which lists seven facts needed to be realized in regard to death. These are:

1. I am an individual with a life therefore I will die.
2. I belong to a species with the characteristic of death.
3. Intellectually, I know death is certain.
4. There are many causes of death; I cannot evade them all.
5. Death will occur in the future, I do not know when.
6. Death is final and certain.
7. Death is the ultimate separation.

Funerals

If the individual can come to the realization that he will die one day, he can begin to examine the factors that are associated with death—in this lesson, namely, planning the funeral. Jessica Mitford's *The American Way of Death* brought to light the many issues which are associated with funerals. Today, the average funeral costs the family of the loved one approximately $2,000. Much of this expense can be reduced if the person, while alive, were to be honest in dealing with his desires about a funeral. However, in some areas a funeral can be arranged for as low as $300.

At this stage, the teacher may wish to provide students the opportunity to plan their own funeral. Most funeral directors are more than happy to provide classes with a tour of the funeral home and a lecture about the process of preparing a funeral. Among the factors that can be examined are:

1. What are the different kinds of caskets available and how much do they cost?
2. What is the process and cost of a cremation, embalming, and cosmetology?
3. Where can services be held?
4. How much do flowers cost?
5. What are the different types of monuments available and how can I go about selecting my own?
6. What happens to my plot after I am buried?

The teacher can point out that often the aforementioned points are not discussed by the dying person and the family, and as a result, unknown expenses are often incurred.

Another method of dealing with these issues is in the form of a will. Students can be asked to write their own will. In this will, the student can be asked to list whatever he feels important for him to have at the time of his death or how he wishes to have his possessions disposed of. The following pages display an example of a last will and testament. The student can read this will and add, modify, and delete passage more apropos.

For example, the student can look at issues such as:

1. What shall be the specifics of his funeral?—i.e. who shall speak, how much money should be spent, etc.
2. What would he prefer done with his body?—i.e. donated to science, buried without donations, organ donations, etc.
3. What role should family and friends play at the funeral?
4. How would he prefer people to remember him?
5. What should be done with his possessions?—money, clothes, house, etc.

Evaluation

Evaluation of this lesson should be on-going. Since this area can be a sensitive one for many students, it is important that assessment be made throughout. The teacher can ask students to hand in a reaction sheet to the assignment before the assignment is made. A reaction paper after the assignments and discussion can provide valuable data concerning alleviation of fears as well as knowledge about the death process.

Last Will and Testament
of
_____

I, _____, residing at _____ Street in the Borough of Brooklyn, County of Kings, City and State of New York, being in good health and of sound and disposing mind and memory and knowing the extent of my property and sensible of the uncertainty of life and desiring to make disposition of my property and effects while in good health and strength, do hereby make publish and declare this to be my Last Will and Testament hereby revoking any and all former Wills and Codicils by me heretofore made.

FIRST: I direct that all my debts which are legally due and owing be paid as soon after my death as may be practicable.

SECOND: I give, will, devise and bequeath to my beloved wife, _____, all of my property, which I may die seized or possessed of, whether real or personal, of whatever kind and description and wherever situated.

THIRD: In the event my beloved wife, should predecease me or die in the same accident, or in the same catastrophe, or other occurrence with me, or in the event it shall be impossible to determine which of us died first, then and in this event, I give, will devise and bequeath all of my property of which I may die seized or possessed of, whether real or personal, of whatever kind and description and wherever situated, to my beloved daughter, _____, and any other children that may be born after the date of this instrument, to be theirs absolutely and forever, and to share equally among them, share and share alike per stirpes and not per capita, and to be held in trust for any of my beloved children who may be minors at said time, said trusts terminating at such time as each child attains the age of eighteen (18) years or sooner dies.

FOURTH: Should the contingencies stated in Paragraph "THIRD" occur, and any of my beloved children be minor at said time, then and in these events, I hereby nominate, constitute and appoint as trustees over the above mentioned trust or trusts and to serve as guardians of said minor child or children my beloved father-in-law, _____, and my beloved mother-in-law, _____, to qualify and serve in both capacities without bond any law to the contrary notwithstanding.

FIFTH: In the event my beloved father-in-law, _____, and my beloved mother-in-law, _____, cannot for any reason whatsoever serve as trustees over the above mentioned trust or trusts or to serve as guardians for said minor child or children, then and in this event I hereby nominate, constitute and appoint as trustees over the above mentioned trust or trusts and to serve as guardians of said minor child or children my beloved brother, _____, and my beloved sister-in-law, _____, to qualify and serve in both capacities without bond any law to the contrary notwithstanding.

SIXTH: I authorize said trustees, if there be more than one minor child, to hold and administer any property in the trusts created hereby, in one or more consolidated funds, in whole or in part, in which the separate trusts shall have undivided interests.

SEVENTH: I authorize said trustees to pay all or any part of the principal and interest of said trusts for the respective education and welfare of each child, at such time and in such manner as said trustees in his and her sole discretion may deem to be in the best interest of each child.

EIGHTH: I hereby nominate, constitute and appoint as Executrix of this my Last Will and Testament my beloved wife, _____, to serve without bond, any law to the contrary notwithstanding.

NINTH: In the event my beloved wife, _____, cannot for any reason whatsoever serve as Executrix of this my Last Will and Testament, than and in this event, I hereby nominate, constitute and appoint as Executor and Executrix of this my Last Will and Testament my beloved father-in-law, _____, and my beloved mother-in-law, _____ to serve without bond, any law to the contrary notwithstanding.

TENTH: I authorize my Executrix or Executor whomsoever qualifies and serves hereunder, whenever in her or his discretion, to retain for such length of time as she or he may deem advisable, without liability for depreciation, any property, real or personal, at any time forming a part of my Estate, to sell or convey, to lease or let for any term, to mortgage or exchange for any purpose, or otherwise generally deal with any such property, whether real or personal, at such time or times, and on such terms and conditions including terms of credit, as my Executrix or Executor, in her or his sole discretion, shall determine; and to distribute such property in kind or in money, or partly in kind or partly in money.

ELEVENTH: It is my intention to conform to the provisions of the Law of the State of New York for testamentary dispositions, but in the event that for any reason any part of my Will or any provisions thereof shall be construed to be invalid, I declare that the invalidity of such part or provision shall not be considered or held to impair any other disposition of my property.

IN WITNESS WHEREOF, I, the undersigned testator have on this 19 day of December, Nineteen Hundred and Seventy-five, subscribed, sealed, published and declared the foregoing instrument as and for my Last Will and Testament.

_____

Witnesseth:

_____

_____

The foregoing instrument, consisting of four pages and this attestation clause, was on the day of the date thereof, subscribed, sealed, published and declared by _____, the testator therein and herein named, as and for his Last Will and Testament, in the presence of us, the undersigned, who at his request, and in his presence and in the presence of each other, have hereunto set our hands and seals as witnesses; this clause having been first read to us and we now certify that the matters herein specified took place in fact and in the order herein stated.

Aging, Dying and Death
Stages of Dying

Objectives

1. The student will identify and describe the five stages of death a dying person will experience.

2. The student will be able to recognize the signs of each stage of death.

Source

Elizabeth Kübler-Ross, *On Death and Dying,* New York: Macmillan Publishing Company, 1969.

Content and Procedures

Introduction

Today's teenagers have grown up in a period where they have been insulated from death. If a family member died while the child was young, that child was often sent to a babysitter and not allowed to attend the funeral. Perhaps the insulation has been increased by the fact that questions or talk about death or an imminent death are avoided.

Stages of Death

When a person dies, the place of death is often a hospital, nursing home, or other site away from home. In any event, many of today's teenagers, due to the isolation of death imposed upon them, do not know much about the many implications of death and dying—implications to the dying person, the family, friends, and above all, to themselves. However, one fact remains—each student will experience the death of someone close to him as well as obviously, his own. Yet, the most difficult experience a person will ever have is *learning* how to face and deal with death. The word "learning" is emphasized since understanding the stages of death, as determined by Elizabeth Kübler-Ross, is a learning process. Based upon her interaction with hundreds of dying patients and their families, the following are the stages one goes through (not all people go through all of the stages in textbook fashion) during the process of dying:

Stage one—denial—During this stage, the person may be in a temporary state of shock and insist that he is not dying. If a terminal disease is diagnosed, the person may not accept the diagnosis and claim he is physically sound.

State two—anger—Once the individual overcomes the denial, he becomes resentful. He may be angered at all healthy people around him and last out at these individuals.

Stage three—bargaining—This stage can take the form of seeking every ray of hope—often in unrealistic manners. The person may wish to make a deal with the doctor.

Stage four—depression—At this stage, the person accepts the fact that he will die and he then becomes isolated. He becomes depressed about the fact he will not be able to complete unfinished tasks. At this point in time, the person needs comfort and understanding from those whom he is close to, whether these persons be professionals or family.

Stage five—acceptance—Once this stage is reached, the person is no longer angry, is no longer seeking unrealistic deals, and is not depressed. He is now resigned to the fact that he will make the remainder of his life meaningful and will participate in all activities with imminent death, as a natural occurrence.

Using role play, the teacher can break the class up into five equal groups. Each group will be responsible for developing a scenario which will depict a stage of death.

Based upon the role play, the class will be responsible for guessing what stage of death was portrayed. In addition, the class would be required to identify the rationale for their selection—i.e. what occurrences took place that enabled you to make your decision concerning the stage of death portrayed?

Evaluation

The following are five statements a dying person may express. Identify the stage of death with the statement.

"Doctor, if you will cure my lung cancer, I will never smoke another cigarette." (Bargaining)

"How can I have leukemia? I feel fantastic! I don't believe you know what you're talking about." (Denial)

"Since I will be dead in one month, I'd like to review the will one more time so that I know the courts will not raise any questions." (Acceptance)

"Get away from me. You doctors only want my money." (Anger)

"I would love to have seen how my ideas would have been incorporated in the business. I'm sorry I will not be around (with tears in his eyes) to see the results." (Depression)

Aging, Dying, and Death

_____ Visit a senior citizens center in your community. Write notes or keep in touch with someone at the center who is not visited frequently by family.

_____ Visit a nursing home in your community. After the visit, write down five things that you learned.

_____ Interview four people over age 65 and learn how they view their lifestyle. What are the major advantages and disadvantages of being their age? What do older people fear the most? What makes them happy? What advice do they have for younger people? Do most of their friends over 65 take an active interest in politics and vote during elections?

_____ Make a list of the agencies in your community concerned with the problems of aging.

_____ Write a three to four page review or critique of a book concerned with the topic of death.

_____ Compare American attitudes toward death with those of other cultures.

_____ Listen to various records that talk about death and classify the songs according to their message (life after death, death is the end, death by drugs, violent death, death of a loved one, etc.).

_____ Learn emergency measures for preventing premature death (CPR, chocking).

_____ Compare and contrast Jewish, Christian, and Eastern beliefs regarding death.

_____ Attend a funeral of someone you do not know, then write a short paper of your overall reaction and evaluation of the funeral. Discuss what suggestions, if any, you would make to improve the meaningfulness or value of the arrangements and service to the survivors.

Index

Benjamin, Alfred, 54
Berkeley Model, curriculum, 78
    see Body Systems Approach Curriculum
Bicycle, safe use of, 366
Birth Control, see Contraceptives
Blood pressure test, 304
Borelli, George, 26
Brainstorming, activity in health teaching, 126
Breslow, Lester, 294, 299
Brown, Dean, 115
Brown, Louise, 220
Brownbag, value activity in health teaching, 128
Burt, John, 10, 74, 88, 398
Business and commercial organizations, 144–46

C

Califano, Joseph, Jr., 277
Candidiasis, 346–47
Cardiovascular fitness, teaching strategies for, 228–34
Carlson, Elof A., 221
Carsten, Arland, 222
Cheating, on tests, 105
Chronic bronchitis, 279
Cigarette smoking
    accidents, 284
    babies, 283
    economics of, 283–84
    government, 284–85
    mouth, 280–81
    reasons for, 285–86
    statistics of, 279
Clark, Leland C., Jr., 222
Classroom
    fear of, 22
    health and education, 100 resources for, 150–54
    as a laboratory, 19
    as a learning environment, 19, 20
    as a positive atmosphere, 20
Cognitive domain, 87
Color the behavior, value activity in health teaching, 128
Communicable disease
    causative organisms, 330–31
    common symptoms, 320–22
    epidemiology of, 335
    immunization for, 322–23
    kinds of, 325–26
    prevention and control of, 66
    and readmitting to classroom, 63
    signs of, 318–27
    study sheets
        symptoms and control measures, 325–26
        transmission of infectious agents, 339–40
    teaching strategies for, 318–42
    treatment of, 334
Communication skills
    in classroom, 23
    defined, 23
    and discipline, 25

and health counseling, 54–56
for mental health, 182–87
teaching about, 181–87
using "I" messages, 24
using messages, 23
Community
    as health counselors, 62–63
    representatives for health curriculum planning, 73
    as resources for referral, 62
Competency Based Approach Curriculum
    design, 78
    WOW Health Education Curriculum Guide, 78
Computing, activity in health teaching, 126
Conceptual curriculum approach
    concepts, 76
    Health Instruction framework for California Public Schools, 77
    New York State Strands Program, 77
    Pennsylvania Department of Education, 77
    School Health Education Study, 76
Connor, William E., 247
Consumer health
    educational resources, 167–68
    teaching strategies, 430–48
Consumer Product Safety Commission (CPSC), 356
Consumer Protection Agencies, 435
Contraceptives, 404–16
    defined, 406
    quiz on, 415–16
Cooper, Kenneth, 235
Counseling, see Health counseling
Counselor-Qualities Matrix, 50 Fig. 3.1
Current events newsletter, activity in health teaching, 126
Curriculum
    contents of, 71
    defined, 71
    developing the, 71–72
        see also Health Education Curriculum

D

Dear helper, activity in health teaching, 126
Death
    by accidents, 4
    causes, 4
    definitions of, 467
    by homicide, 4
    last will and testament for, 469–70
    rate, 4
    seven facts to realize about, 467
    stages of, 470–71
    by suicide, 4
Death, and dying education
    teaching strategies, 463–72
Debates, activity in health teaching, 126
Decision-making
    a healthy process, 21
    as a responsibility, 9
Department of Health, Education and Welfare (HEW), 5, 446
Detective, activity in health teaching, 127

Torre, Carolyn, 252
Travis, John, 309
Trichomoniasis, 343
Trigger films, 122
Trust
    and acceptance of student, 21
    in the classroom, 21
    defined, 21
    discipline, 25
    in teachers, 22

U

Unfinished sentences, value activity in
        health teaching, 130
Unit Approach Curriculum, 79

V

Vaccines, 334
Values clarification
    defined, 127–28
    goals, 128
    health instruction, activities for, 127–30
    implementing, 128

    utilized in health instruction, 66
    utilized in venereal disease education,
        317
    utilizing cognitive and affective
        instruction, 66
Values voting, value activity in health
        teaching, 130
Venereal disease, see STDs
    who's who in, 347
Venereal warts, 345
Vickery, Donald M., 293, Fig. 17.1, 309
Vitamins, 271–72

W

Water pollution, 455
Wayson, William, 25, 29
Winner-loser continuum, values activity in
        health teaching, 130
World Health Organization
    definition of health, 7
WOW (Washington, Oregon, and
        Wisconsin) Health Education
        Curriculum Guide, 78